Toxicology Pearls

Toxicology Pearls

KEVIN C. OSTERHOUDT, MD, MSCE, FAAP, FACMT

Assistant Professor, Department of Pediatrics
University of Pennsylvania School of Medicine
Attending Physician, Division of Emergency Medicine
Associate Medical Director, The Poison Control Center
Children's Hospital of Philadelphia
Philadelphia, Pennsylvania

JEANMARIE PERRONE, MD, FACMT, FACEP

Associate Professor of Emergency Medicine, Laboratory Medicine, and Pediatrics
University of Pennsylvania School of Medicine
Attending Physician, Department of Emergency Medicine
Hospital of the University of Pennsylvania
Staff Toxicologist, The Poison Control Center
Children's Hospital of Philadelphia
Philadelphia, Pennsylvania

FRANCIS DeROOS, MD

Associate Professor, Department of Emergency Medicine
University of Pennsylvania Hospital
Residency Director, Department of Emergency Medicine
Hospital of the University of Pennsylvania
Staff Toxicologist, The Poison Control Center
Children's Hospital of Philadelphia
Philadelphia, Pennsylvania

FRED M. HENRETIG, MD

Professor of Pediatrics and Emergency Medicine
University of Pennsylvania School of Medicine
Medical Director, The Poison Control Center
Director, Section of Medical Toxicology
Division of Emergency Medicine
Children's Hospital of Philadelphia
Philadelphia, Pennsylvania

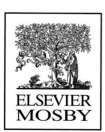

ELSEVIER
MOSBY

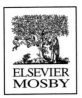

The Curtis Center
170 S Independence Mall W 300 E
Philadelphia, Pennsylvania 19106

TOXICOLOGY PEARLS   ISBN: 1-56053-614-4
Copyright © 2004 Elsevier Inc. All rights reserved.

Notice

Toxicology is an ever-changing field. Standard safety precautions must be followed, but as new research and clinical experience broaden our knowledge, changes in treatment and drug therapy may become necessary or appropriate. Readers are advised to check the most current product information provided by the manufacturer of each drug to be administered to verify the recommended dose, the method and duration of administration, and contraindications. It is the responsibility of the licensed prescriber, relying on experience and knowledge of the patient, to determine dosages and the best treatment for each individual patient. Neither the publisher nor the authors assume any liability for any injury and/or damage to persons or property arising from this publication.

The Publisher

Library of Congress Cataloging-in-Publication Data

Toxicology pearls/[edited by] Kevin C. Osteroudt... [et al.].
   p.; cm
  Includes index.
  ISBN 1-56053-614-4
   1. Toxicology–Case studies. I. Osterhoudt, Kevin C.
  [DNLM: 1. Poisoning–Case Reports. 2. Toxicology–Case Reports. QV 600 T75579 2004]
RA1219.T69 2004
6159'07–dc22

Acquisitions Editor: Jacqueline Mahon
Production Services Manager: Joan Sinclair
Project Manager: Cecelia Bayruns

Printed in the United States of America

Last digit is the print number: 9 8 7 6 5 4 3 2 1

To our children—Jon, Jeff, Spencer, Connor, Annika, Ryan, and Aidan—may we leave their children a world safer form poisons than the one we inherited; and to all the dedicated women and men providing public service and expertise through the poison control center system.

CONTENTS

Patient	Page

CONTRIBUTORS

Sara Abbruzzi, DO
Department of Internal Medicine, Philadelphia College of Osteopathic Medicine, Philadelphia, Pennsylvania

Charlene H. An, MD
Assistant Professor, Department of Emergency Medicine, SUNY Downstate Medical Center, Brooklyn, New York

Jennifer Brandeis, JD, MD
Department of Emergency Medicine, University of Pennsylvania School of Medicine, Philadelphia, Pennsylvania

Craig Savoy Brummer, MD
Physician, Department of Emergency Medicine, Hospital of the University of Pennsylvania, Philadelphia, Pennsylvania

Diane P. Calello, MD
Fellow, Division of Emergency Medicine, Children's Hospital of Philadelphia, Philadelphia, Pennsylvania

Otilia Capellan, MD
Physician, Staff Mary's Hospital, Waterbury, Connecticut

Brendan G. Carr, MD, MA
Department of Emergency Medicine, University of Pennsylvania School of Medicine and Hospital of the University of Pennsylvania, Philadelphia, Pennsylvania

Esther H. Chen, MD
Assistant Professor, Department of Emergency Medicine, University of Pennsylvania School of Medicine, Philadelphia; Attending Physician, Department of Emergency Medicine, University of Pennsylvania Medical Center, Philadelphia, Pennsylvania

Reza J. Daugherty, MD
Instructor in Pediatrics, University of Pennsylvania School of Medicine; Fellow, Pediatric Emergency Medicine, The Children's Hospital of Philadelphia, Philadelphia, Pennsylvania

Francis DeRoos, MD
Associate Professor, Department of Emergency Medicine, University of Pennsylvania Hospital; Residency Director, Department of Emergency Medicine, Hospital of the University of Pennsylvania; Staff Toxicologist, The Poison Control Center, Children's Hospital of Philadelphia, Philadelphia, Pennsylvania

Aaron J. Donoghue, MD
Instructor, Department of Pediatrics, University of Pennsylvania School of Medicine, Philadelphia; Fellow, Critical Care Medicine and Emergency Medicine, Children's Hospital of Philadelphia, Philadelphia, Pennsylvania

Judith M. Eisenberg, MD
Medical Toxicology, Fellow, Drexel University College of Medicine, Philadelphia, Pennsylvania

M. Bradley Falk, MD
Department of Emergency Medicine, University of Pennsylvania Health System, Philadelphia, Pennsylvania

Eron Friedlaender, MD
Instructor and Attending Physician, Department of Pediatrics, Division of Emergency Medicine, Children's Hospital of Philadelphia, Philadelphia, Pennsylvania

Michael I. Greenberg, MD
Professor, Department of Emergency Medicine, Drexel University College of Medicine; Clinical Professor, Department of Emergency Medicine, Temple University School of Medicine, Philadelphia, Pennsylvania

Howard A. Greller, MD
Attending Physician, Department of Emergency Medicine, New York University Medical Center/Bellevue Hospital Center, New York, Senior Fellow—Medical Toxicology, New York City Poison Control Center, New York, New York

Rebecca Guest, MD
Assistant Professor, Jefferson Medical College of Thomas Jefferson University; Attending Physician, Department of Emergency Medicine, Albert Einstein Medical Center, Philadelphia, Pennsylvania

Richard Hamilton, MD
Associate Professor, Department of Emergency Medicine, Drexel University College of Medicine; Emergency Medicine Control, Medical College Hospital, Philadelphia, Pennsylvania

Rachel Haroz, MD
Department of Emergency Medicine, Medical College of Pennsylvania Hospital, Philadelphia, Pennsylvania

Robert G. Hendrickson, MD
Assistant Professor, Department of Emergency Medicine, Oregon Health and Science University; Medical Toxicologist, Oregon Poison Center, Portland, Oregon

Fred M. Henretig, MD
Professor of Pediatrics and Emergency Medicine, University of Pennsylvania School of Medicine; Medical Director, The Poison Control Center; Director, Section of Medical Toxicology, Division of Emergency Medicine, Children's Hospital of Philadelphia, Philadelphia, Pennsylvania

Vivian Hwang, MD
Instructor, Departments of Emergency Medicine and Pediatrics, University of Pennsylvania School of Medicine, Philadelphia; Attending Physician, Department of Emergency Medicine, Hospital of the University of Pennsylvania, Philadelphia; Fellow, Division of Emergency Medicine, Children's Hospital of Philadelphia, Philadelphia, Pennsylvania,

Paul Ishimine, MD
Assistant Clinical Professor, Departments of Medicine and Pediatrics, University of California School of Medicine, San Diego; Attending Physician, Department of Emergency Medicine, UCSD Medical Center, San Diego; Attending Physician, Division of Pediatric Emergency Medicine, Children's Hospital and Health Center, San Diego, California

Paul Kolecki, MD
Assistant Professor, Department of Emergency Medicine, Director of Emergency Medicine Student Education, Thomas Jefferson University; Consultant, Philadelphia Poison Control Center, Philadelphia, Pennsylvania

Thomas Joseph Lydon, MD, PhD
Resident, Department of Emergency Medicine, Hospital of the University of Pennsylvania, Philadelphia, Pennsylvania

Robert Marsan, Jr.
University of Pennsylvania, Philadelphia, Pennsylvania

C. Crawford Mechem, MD
Associate Professor, Department of Emergency Medicine, University of Pennsylvania School of
Medicine and Hospital of the University of Pennsylvania, Philadelphia, Pennsylvania

Zachary F. Meisel, MD, MPH
Department of Emergency Medicine, University of Pennsylvania School of Medicine, Philadelphia,
Pennsylvania

Angela M. Mills, MD
Lecturer, Department of Emergency Medicine, University of Pennsylvania School of Medicine,
Philadelphia; Physician, Department of Emergency Medicine, Hospital of the University of
Pennsylvania, Philadelphia, Pennsylvania

Anthony P. Morocco, MD
Attending Physician and Medical Toxicologists, Departments of Emergency Medicine and Medical
Toxicology; Director, Emergency Medical Services, Guam Memorial Hospital, Tamuning, Guam

Allison A. Muller, PharmD
Adjunct Assistant Professor, Department of Pharmacy Practice, Temple University, Philadelphia;
Clinical Assistant Professor, Department of Pharmacy Practice, University of the Sciences,
Philadelphia; Clinical Managing Director, The Poison Control Center, Children's Hospital of
Philadelphia, Philadelphia Pennsylvania

Susan A. O'Malley, MD
Associate Emergency Medical Services Coordinator, Department of Emergency Medicine,
Brookhaven Memorial Hospital Medical Center, Patchogue, New York

Kevin C. Osterhoudt, MD, MSCE, FAAP, FACMT
Assistant Professor, Department of Pediatrics, University of Pennsylvania School of Medicine;
Attending Physician, Division of Emergency Medicine; Associate Medical Director, The Poison
Control Center, Children's Hospital of Philadelphia, Philadelphia, Pennsylvania

Chirag Patel, MD
Resident, Department of Emergency Medicine, Hospital of the University of Pennsylvania,
Philadelphia, Pennsylvania

Jeanmarie Perrone, MD, FACMT, FACEP
Associate Professor of Emergency Medicine, Laboratory Medicine, and Pediatrics, University of
Pennsylvania School of Medicine; Attending Physician, Department of Emergency Medicine,
Hospital of the University of Pennsylvania; Staff Toxicologist, The Poison Control Center, Children's
Hospital of Philadelphia, Philadelphia, Pennsylvania

Ronald Perry, MD, PhD
Physician, Department of Emergency Medicine, University of Pennsylvania, Philadelphia,
Pennsylvania

Robert H. Poppenga, DVM, PhD
Associate Professor, Department of Pathobiology; Chief, Toxicology Laboratory, University of
Pennsylvania School of Veterinary Medicine, Kennett Square, Pennsylvania

Amy L. Puchalski, MD
Assistant Professor, Department of Emergency Medicine, Medical College of Georgia, Augusta;
Attending Physician, Department of Emergency Medicine, Children's Medical Center, Augusta,
Georgia

Anthony W. Rekito, MD
Resident, Department of Emergency Medicine, Hospital of the University of Pennsylvania,
Philadelphia, Pennsylvania

James R. Roberts, MD
Chair, Department of Emergency Medicine, Mercy Health Systems, Philadelphia, Pennsylvania

Sandra H. Schwab, MD
Clinical Instructor, University of Pennsylvania School of Medicine, Philadelphia; Fellow, Division of
Emergency Medicine, Children's Hospital of Philadelphia, Philadelphia, Pennsylvania

Todd C. Severson, MD
Formerly, Resident, Department of Emergency Medicine, Hospital of the University of Pennsylvania,
Philadelphia, Pennsylvania; *Currently,* Attending Physician, Department of Emergency Medicine,
Central Maine Medical Center, Lewiston, Maine

Leslie M. Shaw, PhD
Department of Pathology and Laboratory Medicine, Hospital of the University of Pennsylvania,
Philadelphia, Pennsylvania

Philip R. Spandorfer, MD, MSCE
Assistant Professor, Departments of Emergency Medicine and Pediatrics, University of Pennsylvania
School of Medicine, Philadelphia; Attending Physician, Division of Emergency Medicine, Children's
Hospital of Philadelphia, Philadelphia, Pennsylvania

Jason C. Stillwagon, MD
Attending Emergency Physician, Department of Emergency Medicine, Memorial Health University
Medical Center, Savannah, Georgia

Nancy N. Sun, MD
Chief Resident, Department of Emergency Medicine, Hospital of the University of Pennsylvania,
Philadelphia, Pennsylvania

Nancy Vinca, MD
House Officer, Department of Emergency Medicine, Hospital of the University of Pennsylvania,
Philadelphia, Pennsylvania

Constance M. Yuan, MD, PhD
Clinical Assistant Professor, Department of Pathology, Immunology, and Laboratory Medicine,
University of Florida College of Medicine, Gainesville, Florida

PREFACE

It is better to know some of the questions than all of the answers.
                                        –James Thurber

Poisons and poisoning have fascinated humankind for thousands of years. More recently, environmental pollution and medication errors have become prominent public concerns. Perhaps because of the enormous numbers of drug, chemical, and venom exposures lurking in the world, the medical management of poisoned patients has remained somewhat daunting to many clinicians.

We are pleased to introduce the first edition of *Toxicology Pearls* to The Pearls Series®. This book represents the collaborative efforts of the Philadelphia Poison Control Center team. The four editors are consultant toxicologists to the Poison Center, and each of the authors is or has been associated with the Center either as a consulting toxicologist or as a fellow, resident, or student training in medical toxicology.

Befitting the proud history of Philadelphia and its identification with the "spirit of 1776," we offer 76 case studies. These presentations represent our serving of "oysters," which we hope that readers will open in their minds in a quest to discover useful clinical pearls. It is our intention that this book will demystify medical toxicology by teaching a common approach applicable to all poisoned patients (even to the three veterinary patients we have included). Although several excellent, encyclopedic textbooks of medical toxicology exist, we offer this book as a unique case-based resource with the optimal scope for stimulating students and residents during educational rotations at poison control centers. This book also provides a succinct review of the toxic exposures likely to be encountered by practitioners in the office, clinic, or emergency department.

Clinicians caring for patients with poisoning exposures are encouraged to utilize their regional poison control centers in their efforts to derive answers to toxicological questions. The American Association of Poison Control Centers maintains a single toll-free number throughout the United States (1-800-222-1222).

KEVIN C. OSTERHOUDT, MD, MSCE, FAAP, FACMT
JEANMARIE PERRONE, MD, FACMT, FACEP
FRANCIS DEROOS, MD
FRED M. HENRETIG, MD
EDITORS

Kevin C. Osterhoudt, MD
Fred M. Henretig, MD

PATIENT 1

A 17-month-old boy found unresponsive

A 17-month-old boy appeared well during a small party of his parents' friends and neighbors, and at bedtime at 10:30 PM. He awoke at 7:30 AM the next day, but seemed sluggish, and at 8:30 AM was found to be unresponsive. There is no history of trauma or infectious prodrome. The parents reported that no prescription medications were available in the home. Alcoholic beverages were served at the party (see figure), but the family denied illicit drug use.

Physical Examination: Temperature 36.0° C, pulse 158/min, respirations 16/min, blood pressure 91/60 mmHg. General: obtunded. HEENT: pupils 5 mm and reactive. Chest: stertorous respirations improve with jaw-thrust positioning. Heart: normal. Abdomen: normal. Extremities: normal. Skin: mildly diaphoretic. Neuromuscular: reacts to painful stimuli, cranial nerve functioning intact, deep-tendon reflexes normal and symmetrical.

Laboratory Findings: None

Question: What are the priorities in the clinical stabilization of the acutely poisoned patient?

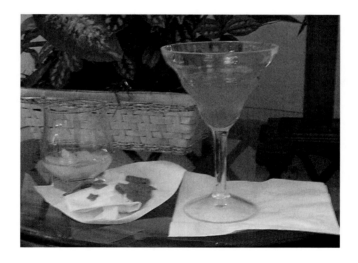

Treatment: Attention to and support of the airway, breathing, and circulation are of paramount importance. Oxygen and glucose are the substrates necessary for brain function, and their blood concentrations should be evaluated in any patient with neurological disability.

Discussion: Popular movies and television programs often portray poisonings as insidiously progressive illnesses that can be cured with a single administration of an antidote. Actually, very few poisoning syndromes fit such a description. Specific antidotes are available for a minority of poisoning scenarios. Since physiological elimination systems exist for most drugs and chemicals, good supportive medical care is effective treatment for most poisonings.

The American College of Surgeons uses an "ABCDE" paradigm to teach the structured initial assessment of the patient with traumatic injury, and such a model is also well-suited for the evaluation of the poisoned patient (see table below). Many poisons can produce respiratory depression, and ingested or inhaled foreign bodies or caustic chemicals can lead to anatomic airway disturbances. Cardiac dysrhythmia and shock are dangerous cardiovascular complications of many poisons. Interference with the oxygen-binding capability of hemoglobin, or interruption of cellular oxidative phosphorylation, can also lead to life-threatening cardiorespiratory failure. Neurological disability may manifest as seizures, agitation, delirium, hallucination, somnolence, obtundation, or coma. During the "secondary survey" of toxicological assessment, other perils of poisoning such as metabolic acidosis and renal, hepatic, or other organ system injury should be considered.

In the present patient, airway insufficiency was improved with basic medical airway positioning measures, and supplemental oxygen was administered. Although the child's heart rate and blood pressure seemed appropriate, intravenous access was obtained to allow for easy fluid and drug administration. The child's neurological disability mandated emergent assessment of two substrates necessary for neuronal function: oxygen and glucose. The blood dextrose was measured at the bedside to be 24 mg/dL. Five cc/kg of 10% dextrose in water was administered intravenously, resulting in a rapid return to lucidity.

Several poisons can cause hypoglycemia (see table below), but this patient's history suggested ethanol intoxication. His blood alcohol level was now 38 mg/dL. Young children, with relatively smaller hepatic glycogen stores compared to adults, are prone to ethanol-induced hypoglycemia, especially during the overnight fast. The accumulation of reduced nicotine adenine dinucleotide (NADH) during metabolism of ethanol tends to shunt pyruvate away from its role as the precursor for gluconeogenesis. With good supportive care including additional intravenous fluids, the child recovered fully. Poisoning prevention counseling was provided to the family.

Structured Initial Approach to the Poisoned Patient

Airway
  Maintain airway, check protective reflexes
Breathing
  Check ventilatory status
Circulation
  Obtain vascular access, check heart rhythm and
    blood pressure
Disability
  Altered consciousness merits consideration of
    O$_2$, glucose, naloxone (0.4–2 mg initially,
    may repeat)
Exposure
  Evaluate toxidrome

Oral Drugs that May Predispose to Hypoglycemia

Beta-adrenergic antagonists (propranolol)
Ethanol or other toxic alcohols
Salicylate
Sulfonylurea hypoglycemic medications
Valproic acid

Clinical Pearls

1. Attention to the airway, breathing, circulation, and neurological function is of critical importance to the poisoned patient.
2. Specific antidotal therapy is available for a minority of poisoned patients.
3. Assessment of the blood glucose content is a vital step in the assessment of neurological dysfunction.
4. Ethanol intoxication may lead to hypoglycemia, especially among young children or malnourished adults.

REFERENCES

1. Yip L: Ethanol. In Goldfrank L, Flomenbaum N, Lewin N, et al (eds): Goldfrank's Toxicological Emergencies, 7th ed. New York, McGraw-Hill; 2002, pp 952-965.
2. Osterhoudt KC, Shannon M, Henretig FM: Toxicological emergencies. In Fleisher G, Ludwig S (eds): Textbook of Pediatric Emergency Medicine, 4th ed. Philadelphia, Lippincott, Williams, and Wilkins, 2000, pp 887-942.
3. Henretig FM: Special considerations in the poisoned pediatric patient. Emerg Med Clin North Am 12:549-567, 1994.

PATIENT 2

A 14-year-old girl with headache and vomiting

An agitated, somnolent, and tearful 14-year-old girl is vomiting and suffers from the "worst headache of her life." She was previously healthy and does not take any medication or vitamin on a regular schedule. She had argued with her boyfriend the night before, and had taken some "sinus pills" to relieve a minor headache and to help her get to sleep. Her parents had given her some acetaminophen several hours later after her headache had worsened. She denies recreational drug abuse, thoughts of self-harm, or drug overdose.

Physical Examination: Temperature 37.2° C, pulse 52/min, respirations 18/min, blood pressure 196/97 mmHg. General: somnolent, but briefly arousable; tearful. HEENT: mydriatic but equal pupils, no papilledema, mucous membranes moist. Chest: normal. Cardiovascular: bradycardia, no murmurs. Abdomen: normal bowel sounds. Skin: mildy diaphoretic. Neuromuscular: depressed consciousness, oriented, cranial nerve function intact.

Laboratory Findings: Hemogram: WBC 9200/μL hemoglobin 12.4 g/dL, platelets 262,000/μL. Serum chemistries: normal. Urinalysis: normal. Urine pregnancy test: negative. Electrocardiogram: sinus bradycardia. Computed tomography (CT) of brain: normal. Urine immunoassay for drugs of abuse: positive for amphetamines. Serum acetaminophen level: < 10 mcg/ml.

Question: Does this patient's medical history and physical exam suggest any type of poisoning syndrome?

Diagnosis: Careful perusal of this girl's "toxidrome" might suggest toxicity from an alpha-adrenergic sympathomimetic agent such as phenylpropanolamine.

Discussion: After careful attention to a poisoned patient's airway, breathing, circulation, and neurological disability, a prudent next step might be to examine the patient carefully for clues to the underlying toxic syndrome. Many toxic syndromes, or toxidromes, can be defined by attention to a patient's mental status, vital signs, pupil size and reactivity, bowel and bladder function, and skin (see table, top).

In the present patient, the combination of severe headache, vomiting, central nervous system depression, hypertension, and bradycardia is most ominous for increased intracranial pressure. Fortunately, CT imaging did not provide any evidence of intracranial hemorrhage. In the consideration of poisoning, "sinus pills" are often a combination of sympathomimetic decongestant agents and/or drying anticholinergic antihistaminic agents. Mental status changes, hypertension, mydriatic pupils, and diaphoresis are all consistent with the sympathomimetic toxidrome. However, despite the positive urine immunoassay for amphetamines, at first glance the girl's bradycardia seems counterintuitive to a sympathomimetic poisoning syndrome.

In this case, it is important to consider that the varied alpha-adrenergic and beta-adrenergic receptors within the sympathetic nervous system response are associated with distinct features of the sympathomimetic toxidrome (see table, bottom) below illustrates that this girl's toxic syndrome is completely consistent with alpha-adrenergic sympathetic stimulation accompanied by a baroreceptor reflex–mediated bradycardia. Indeed, the sinus pills she had taken in mild excess, without intent of overdose, were found to be phenylpropanolamine—a selective alpha-adrenergic agonist. She recovered uneventfully from this illness over the course of the subsequent 6 hours. It is interesting to note that due to a recurrent association between phenylpropanolamine use and hypertensive crisis, phenylpropanolamine was recalled from over-the-counter cold remedies by the U.S. Food and Drug Administration in 2000.

Toxidrome analysis is an important tool for the healthcare provider. Indeed, the depressed consciousness and pin-point pupils of a heroin overdose, or the agitation, tachycardia, and hypertension of a cocaine overdose, can be suspected clinically well before the results of urine drug testing are available.

Common Toxidromes

	Opioid (Heroin, Etc)	Sympathomimetic (Cocaine, Amphetamine)	Anticholinergic (Atropine, Jimson Weed)	Cholinergic (Organophosphates)
Mental Status:	Depressed	Agitated	Delirious	Depressed
Blood Pressure:	– (↓)	↑	↑	↓ (↑)
Heart Rate:	– (↓)	↑	↑	↓ (↑)
Temperature:	– (↓)	↑	↑	– (↓)
Pupil Size:	↓	↑	↑	↓
Bowel Activity:	↓	–	↓	↑
Skin:	–	Diaphoresis	Flushed, dry	Diaphoresis

↑ = increased, ↓ = decreased, – = no effect, () = less common effect

Contribution of Distinct Adrenergic Receptor Types to Sympathomimetic Toxidrome

	Alpha$_1$	Alpha$_2$	Beta$_1$	Beta$_2$
Blood Pressure:	↑*	↓	– (↑)	↓
Heart Rate:	– (↓)	↓	↑*	– (↑)
Pupil Size:	↑*	– (↓)	–	–

↑ = increased, ↓ = decreased, – = no effect, () = less common effect
*Denotes predominant effect in classic sympathomimetic toxidrome

Clinical Pearls

1. Toxidrome analysis is vital to the initial care of the poisoned patient and may be more clinically useful than urine drug screens.

2. Phenylpropanolamine and phenylephrine are selective alpha-adrenergic agonist drugs that may cause hypertension without tachycardia.

REFERENCES

1. Osterhoudt KC, Fein JA: A high-pressure situation. Pediatr Annals 30:621-624, 2001.
2. Osterhoudt KC, Shannon M, Henretig FM: Toxicologic emergencies. In Fleisher G, Ludwig S (eds): Textbook of Pediatric Emergency Medicine, 4th ed. Philadelphia, Lippincott, Williams, and Wilkins, 2000, pp 887-942.
3. Bale JF Jr, Fountain MT, Shaddy R: Phenylpropanolamine-associated CNS complications in children and adolescents. Am J Dis Child 138:683-685, 1984.

Brendan G. Carr, MD
Jeanmarie Perrone, MD

PATIENT 3

A 37-year-old man with an unusual intravenous injection

A 37-year-old man presents to the emergency department after being involuntarily committed to psychiatric care by police officers. The patient's friend had summoned the officers after the patient reported that he was attempting to kill himself. The patient had injected three syringes of a silver-colored liquid intravenously into his antecubital fossa. Upon hearing the police at the door he swallowed the fourth syringe of the liquid. He reports that he has collected the liquid over several years at construction sites where he removed it from thermostats and switches. His medical history is significant for depression, arthritis, alcohol abuse, and alcohol withdrawal. He has taken celecoxib occasionally for arthritis pain. He has a remote history of intravenous drug abuse and admits to current heavy alcohol use (approximately 12–18 beers per day).

Physical Examination: Temperature 38.1° C, pulse 87/min, respirations 16/min, blood pressure 144/93 mmHg, oxygen saturation 98% in room air. General: no distress. HEENT: pupils equal and reactive, anicteric sclera, no pharyngeal erythema or exudates. Chest: clear bilaterally. Cardiovascular: normal; no murmurs, rubs, or gallops. Abdomen: soft, nontender. Extremities: multiple tattoos; left antecubital fossa warm and erythematous, erythema extends distally to wrist; no subcutaneous air appreciated, compartments soft and minimal pain with passive movement, + distal pulses, cap refill < 2 seconds. Neuromuscular: alert and oriented, non-focal.

Laboratory Findings: Hemogram: WBC 7900/μL, hemoglobin 15.1 g/dL, platelets 298,000 μL. Serum chemistries: Na^+ 143 mEq/L, K^+ 4.5 mEq/L, Cl^- 105 mEq/L, HCO_3^- 26 mEq/L, BUN 8 mg/dL, creatinine 1.0 mg/dL. Urinalysis: normal. Urine immunoassay for drugs of abuse: positive for marijuana. Serum ethanol: 160 mg/dL; serum negative for acetaminophen and salicylate. Radiograph left arm, antecubital fossa (see figure below): metallic density extensively involving soft tissues and venous system. Radiograph abdomen (see figure on next page): intraluminal metallic density in GI tract.

Question: What did this patient ingest and inject that lead to these radiographic and clinical findings?

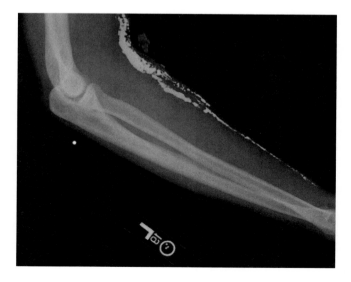

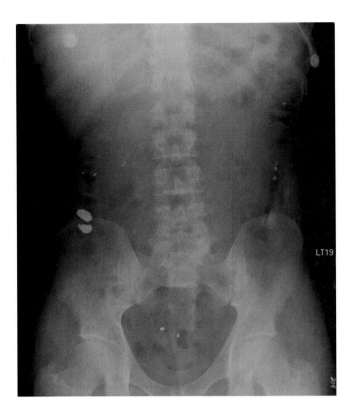

Diagnosis: Mercury is the only metal that is a liquid at room temperature and has long been used in thermometers because of this unique property. The silver liquid used by this man was elemental mercury.

Discussion: Essential in the diagnosis and treatment of mercury poisoning is recognition of the different forms of mercury and their individual toxicities. Mercury exists in three forms: (1) elemental mercury ("quicksilver"), (2) organic mercury (complexed with carbon chains), and (3) inorganic mercury (mercury salts).

Elemental mercury exposures, as described in this case, pose greatest danger when the liquid metal is aerosolized and inhaled. Chronic mercury inhalation is associated with a classic triad of tremor, neuropsychiatric disturbance, and gingivostomatitis. Acute inhalation of aerosolized mercury can also lead to chemical pneumonitis that can progress to hypoxia and respiratory failure. Ingestion of elemental mercury is less worrisome as systemic absorption is minimal. Intramuscular or intravenous injection of elemental mercury is associated with risk for pulmonary complications from embolization, local skin irritation at the injection site, and long-term effects from chronic exposure.

Exposures to short-chain *organic* mercury compounds are responsible for the majority of human mercury burden. These agents (methyl and ethyl mercury) are rapidly absorbed from the gastrointestinal (GI) tract and readily cross into the central nervous system (CNS), causing tremor, ataxia, dysarthria, constriction of visual fields, and extremity paresthesias. Organic mercury contamination in Minimata Bay, Japan, in the 1940s caused an epidemic of profound neurological deficits in the children of families consuming a fish diet with high levels of methyl mercury from the bay. Exposures to longer-chain organic mercury compounds are less associated with acute toxicity and more often induce chronic symptoms.

A phenomenon of primarily historic note is "acrodynia" or "pink" disease. This is a syndrome of swollen pink hands and feet sometimes followed by more severe dermal symptoms (including rash and desquamation) that resulted from use of mercury containing calomel teething powder in children. It was often initially diagnosed as Kawasaki's disease due to overlapping findings.

Inorganic mercury ingestions are notable due to the caustic nature of mercury salts. Nausea, vomiting, and abdominal pain are typical presentations and occur as a result of esophageal and gastric erosions. Renal failure and shock occur frequently and early after mercury salt (especially mercuric chloride) ingestions.

Chronic mercury exposure is associated with classic neurological findings including tremor and peripheral neuropathy. In addition, oral lesions, rash, salivation, headaches, and diaphoresis can occur. **Erethism** is a syndrome of chronic mercury exposure consisting of emotional lability, insomnia, poor concentration, and memory deficits. These are the personality changes described in the "**mad hatters**" who were exposed chronically to mercury salts in the felt-making and hatting industry of the late 1800s.

The diagnosis of mercury poisoning is best confirmed by element-specific assays. Both blood and urine assays exist for quantifying mercury exposure. Elemental and inorganic exposures can be detected with whole blood or urine assays acutely. Organic mercury exposures can only be performed with whole blood assays. Twenty-four-hour urine collections are necessary to adequately estimate degree of exposure and to guide duration of therapy.

Most non-poisoned adults have undetectable serum mercury levels. Levels less than 10 µg/L in whole blood and 20 µg/L in urine are considered normal. Symptoms are not well correlated with blood mercury levels, in part because of redistribution of toxin to the CNS. Aside from assisting with diagnosis, blood and urine levels play a role in serial measurements to evaluate duration of therapy with chelation.

Treatment for mercury exposure is dependent on the type of mercury that the patient was exposed to as well as the route of exposure. Treatment is typically divided into initial decontamination and long-term chelation. **Decontamination** after acute exposure begins with responsible decontamination of the scene of the exposure. Care should be taken not to unintentionally aerosolize spills of elemental mercury (i.e., by vacuuming) and to minimize duration of exposure to the offending agent.

Decontamination of the GI tract after ingestion of elemental mercury is usually not necessary since it is poorly absorbed and will pass through the intact GI tract without complications. In contrast, mercuric salt ingestion is similar to a caustic, and although vomiting and hematemesis are fre-

quent, further decontamination should be withheld to prevent obscuring endoscopy of the injured GI tract. Inhalation or aspiration of mercury-containing compounds presents a difficult problem. Postural drainage and endotracheal suction have been suggested, but are of unclear value.

Injection of mercury-containing compounds (especially quicksilver) subcutaneously, intramuscularly, or intravenously is a rare event. Acute toxicity is primarily via venous embolization to the pulmonary and renal systems. Sterile soft-tissue abscesses are frequently noted. Long-term toxicity occurs from endogenous conversion of elemental mercury to compounds capable of crossing into the CNS. Surgical debridement can be utilized to decrease long-term exposure by decreasing the volume of toxin, but care should be taken to protect operating personnel from vapor release.

Once initial decontamination has been achieved, the indications for **chelation** must be addressed. Traditional chelation of mercury compounds can be achieved with either dimercaprol (BAL) or DMSA (2,3-dimercaptosuccinic acid: succimer). These agents work by providing thiol groups to compete with endogenous binding of mercury compounds. BAL is available as an intramuscular injection and DMSA is an oral therapy. Although chelation is effective in decreasing blood and urine mercury levels, neurological consequences of mercury (especially methyl mercury) exposure may not be reversible.

The present patient had no pulmonary, GI, or neurological symptoms upon admission to the hospital. The radiograph of his antecubital fossa revealed a large burden of mercury in the soft tissue and venous system. The chest radiograph was obtained to determine whether any of the injected mercury had embolized to the pulmonary tree. Fortunately for this patient, there was no significant embolization to the lungs. The abdominal radiograph was a rough assessment of the enteral burden of mercury following the ingestion. There was evidence of localized cellulitis in the antecubital fossa, but very little evidence of venous embolization of the mercury injection. The patient was taken for surgical debridement (without suction or electrocautery to limit vaporization of the elemental mercury), which was effective in decreasing the mercury burden as estimated by plain radiography. Prior to enteral chelation, the gastrointestinal tract was decontaminated with whole bowel irrigation. Chelation therapy was initiated with DMSA (succimer). Baseline whole blood and 24-hour urine levels were measured and followed serially to guide further therapy.

Clinical Pearls

1. Mercury exists in three different forms—elemental, organic, and inorganic. Each exposure has unique characteristics.

2. Elemental mercury ingestions are fairly benign, and pass spontaneously without complications through an intact GI tract. Some health-food stores sell elemental mercury–filled capsules for "cleansing purposes."

3. Elemental mercury is most dangerous if vaporized. This can occur if it is warmed even slightly above room temperature and can cause significant pulmonary toxicity and pneumonitis. Care should be taken to avoid heating or vaporizing elemental mercury when cleaning up a broken thermometer or sphygnomanometer.

4. Chelation therapies exist for mercury poisoning, although their clinical utility is often uncertain.

REFERENCES

1. Ho BS, Lin JL, Huang CC, Tsai YH, Lin MC: Mercury vapor inhalation from Chinese red (Cinnabar). J Toxicol Clin Toxicol 41:75-78, 2003.
2. Winker R, Schaffer AW, Konnaris C, et al: Health consequences of an intravenous injection of metallic mercury. Int Arch Occup Environ Health 75:581-586, 2002.
3. Deschamps F, Strady C, Deslee G, et al: Five years of follow-up after elemental mercury self-poisoning. Am J Forensic Med Pathol 23:170-172, 2002.
4. Sue YJ: Mercury. In Goldfrank LR, Flomenbaum NE, Lewin NA, et al (eds): Goldfrank's Toxicological Emergencies, 7th ed. New York, McGraw Hill, 2002.
5. Ruha AM, Tanen DA, Suchard JR, Curry SC: Combined ingestion and subcutaneous injection of elemental mercury. J Emerg Med 20:39-42, 2001.

PATIENT 4

A 3-year-old boy with exploratory drug ingestion

A previously healthy 3-year-old boy was found exploring his grandparents' medications. Several pill bottles were opened, and the residue of at least one pill was discovered on his teeth and tongue. The implicated medications include: alprazolam, aspirin, digoxin, furosemide, paroxetine, and verapamil. He had also opened several capsules of verapamil and poured the drug over his (and his brother's) breakfast cereal (see figure). The child arrives in the emergency department 30 minutes after drug exposure and is acting normally.

Physical Examination: Normal.

Laboratory Findings: Electrocardiogram: normal rate with normal intervals.

Questions: Would gastrointestinal decontamination be appropriate for this child? If so, which modality should be used?

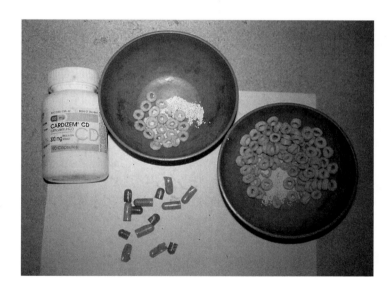

Treatment: The clinical application of gastrointestinal decontamination therapy is a basic tenet of medical toxicology, but remains hotly controversial. A single dose of activated charcoal seems prudent for this child.

Discussion: Over half of poison-exposure cases reported to American Poison Control Centers occur among children aged less than 5 years, but poisoning deaths are rare within this group. Ingestions with intent of self-harm, typical among adolescents and adults, are considerably more lethal than ingestions arising from curious exploration. In the present case, it is impossible to quantify the total amount of drug ingested or to clearly define risk. Verapamil should be considered a serious poisoning exposure in this setting, and several of the implicated drugs are capable of causing significant toxicity. The secondary prevention of poisoning morbidity, via gastrointestinal (GI) decontamination, seems a laudable goal.

GI decontamination can be achieved via gastric emptying with syrup of ipecac-induced emesis or orogastric lavage, poison adsorption via activated charcoal, or catharsis via whole bowel irrigation with polyethylene glycol. Each of these decontamination strategies is supported by sound theory and some scientific investigation employing a combination of *in vitro*, animal, and human volunteer study models. Unfortunately, little evidence has been gathered to demonstrate improved outcomes among poisoned patients treated with GI decontamination.

Prior to prescription of GI decontamination it is important to deem that the poisoning exposure is likely to cause illness if untreated, that significant amounts of the drug are still within the GI tract and amenable to decontamination, and that no therapeutic contraindications exist. Current expert opinion suggests that induction of emesis should be reserved for out-of-hospital first-aid, in situations where definitive medical care is likely to be delayed. Orogastric lavage should be reserved for life-threatening ingestions that are treated early after exposure, in which charcoal alone is deemed to be insufficient. Several theoretical indications for whole bowel irrigation are presented in the table. For most poison ingestions, activated charcoal is believed to be the single best choice of decontamination strategy, although ethanol, iron, and lithium are poorly adsorbed.

Activated charcoal is administered orally as a slurry in a typical dose of 1 g/kg up to a maximum of 75 g. Some patients, especially young children and depressed adults, will refuse to drink the slurry, which may be administered via a nasogastric tube if desired. Approximately 1 in 5 patients given activated charcoal will vomit during or after its administration. Pulmonary aspiration of charcoal, which has been lethal, is the most worrisome rare complication of activated charcoal administration, and is most common after nasogastric tube administration. To be effective, activated charcoal should be administered proximate to poison ingestion while drug is still present within the stomach. Current evidence suggests that charcoal administration within emergency departments is uncommonly accomplished within 1 hour of ingestion, and such practice certainly limits its effectiveness.

The present patient was given 1 g/kg of activated charcoal, and he remained well. It is unknown whether this was because of, or in spite of, the GI decontamination efforts. Poisoning prevention guidance was provided to the family.

Ingestions for Which Whole Bowel Irrigation Might Be Considered

Body packers
Massive overdoses
Metals/lithium
Patch drug-delivery systems
Pill concretions
Sustained-release drug preparations

Clinical Pearls

1. For most poisoning exposures by ingestion, activated charcoal is believed to be more efficacious than ipecac-induced emesis or orogastric lavage.

2. Pulmonary aspiration of charcoal is a rare, but dangerous, complication of charcoal therapy—especially after nasogastric administration.

3. A risk vs. benefit analysis should be carefully considered before the prescription of GI decontamination for any potentially poisoned patient.

REFERENCES

1. Bond GR: The role of activated charcoal and gastric emptying in gastrointestinal decontamination: A state-of-the-art review. Ann Emerg Med 39:273-286, 2002.
2. Osterhoudt KC: Toxic topic – Ipecac for the treatment of pediatric poisonings. Pediatr Case Rev 1:47-49, 2001.
3. Burns MM: Activated charcoal as the sole intervention for treatment after childhood poisoning. Curr Opin Pediatr 12: 166-171, 2000.

Craig Savoy Brummer, MD
Jeanmarie Perrone, MD

PATIENT 5

A 44-year-old man with altered mental status and hypotension

A woman returned home from a brief outing to find her 44-year-old husband mumbling and confused with a bottle of wine and an empty medication container. She had seen him approximately 1 hour earlier, and he had been fine. He was uncooperative with paramedics en route to the hospital, and they were unable to obtain vital signs or initiate an intravenous line.

Physical Examination: Temperature: 36.1° C, pulse 125/min, blood pressure 80/40 mmHg, respirations 14/min, oxygen saturation 97% on 2 L O_2 via nasal cannula. General: agitated confused, uncooperative, mumbling speech. HEENT: dry mucous membranes, 5-mm pupils, poorly reactive to light. Chest: clear. Cardiovascular: tachycardic, normal auscultation. Abdomen: diminished bowel sounds. Extremities: multiple track marks. Skin: dry, no diaphoresis, no flushing.

Laboratory Findings: Arterial blood gas (100% Fio_2): pH 7.39, $Paco_2$ 50 mmHg, Pao_2 154 mmHg. Hemogram: normal. Serum chemistries: blood glucose 120 mg/dL, normal. EKG: sinus tachycardia, 127 beats/min, QRS 128 ms, right axis deviation with a positive deflection of the R wave in lead aVR (see figure below).

Question: The clinical and electrocardiographic findings suggest what type of medication poisoning?

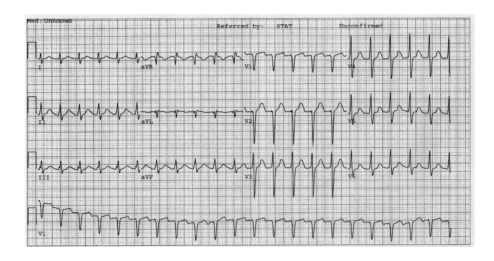

Diagnosis: Lethargy, anticholinergic findings, tachycardia, QRS widening, and the right axis deviation of the terminal R wave in lead aVR suggests tricyclic antidepressant overdose.

Discussion: Tricyclic antidepressant (TCA) poisoning continues to be a leading cause of hospitalization and death due to ingestion of prescription drugs. The term "tricyclic antidepressants" refers to a class of antidepressants characterized by a three-ringed structure. Cyclic antidepressants (CAs) refer to the group of antidepressant drugs including TCAs and heterocyclic antidepressants, such as amoxapine and maprotiline, considered less cardiotoxic.

TCAs have well-studied effects on the myocardium and on certain neurotransmitters and receptors, which explain the varied clinical presentations of TCAs. Central anticholinergic effects may account for the agitation, delirium, and lethargy and may be a factor contributing to seizures. TCAs are competitive antagonists at peripheral muscarinic acetylcholine receptors, causing dry mouth, urinary retention, dilated pupils, and sedation. Antihistaminic effects also contribute to sedation. Seizures may result from an inhibitory effect on GABA receptors. Alpha-adrenergic blockade induces peripheral vasodilation, which contributes to hypotension. CAs block intrasynaptic reuptake of catecholamines, resulting in intracellular depletion and decreased responsiveness to indirect-acting pressors such as dopamine. CAs have Type IA antidysrhythmic properties and block sodium channels in the heart. This results in prolongation of phase 0 of the action potential and delays the rapid upstroke of depolarization. This effect is noted on the EKG as prolonged QRS and a rightward axis deviation (RAD) seen best as a positive deflection of the R wave in lead aVR.

TCAs are highly lipophilic and readily cross the blood-brain barrier, rapidly affecting the central nervous system after ingestion. TCAs have a large volume of distribution throughout the body and high protein binding; neither hemodialysis nor hemoperfusion is clinically effective. TCA toxicity should be considered a clinical diagnosis; bedside tests such as the EKG are more predictive than TCA-levels in predicting toxic effects. Among TCA-poisoned patients presenting to emergency departments, one-third of patients with QRS duration greater than 100 milliseconds develop seizures, and half of patients with QRS duration greater than 160 milliseconds develop ventricular dysrhythmias or ectopy. In EKG lead aVR, an upright R wave greater than 3 mm is predictive of a more serious clinical course (seizures and dysrhythmias).

TCAs are rapidly absorbed, and central nervous system depression is typically the first manifestation of overdose. Tachycardia, hypotension, seizures, and dysrhythmias may ensue. Patients remaining asymptomatic, with normal EKG intervals, are unlikely to deteriorate after several hours of observation.

Initial assessment of TCA overdose includes standard measures of cardiorespiratory monitoring and support, and consideration of gastrointestinal decontamination. Sodium bicarbonate therapy is considered a specific antidote for the cardiac conduction delays of TCA poisoning. Sodium therapy (either hypertonic saline or sodium bicarbonate) competitively antagonizes the myocardial sodium channel blockade, and alkalinization may further reduce toxic effects. Potential indications for sodium bicarbonate therapy include QRS widening greater than 100 ms, acidemia, hypotension refractory to fluids, and ventricular dysrhythmias. Sodium bicarbonate is commonly given as an initial bolus of 1 to 2 mEq/kg, followed by an infusion or serial bolus doses until a blood pH of 7.5 to 7.55 is achieved. The effectiveness of therapy can be monitored via the QRS duration and vital signs. Direct-acting vasopressors, such as norepinephrine, are recommended for refractory hypotension, since TCA-induced blockade of catecholamine reuptake may decrease the efficacy of indirect-acting agents such as dopamine. Seizures, which may contribute to acidosis and exacerbate cardiotoxicity, should be treated aggressively with benzodiazepines or barbiturates.

Tricyclic antidepressant toxicity was suspected in the present patient due to his rapidly declining mental status, hypotension, tachycardia, and anticholinergic signs. Initial EKG findings confirmed the diagnosis with a prolonged QRS interval (128 msec) and a slight right axis deviation of the terminal R wave in lead aVR (+R wave in aVR). All of these symptoms warranted aggressive medical stabilization, and endotracheal intubation and gastrointestinal decontamination were performed. Orogastric lavage did yield pill fragments, likely secondary to anticholinergic-delayed gastric emptying. Activated charcoal was subsequently administered via the orogastric tube. QRS prolongation noted on the EKG was treated with a sodium bicarbonate bolus. Serial EKGs demonstrated widening QRS intervals (128–140 msec), and a sodium bicarbonate infusion was started (3 ampules sodium bicarbonate in 1 liter D5W). Blood pressure improved with IV fluids and the sodium bicarbonate therapy. Narrowing of the QRS interval with bicarbonate therapy is evident in the figure on the next page.

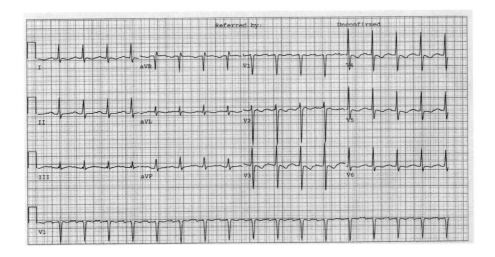

The patient was admitted to the medical intensive care unit, where he steadily improved. The EKG changes resolved over the next 12 hours; the patient awakened; and the bicarbonate infusion was stopped. The patient's wife subsequently brought in an empty bottle of amitryptiline (Elavil).

Clinical Pearls

1. Suspect TCA overdose in patients with altered mental status, hypotension, seizures, and characteristic EKG changes of widened QRS and +R in lead aVR.

2. Poisoned patients with wide complex cardiac dysrhythmias should be treated with sodium bicarbonate titrated to narrowing of the QRS complex and alkalinization of serum to pH 7.5–7.55.

3. TCA-induced hypotension may be treated with intravenous fluids, sodium bicarbonate therapy, and, in refractory cases, with direct-acting vasopressors. Extracorporeal cardiovascular support may be lifesaving in severe cases.

4. Treat seizures quickly to prevent worsening metabolic acidosis and exacerbation of cardiac toxicity. Consider endotracheal intubation, sodium bicarbonate therapy, and hyperventilation for any patient with suspected TCA poisoning who has a seizure.

REFERENCES

1. Legome E: Tricyclic antidepressant overdose. Emedicine, 2001 Aug 2 (8), www.emedicine.com/EMERG/topic37.htm
2. McCabe JL, Cobaugh DJ, Menegazzi JJ, Fata J: Experimental tricyclic antidepressant toxicity: A randomized, controlled comparison of hypertonic saline solution, sodium bicarbonate, and hyperventilation. Ann Emerg Med 32:329-333, 1998.
3. Tran TP, Panacek EA, Rhee KJ, Foulke GE: Response to dopamine vs norepinephrine in tricyclic antidepressant-induced hypotension. Acad Emerg Med 4:864-868, 1997.
4. Liebelt EL, Ulrich A, Francis PD, Woolf A: Serial electrocardiogram changes in acute tricyclic antidepressant overdoses. Crit Care Med 25:1721-1726, 1997.
5. Liebelt EL, Francis PD, Woolf AD: ECG lead aVR versus QRS interval in predicting seizures and arrhythmias in acute tricyclic antidepressant toxicity. Ann Emerg Med 26:195-201, 1995.
6. Taboulet P, Michard F, Muszynski J, et al: Cardiovascular repercussions of seizures during cyclic antidepressant poisoning. J Toxicol Clin Toxicol 33:205-211, 1995.
7. Litovitz TL, Schmitz BF, Bailey KM: 1989 Annual Report of the American Association of Poison Control Centers National Data Collection System. Am J Emerg Med 8:394, 1990.
8. Frommer DA, Kulig KW, Marx JA, Rumack B: Tricyclic antidepressant overdose. A review. JAMA 211:521-526, 1987.
9. Boehnert MT, Lovejoy FH Jr: Value of the QRS duration versus the serum drug level in predicting seizures and ventricular arrhythmias after an acute overdose of tricyclic antidepressants. N Engl J Med 313:474-479, 1985.

Todd C. Severson, MD
Jeanmarie Perrone, MD

PATIENT 6

A 29-year-old man with decreased consciousness and bradycardia

A previously healthy 29-year-old man is brought to the emergency department (ED) by friends who report that he had become very sleepy while at a party. They admitted to drinking alcohol earlier in the evening, but were surprised when the patient became abruptly lethargic and unarousable. His friends did not witness any seizure activity and were unaware of any illicit recreational drug use. Upon arrival to the ED, the patient is somnolent.

Physical Examination: Temperature 35.9° C, pulse 56/min, respirations 12/min, blood pressure 108/74 mmHg, pulse oximetry 97% in room air. General: thin, well-developed, markedly lethargic, moaning occasionally, with spontaneous unlabored respirations. HEENT: pupils mid-position, equal and reactive; no tongue or oral trauma; neck supple, no JVD, passive full range of motion. Chest: normal. Cardiovascular: bradycardia, regular rhythm. Abdomen: soft, nontender, normoactive bowel sounds. Skin: warm, well-perfused, no diaphoresis, no lesions. Neuromuscular: lethargic and minimally responsive, no focal deficits.

Laboratory Findings: Hemogram: WBC 8000/μL, hemoglobin 14.2 g/dL, platelets 127,000 / μL. Serum chemistries: sodium 141 mEq/L, potassium 4.7 mEq/L, chloride 101 mEq/L, bicarbonate 25 mEq/L, glucose 117 mg/dL. Arterial blood gas (room air): pH 7.34, $Paco_2$ 45 mmHg, Pao_2 92 mmHg. Urine immunoassay for drugs of abuse: negative. Electrocardiogram: sinus bradycardia, rate 56, otherwise normal.

Question: What substance(s) would be most consistent with this patient's presentation?

Diagnosis: Excluding any causative medical condition, the current presentation is most consistent with central nervous system (CNS) depression from barbiturate or sedative-hypnotic overdose. The negative urine drug screen suggests a less common drug not detected by typical commercial immunoassays.

Discussion: Routine medical management for the poisoned patient with altered mental status involves support of the patient's airway, breathing, and circulation, including supplemental oxygen, monitoring, and intravenous access, as necessary. A bedside fingerstick glucose determination must not be overlooked. Adjunctive studies including serum chemistries, arterial blood gas analysis, an electrocardiogram, urinalysis, and serum or urine toxicology screens may contribute to the diagnosis. Computed tomographic imaging of the head and/or lumbar puncture may also be indicated if the history of ingestion is not substantiated.

In the present patient, the negative medical history, preceding good health, lack of evident trauma or seizure activity, non-focal neurological exam, and generally unremarkable laboratory findings argue against alternative medical diagnoses and suggest a drug overdose. The patient has CNS depression, mild respiratory depression (respiratory acidosis on his arterial blood gas), bradycardia, and hypothermia. An opioid overdose could cause such symptoms; however, one would anticipate miotic pupils and more respiratory depression than observed in this patient. Nonetheless, there is little downside to an empiric trial of the opioid antagonist naloxone, since pupillary findings are not absolute. This patient received a total of 2 mg of naloxone (starting at a dose of 0.2 mg since opioid dependence cannot be excluded, and precipitous opioid withdrawal must be avoided) without response.

Other drugs that may induce lethargy and bradycardia include skeletal muscle relaxants such as baclofen and centrally acting antihypertensive drugs such as the alpha-2 agonists clonidine and guanabenz. Benzodiazepine overdose would also provide a reasonable explanation for the patient's symptoms. The benzodiazepine toxidrome is often described as "coma, with normal vital signs." Bradycardia and respiratory depression are less likely, but may be found in the setting of co-ingestion with ethanol as in this case. Toxicology screens were negative for benzodiazepines, and the serum ethanol level was 0.104 mg/dL, a level unlikely to cause such a profound decrease in level of consciousness. Other sedative-hypnotic agents, such as methaqualone, zolpidem, or gamma-hydroxybutyrate (GHB), are also important considerations. Upon further questioning, the patient's friends reluctantly reported that the patient was using "Liquid Nitro," also known as GHB, at the party.

GHB is a metabolite of the neurotransmitter gamma-aminobutyric acid (GABA) and is found endogenously in the CNS in trace concentrations. It has been used clinically as an anesthetic agent outside of the United States since the 1960s, and was introduced in the U.S. around 1990 as a "dietary supplement" popular with weight lifters. In the past decade, GHB has emerged as a popular recreational drug and as a "club drug" popular at "rave" dance parties. It has also been implicated as a "date-rape" drug used to incapacitate potential victims of sexual assault. It was reclassified as a schedule I controlled substance in early 2000. Illicit GHB is typically supplied as liquid solution and has a characteristically unpleasant salty or "soapy" taste. It is not detected by routine urine or serum toxicology screens.

The main clinical effect of GHB is dose-related CNS depression, which may include euphoria, relaxation, drowsiness, amnesia, and hypotonia. With higher doses respiratory depression, obtundation, coma, and death can occur. Hypothermia and bradycardia are commonly associated with GHB overdose. The bradycardia is usually transient and mild without hemodynamic consequences. Mechanical ventilation may be necessary to support respiratory depression or loss of airway protective reflexes in severe poisonings. The hallmark of even the most significant poisonings is a very brief intoxication, with improvement to normal mental status in 30–120 minutes.

As with most sedative-hypnotic poisonings, management is supportive. There is no antidote for GHB, although some case reports suggest a favorable response to low-dose physostigmine. Charcoal is of limited utility owing to GHB's rapid absorption but may be worthy of consideration if co-ingestants are present. Because of GHB's short duration of effect, the intoxication is self-limited and most patients regain full consciousness within a few hours. However, the presence of significant co-ingestants may alter or prolong the recovery course. This patient awakened approximately 1 hour after arrival and was more alert and able to answer questions. He denied intentionally trying to harm himself but admitted to using more GHB than he had in the past.

Clinical Pearls

1. GHB intoxication should be considered in young patients with rapid onset of stupor or coma followed by rapid resolution.

2. Vital sign abnormalities including mild bradycardia, hypothermia, and sometimes respiratory depression are early clues to GHB intoxication. Laboratory studies are unhelpful since GHB is not detected on routine toxicological screens.

3. Chronic GHB use leads to dependence and a serious GHB abstinence syndrome. It is comparable to ethanol withdrawal producing diaphoresis, tremor, insomnia, autonomic instability, and delirium.

REFERENCES

1. Osterhoudt KC, Henretig FM: Toxic topic: Comatose teenagers at a party—What a tangled web we weave. Pediatr Case Rev 3:171-173, 2003.
2. Mason PE, Kerns WP: Gamma-hydroxybutyric acid (GHB) intoxication. Acad Emerg Med 9:730-739, 2002.
3. Dyer JE, Roth B, Hyma BA: Gamma-hydroxybutyrate withdrawal syndrome. Ann Emerg Med 37:147-153, 2001.
4. Chin RL, Sporer KA, Cullison B, et al: Clinical course of gamma-hydroxybutyrate overdose. Ann Emerg Med 31:716-722, 1998.
5. Li J, Stokes SA, Woeckener A: A tale of novel intoxication: Seven cases of gamma-hydroxybutyric acid overdose. Ann Emerg Med 31:723-728, 1998.
6. Li J, Stokes SA, Woeckener A: A tale of novel intoxication: A review of the effects of gammahydroxybutyric acid with recommendations for management. Ann Emerg Med 31:729-736, 1998.
7. Dyer JE, Andrews KM: Gamma hydroxybutyrate withdrawal. Clin Toxicol 35:553, 1997.

Rachel Haroz, MD
James R. Roberts, MD

PATIENT 7

A 29-year-old camper with bruising, swelling, and severe leg pain

A 29-year-old woman, while camping in the Arizona Desert, strayed from the campsite and brushed against some vegetation. She experienced burning pain in her left ankle that quickly became increasingly severe. She noted redness, swelling, and two small puncture marks above her lateral malleolus. Worried about a possible snakebite, her friends took her to the nearest hospital, arriving approximately 2 hours after the event. No first aid was administered.

On arrival the patient has worsening pain in her entire left leg, with swelling to her knee. She also has nausea, generalized weakness, and tingling around the mouth.

Physical Examination: Temperature 37.6°C, pulse 130/min, respirations 28/min, blood pressure 95/50 mmHg. General: very anxious, slightly pale, in severe pain. HEENT: diaphoresis, otherwise normal. Chest: normal. Cardiovascular: tachycardia with no murmur. Abdomen: mild diffuse tenderness with normal bowel sounds. Extremities: left lower extremity markedly edematous from the ankle to approximately 2 inches above the knee; several areas of ecchymoses, particularly around the puncture wounds (see figure below).

Laboratory Findings: Hemogram: WBC 21,000 /μL, hemoglobin normal, platelets 125,000/μL. INR: normal. Serum chemistries: normal. Urinalysis: normal. EKG: sinus tachycardia, otherwise normal. Chest radiograph: normal.

Questions: What kind of bite accounts for this presentation? What is the treatment?

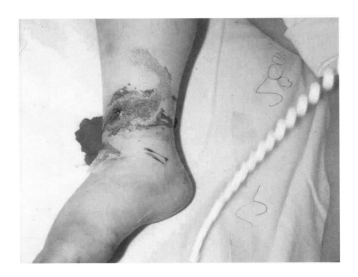

Diagnosis and Treatment: This scenario demonstrates moderate envenomation by a rattlesnake. Management should include stabilization and support of vital signs, evaluation for coagulopathy, hospitalization in a monitored setting, and administration of antivenom.

Discussion: Venomous snakebites occur approximately 8000 times each year in the United States and lead to 9–15 deaths annually. The majority of snakebite victims are white males between 19 and 30 years of age with a blood alcohol level of 0.1% or greater. Most bites occur on the extremities, between the months of April and October.

Crotalids comprise the vast majority of American venomous snakes. These include the rattlesnakes (such as the Eastern and Western diamondback, Massasauga, timber rattlesnake, prairie and Pacific rattlesnake, pygmy rattlesnake, the Mojave rattlesnake, and others) and the moccasins (cottonmouths and copperheads). Crotalids, or pit vipers, have a depressed area or pit, a heat-sensitive organ, located between the nostril and eye. This organ allows the snake to sense warm-blooded prey. Two (although occasionally more or less) retractable curved fangs are located in the upper jaw that can withdraw posteriorly as the mouth is closed. Crotalids also have elliptical pupils.

Among Crotalid envenomations, copperhead bites (see figure below) produce the fewest local and systemic symptoms of the native snakes, and are usually not serious enough to require antivenom. The severity of a cottonmouth bite seems between that of the copperhead and the rattlesnake. Another group of North American venomous reptiles are the coral snakes (Elapids), but this discussion focuses on Crotalid envenomations.

Crotalid venom composition is extremely complex, and varies with the species, time of year, diet, size, and age of the snake. Venoms contain multiple hemotoxic, neurotoxic and cardiotoxic peptides and enzymes, such as phospholipases, hyaluronidases, esterases, and proteolytic enzymes. Snake venom can cause severe tissue necrosis, increased vascular permeability with extravasation, coagulopathy, hemolysis, pulmonary edema, diffuse hemorrhage, lactic acidosis, hypovolemic and/or cardiogenic shock, coma, and renal failure. Although venom does not cross the blood-brain barrier, Mojave rattlesnake venom blocks presynaptic neuromuscular junction transmission and may result in decreased respiratory effort and flaccid paralysis. Coral snakes are also primarily neurotoxic.

Envenomation occurs when the fangs penetrate the skin and venom is injected, usually into the subcutaneous tissue. However, 25% of all pit viper bites and 50% of coral snake bites are "dry," resulting in no envenomation. Two fang marks usually characterize pit viper bites, and envenomation results in local swelling and pain, usually within 5 minutes to an hour of the bite. Mojave rattlesnake strikes are an exception—bites are much less painful and envenomation results in neurotoxic rather than hemotoxic symptoms. Other **signs of crotalid envenomation** include anxiety, agitation, confusion, petechiae, hemorrhagic blebs, ecchymoses, lymphangitis, nausea, vomiting, lethargy, paresthesias, a "minty" or "metallic" taste, and severe generalized weakness. In severe envenomations, local symptoms rapidly progress to **systemic symptoms** characterized by tachypnea and respiratory distress, hypotension, tachycardia, and changes in mental status. Pit viper envenomations may also result in a severe consumptive coagulopathy with prolonged clotting times and frank bleeding. Low platelets, low fibrinogen, and high fibrin degradation products are commonly encountered.

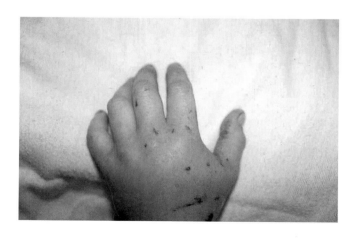

The present patient most likely suffered envenomation by a rattlesnake, although she could not recall hearing a rattle. The envenomation was significant, since both local and systemic symptoms developed. Much has been written about first aid for snakebite victims. Treatments in the past have included incision and suction, ice, electric shock therapy, and tourniquets. These do not benefit survival and are highly discouraged. A victim should be removed from further danger, kept warm, placed at rest, reassured, and transported as quickly as possible to the nearest hospital. The affected extremity should be immobilized at or below the level of the heart. The victim should not be given alcohol or stimulants, and any constricting items such as rings should be removed. If the transport time is 2 or more hours, a constriction band may be used, loosely placed proximal to the bite to restrict lymphatic, but not venous, flow.

Emergency evaluation and stabilization are standard, and specific treatment is based on the severity of the envenomation. Appropriately clean all wounds, and administer tetanus prophylaxis. Wound infections are rare, and antibiotics are reserved for definitive signs of infection (albeit difficult to differentiate from envenomation). However, broad-spectrum antibiotics are widely used empirically. Establish intravenous (IV) access in two locations, start IV fluids, and have laboratory studies drawn. Coagulopathy is the main concern that can be identified by the laboratory. Useful initial laboratory tests might include complete blood count, serum chemistries with aminotransferases and creatine kinase, coagulation profile with fibrinogen and fibrin split products, blood typing, and urinalysis. The blood fibrinogen and platelet count are the most sensitive hematological markers of systemic toxicity. Assess and mark the affected area, and repeat the exam every 20–30 minutes to assess for progression and complications of swelling. Serial physical exams are vital because symptoms can progress after an initial period of delay. An asymptomatic patient that has been bitten by a Crotalid can be observed for 8–12 hours and discharged with careful outpatient instructions.

Antivenin (Crotalidae) Polyvalent (ACP) traditionally has been recommended for severe rattlesnake, cottonmouth, and occasionally copperhead bites. This is a hyperimmunized horse serum, most effective if administered within 4 hours of envenomation. Adverse reactions to ACP range from anaphylaxis (23–56%) to serum sickness (18–86%). For this reason, some suggest that a skin test be done prior to administration of the antivenom, although a 20% false-negative rate and a lesser false-positive rate are reported. Others argue that skin testing is unnecessary once the decision to administer antivenom has been made. The first dose of antivenom is administered by slow IV infusion. At all times, resuscitation equipment including epinephrine, corticosteroids, and diphenhydramine should be kept readily available.

In October 2000, **Crotalidae Polyvalent Immune Fab (CroFab)** became available, and ACP supplies became severely limited. CroFab is a sheep-derived antivenom that may be more potent than ACP, although at present the exact efficacy and clinical use of this product is still being clarified. CroFab may have fewer adverse reactions (acute reactions 14%, serum sickness 16 %), but initial large doses and repeated doses are often required.

The **indications** for the administration of Crotalid antivenom are based on an envenomation scale. However, the use of antivenom varies widely among experts—not only in dose, but also in whether or not antivenom is given at all. The scale ranges from no envenomation to severe/life-threatening envenomation, but the specific antivenom regimen is more empiric than proven. Initial therapy with up to 5 vials of ACP are suggested for mild envenomation, and up to 25–40 vials for severe or life-threatening envenomation. There is no maximum dose, and clinical practice varies widely. Doses are not reduced for children or smaller patients since the antivenom is based on venom amount, not patient size. Unlike ACP, CroFab is given as a loading dose to gain control of the envenomation (about 6 vials), followed by maintenance doses at 6, 12, and 18 hours. Although antivenom is the mainstay for treating coagulopathies and severe systemic toxicity, the ability of anitvenom to markedly reduce local tissue injury has been questioned.

Several **complications** can ensue from the envenomation or from the treatment itself. Local tissue loss, persistent or permanent stiffness, and other dysfunction can be seen after a severe rattlesnake bite. Pit viper envenomation may result in a disseminated intravascular coagulopathy. Although blood components and fresh frozen plasma should be available, administer antivenom for a significant coagulopathy. Compartment syndrome is uncommon because the myofascial plane is rarely penetrated by the fangs, but may result from the local necrosis and edema. Fasciotomy is rarely required, but should not be prohibited. Serum sickness is common after ACP therapy, occurs 7–14 days after antivenom administration, and generally responds to antihistamines and/or a tapering dose of prednisone.

The present patient was experiencing moderate envenomation. She was treated with 15 vials of ACP and given tetanus prophylaxis, broad-spectrum antibiotics, fluid resuscitation, and analgesics. In addition, she was monitored for compartment syndrome. The patient experienced mildal thrombocytopenia as her only hematological complication. No blood products or additional antivenom were required. The ankle remained swollen and stiff for 2 weeks, but with physical therapy it exhibited only mild stiffness 2 months later. There was no tissue loss. One week after discharge she experienced urticaria and mild arthralgias (serum sickness) that responded to antihistamines.

Clinical Pearls

1. No form of first aid or field treatment has been demonstrated to reduce morbidity or mortality from snakebite in the U.S.

2. Crotalid venom has hemotoxic, cardiovascular, and neurological effects and tends to have a rapid onset of action and progression.

3. The use of antivenom is largely empirical, and although recommended for severe envenomation, systemic toxicity, and coagulopathies, the benefit of antivenom for local tissue injury is unproven.

4. The most striking laboratory abnormalities after pit viper envenomation are disorders of coagulation.

5. Most patients treated with antivenom of equine origin will develop serum sickness.

6. The role of CroFab therapy is still being defined, but it may be superior to horse serum preparations.

REFERENCES

1. Gold BS, Dart RC: Current concepts: Bites of venomous snakes. N Engl J Med 347:347-356, 2002.
2. Juckett G, Hancox J: Venomous snakebites in the United States: Management review and update. Am Fam Physician 7:1367-1377, 2002.
3. Roberts JR, Otten EJ: Snakes and other reptiles. In Goldfrank LR, Flomenbaum NE, Lewin NA, et al (eds): Goldfrank's Toxicological Emergencies, 7th ed. Stamford, Appleton and Lange, 1998, pp 1552-1572.
4. Gold BS, Wingert W: Snake venom poisoning in the United States: A review of therapeutic practice. South Med J 87:579-589, 1994.
5. Kurecki BA, Brownlee J: Venomous snakebites in the United States. J Fam Practice 25:386-392, 1987.

Robert Marsan, Jr., BS
Francis DeRoos, MD

PATIENT 8

A 45-year-old woman passed out in the back seat of a car

A 45-year-old woman was driven to the hospital by her friend; she was lying unconscious in the back seat of his car. The driver reports that they had been in traffic on a busy freeway and had only moved a few miles over the past hour. The patient had complained of an upset stomach and headache to her friend and was "not acting herself" just prior to passing out. The driver also had an upset stomach and headache, which he attributed to the stress of traffic and a fast-food meal. Upon entering the emergency department the patient regains consciousness, but remains lethargic and confused.

Physical Examination: Temperature 37.6° C, pulse 112/min, respirations 24/min, blood pressure 134/88 mmHg. Pulse oximetry 98% (in room air). General: lethargic, confused but cooperative, oriented to herself and her friend but not to the date or situation. HEENT: normal. Chest: normal. Lungs: normal. Neurological: depressed consciousness, normal cranial nerve function, normal peripheral motor and sensory function, symmetric deep tendon reflexes.

Laboratory Findings: Hemogram: WBC 11,000/µL, hemoglobin 13.4 g/dL, platelets 182,000/µL. Serum chemistries: normal, including glucose 114 mg/dL. Arterial blood gas (room air): pH 7.5, P_{CO_2} 29 mmHg, P_{O_2} 98 mmHg. EKG: sinus tachycardia, normal intervals, no ischemic changes.

Question: What test will confirm the etiology of this patient's altered mental status?

Diagnosis: Symptoms of nausea, headache, poor energy, and confusion, particularly if experienced by multiple individuals, suggest carbon monoxide (CO) toxicity and should be investigated with both a detailed exposure history and co-oximetric measurement of carboxyhemoglobin (COHb).

Discussion: Headache, dizziness, and nausea are extremely common complaints in any emergency department and may easily be attributed to benign diseases such as viral illness. Yet these vague complaints are also common manifestations of CO poisoning, forcing the clinician to maintain a high degree of suspicion. CO poisoning is the number one cause of both acute poisoning deaths and fire-related deaths in the United States, causing approximately 600 unintentional deaths and 3000 to 6000 intentional deaths annually. Carbon monoxide is a clear, odorless, and nonirritating gas. It is produced during combustion of carbonaceous fuels such as wood, gasoline, and oil. Common sources include home fires, dysfunctional heating systems, and vehicle exhaust fumes. The highest incidence of CO poisoning occurs in the cooler northern states and peaks during the winter months. In this case, the car's exhaust system had significant corrosion and deterioration and was venting exhaust through a hole directly into the back seat of this poorly maintained automobile.

Carbon monoxide readily diffuses across alveolar membranes into systemic circulation. The amount of CO that is absorbed by the body depends on the concentration of CO inhaled, the duration of exposure, and the victim's minute ventilation. Once in the blood stream, CO has approximately 250 times greater affinity for hemoglobin than O_2, thus displacing it and decreasing the O_2 carrying capacity of blood. Heavy cigarette smokers may have COHb concentrations as high as 10%. Fetal hemoglobin has an even higher affinity for CO than adult hemoglobin, raising concerns that if the mother is exposed, the fetus may be subjected to even higher levels of COHb. Carbon monoxide is eliminated from the body by ventilation via the lungs, although approximately 1% is converted into CO_2.

While the mechanisms of tissue injury during CO poisoning are still being investigated, most agree multiple pathways are involved. Tissue hypoxia occurs because of the decreased blood oxygen content and by CO's ability to shift the hemoglobin-O_2 dissociation curve to the left, making it more difficult for oxygen to dissociate from hemoglobin at the tissue level. In addition, CO binds to and inhibits the enzyme cytochrome oxidase. This leads to a cascade of events that ultimately results in neuronal cell death. Nitric oxide, oxygen free radicals, and excitatory amino acids all appear to play a role in this delayed neurological injury. Preventing this biochemical cascade toward neuronal death is thought to be the primary mechanism by which **hyperbaric oxygen (HBO) treatments** may prevent delayed neurological morbidity.

CO-induced cerebral hypoxia can lead to pre-syncope, syncope, seizures, and coma. Angina may occur in patients with severe coronary artery disease, and pulmonary edema or dysrhythmias may be noted on presentation. Moderately to severely poisoned patients are typically tachycardiac and tachypneic due to the hypoxia. The classically taught findings of cherry-red lips, cyanosis, and retinal hemorrhages are rarely seen. Clinical manifestations of poisoning do not correlate well with COHb levels. In addition, because of the destructive cascade of events that leads to delayed neuronal injury, patients may develop numerous types of neurological impairment days after exposure and treatment. These are termed **delayed neuropsychiatric sequelae** and may include dementia, parkinsonism, focal paralysis, movement disorders, depression, or amnestic syndromes. They may manifest days to months after exposure and can be prevented with early HBO therapy.

In the present case, two people in the same car shared non-specific symptoms. The "coincidence" of seeing two individuals with symptoms such as these triggered the physician to consider environmental toxins such as CO and inquire about any possible exposures. Pulse oximetry cannot distinguish between oxyhemoglobin and COHb and is typically normal in mildly to moderately CO-poisoned patients. Therefore only co-oximetry for COHb can be used to determine CO exposure. This can be preformed on either arterial or venous blood samples. In this patient, co-oximetry revealed a COHb level of 34%.

When treating patients with CO poisoning, the first priorities include removing the patient from the source of the CO and initiating 100% oxygen via non-rebreather mask. Once removed from the CO source, the half-life of COHb at room air is 4 to 6 hours and is reduced to 40 to 90 minutes with 100% O_2. Suicide remains the most common source of exposure, so vigilance for clues of possible co-ingestants should always be maintained. In addition, some fires may create significant amounts of cyanide gas, complicating management (see Case 9).

While the initial symptoms tend to resolve as the COHb level drops, delayed neuropsychiatric sequelae may present anywhere from 3 to 60 days after exposure. Elderly patients and those who have suffered a loss of consciousness are at greatest risk. These maladies are difficult to treat once clinically present and may become permanent; therefore it is essential to identify and treat those patients at greatest risk of delayed neuropsychiatric sequelae. While the treatment parameters for HBO are still debated, most physicians agree that any patient with severe CO poisoning who presents with significant neurological symptoms, including syncope or altered mental status, is a candidate for HBO therapy. Significant theoretical, animal-model, and clinical evidence exists to suggest that HBO may be of value in reducing the risk of delayed neuropsychiatric sequelae. Because of the potential for greater exposure to the fetus, physicians have a lower threshold for HBO therapy among pregnant patients. Transport of critically ill patients to HBO chambers (see figure below) can be logistically difficult and dangerous, but HBO therapy is otherwise relatively well tolerated with limited risks. Risks include aural barotrauma and, rarely, hyperoxic seizures.

The present patient was initially treated with 100% O_2 via a non-rebreather mask and then transferred to a nearby hospital for HBO treatment. She had no complaints and a grossly normal neurological examination at 4-week follow-up.

Clinical Pearls

1. CO poisoning should be suspected in any patient with vague neurological or viral-like illnesses, especially when there are multiple patients with similar symptoms.

2. Pulse oximetry and ABG measurements cannot distinguish COHb from Hb. Obtain a co-oximetry measurement specific for COHb using either venous or arterial blood.

3. 100% O_2 and hyperbaric oxygen (HBO) are the treatments for CO poisoning. Consideration of HBO is typically reserved for those with syncope, altered mental status, coma, and/or high-risk conditions such as pregnancy or advanced age.

4. Current theory suggests that the benefit of HBO is cessation of the inflammatory vasculitis that often follows significant CO exposure.

5. An HBO treatment facility can be located by calling your regional poison center at 800-222-1222.

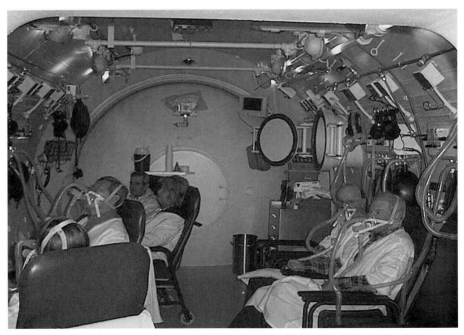

The hyperbaric oxygen treatment chamber at the University of Pennsylvania.

REFERENCES

1. Weaver LK, Hopkins RO, Chan KJ, et al: Hyperbaric oxygen for acute carbon monoxide poisoning. N Engl J Med 347: 1057-1067, 2002.
2. Thom SR: Hyperbaric-oxygen therapy for acute carbon monoxide poisoning. N Engl J Med 347:1105-1106, 2002.
3. Hoffman RS: Inhaled toxins. In Marx JA (ed): Rosen's Emergency Medicine: Concepts and Clinical Practice, 5th ed. St. Louis, Mosby, Inc., 2002, pp 2163-2171.
4. Ernst A, Zibrak, JD: Carbon monoxide poisoning. N Engl J Med 339:1603-1608, 1998.
5. Thom SR, Taber RL, Mendiguren II, et al: Delayed neuropsychologic sequelae after carbon monoxide poisoning: Prevention by treatment with hyperbaric oxygen. Ann Emerg Med 25:474-479, 1995.
6. Thom SR, Keim L: Carbon monoxide poisoning, a review: Epidemiology, pathophysiology, clinical findings, and treatment options including hyperbaric oxygen therapy. Clin Toxicol 27:141-150, 1989.

PATIENT 9

A 27-year-old woman who has collapsed

A 27-year-old student collapsed, and possibly had a seizure, one afternoon on the university campus near the laboratory research building where she works. In the ED, she is initially combative and agitated, but rapidly becomes somnolent. She has no medical history and is on no medication. Since no other history is available, her book bag is searched, and three bottles of over-the-counter analgesics, containing acetaminophen and salicylates, and a vial of a white crystalline substance are found (see figure).

Physical Examination: Temperature 37.8° C, pulse 130/min, respirations 30/min and labored; blood pressure 100/60 mmHg. General: comatose with prominent respiratory effort. HEENT: pupils 5 mm, sluggishly reactive. Chest: hyperpneic, lungs clear to auscultation. Abdomen: normal. Skin: no cyanosis. Neuromuscular: withdrawal to painful stimuli.

Laboratory Findings: Hemogram: normal. Serum chemistries: sodium 151 mEq/L, potassium 3.3 mEq/L, chloride 101 mEq/L, bicarbonate 8 mEq/L, BUN 28 mg/dL, creatinine 0.8 mg/dL, anion gap 47 mEq/L. Arterial blood gas (100% Fio_2): pH 7.32, pco_2 18 mmHg, po_2 264 mmHg. Chest radiograph: normal. EKG: sinus tachycardia.

Question: What types of toxins can produce a large anion gap metabolic acidosis?

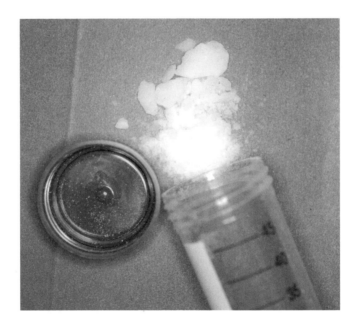

Diagnosis: Several toxins can produce a wide anion gap metabolic acidosis. Many clinicians use the mnemonic MUDPILES to help remember this differential diagnosis (see table).

Discussion: A wide anion gap metabolic acidosis is a significant laboratory finding that requires careful consideration and should not be ignored. When evaluating and refining the differential diagnosis of a wide anion gap metabolic acidosis there are several important sources of information that need to considered, including the history and physical examination, electrolytes, urinalysis, serum lactate level, and, if indicated, ethylene glycol, methanol or salicylate levels.

Without a history of significant gastrointestinal (GI) symptoms, iron poisoning can almost certainly be excluded. The acidosis produced by isoniazid overdose is caused by seizures, and their absence from the history and the lack of clues on physical examination, such as tongue biting or urinary incontinence, make this unlikely as well. Other historical clues include heavy alcohol use, which should raise suspicion for alcoholic ketoacidosis. Ethylene glycol and methanol, which are sometimes used as ethanol substitutes, may also be the cause of ketoacidosis. In addition, a careful medication history may uncover the use of metformin in a diabetic patient or salicylates that can be found in numerous over-the-counter preparations.

A normal BUN excludes uremia from the differential diagnosis. While an elevated glucose may suggest diabetic ketoacidosis, other ketoacidoses associated with ethanol or starvation typically have normal glucose levels. Urinalysis may reveal ketosis, which can be seen in various ketoacidoses, but remember that alcoholic ketoacidosis may have a falsely negative urine dip because the dip-sticks only identify ketones (acetone and acetoacetate); because ethanol produces a low redox state, the acetoacetate is converted into undetected beta-hydroxybutyrate. A serum lactate level is extremely useful in patients presenting with limited history or when the other lab tests are unyielding. Several toxins, including metformin, cyanide, hydrogen sulfide, and carbon monoxide, may produce a lactic acidosis. In patients for whom there is a strong suspicion of a toxic alcohol ingestion, ingestion of unknown automobile products, a large and unexplained osmolar gap, or a profound anion gap metabolic acidosis without a significant lactate, specific methanol and ethylene glycol levels should be ordered.

In the present patient, the combination of clues—the **occupational history** of working in a research laboratory, being found critically ill midday, the altered mental status and large anion gap metabolic acidosis, a significant lactate level of 12 mEq/L, a negative salicylate screen, and the crystals found in her bag—strongly supported a diagnosis of cyanide poisoning. Her serum acetaminophen and salicylate assays were negative.

Cyanide is found in numerous unique occupations and industries, such as the jewelry industry, electroplating, and basic science research laboratories. It is also naturally occurring in various forms in several plants, including the cassava, the seeds of several fruits in the prunus genus like apricots and peaches, and tobacco, and is commonly produced, in addition to carbon monoxide, in many home fires. It is rapidly absorbed via the mucosa and respiratory and GI tracts. It has an extremely high affinity for cationic metals and binds to several important enzymes throughout the body; the most physiologically devastating is its binding to the ferric (Fe^{3+}) iron found in the mitochondria within cytochrome a-a_3. This enzyme is the final step in the oxidative phosphorylation cascade aiding in the electron transfer to oxygen. The binding of cyanide renders this enzyme useless, inhibits the cell's ability to use oxygen, and impedes the cell's ability to utilize pyruvate in the tricarboxylic acid (TCA) or Krebs cycle, instead shunting pyruvate into lactate (see figure on next page). This effect is rapid, potent, and produces a profound lactic acidosis. Fortunately it is also fairly unstable, and the body has physiological methods of reversing this process that can be exploited with antidotal therapy.

The onset of the clinical effects of cyanide poisoning is rapid and dramatic and depends almost exclusively on the amount rather than the route or source of the exposure. Severely poisoned patients present with any of the physiological manifestations associated with a severe metabolic acidosis and hypoxia, including tachypnea and hyperpnea, tachycardia, diaphoresis, anxiety, agitation, seizures, and coma. Despite the impressive symptoms of dyspnea and work of breathing, these patients are rarely cyanotic (unless in concomitant

MUDPILES Mnemonic for Anion Gap Metabolic Acidosis

Methanol
Uremia
DKA, AKA, starvation ketoacidosis
Phenformin, metformin
Isoniazid, iron, inborn errors of metabolism
Lactate—CN, CO, H_2S
Ethylene glycol
Salicylate

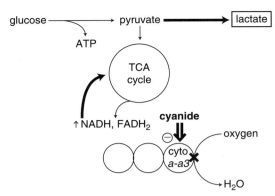

glucose → pyruvate → lactate
ATP
TCA cycle
↑ NADH, FADH$_2$
cyanide ⊖
cyto a-a3 ✗
oxygen
→ H$_2$O

Cyanide inhibits cytochrome a-a3, which blocks oxidative phosphorylation, causes a buildup of reduced substances like NADH, which inhibit the TCA cycle, forcing pyruvate to be shunted into lactate and producing a lactic acidosis.

pulmonary edema or apnea), and their pulse oximetry readings are typically normal. This swift onset of effects is only compounded by the rapidity of the progression and deterioration of cyanide-poisoned patients and necessitates early diagnosis.

The diagnosis of cyanide poisoning is critical in effectively treating these patients and rests upon a careful exposure history that includes recent meals, hobbies, occupations, and location of event. Diagnosis also depends on a recognition of the clinical presentation of a previously well person with rapid-onset altered mental status and a profound lactic acidosis. Some routine studies including an arterial blood gas (ABG), co-oximetry measurement of carbon monoxide, serum electrolytes, and lactate level are helpful in diagnosing cyanide poisoning. The ABG often reveals a profound metabolic acidosis with adequate oxygenation. Since cyanide inhibits peripheral tissue use of oxygen, the oxygen content in the arterial and venous systems remains unchanged. This arteriovenous oxygen difference has been exploited to aid in diagnosing cyanide poisoning in patients in intensive care units receiving sodium nitroprusside infusions, but is, unfortunately, impractical in the ED because it requires pulmonary artery sampling for accuracy. Specific laboratory assays for cyanide in either the serum or erythrocytes, where it concentrates because of the iron moiety, are used to retrospectively confirm a poisoning because of the long turnaround times required for these assays and the rapid treatment decisions that are required.

Treatment of cyanide-poisoned patients should focus on aggressive supportive care, improving oxygenation and acidosis, and use of the **Taylor Cyanide Antidote Kit**. GI decontamination with orogastric lavage and oral activated charcoal may be beneficial due to the potent toxicity and lethality, and should be considered after initial resuscitation. Intravenous access, 100% oxygen supplemented via nonrebreather or endotracheal tube, and continuous cardiac monitoring should be initiated immediately, and crystalloid fluid boluses for hypotension and sodium bicarbonate boluses for profound acidosis should be administered as needed. The Taylor Cyanide Antidote Kit contains three specific agents. The first two, **amyl nitrite** and **sodium nitrite**, are used to induce methemoglobinemia. This oxidized iron moiety (Fe^{3+}) has a much higher affinity for cyanide than normal hemoglobin and thus acts as a sink or reservoir to promote dissociation from the cytochrome a-a_3 enzyme. Amyl nitrite is administered by inhalation and is only needed in unique "in the field" resuscitations; sodium nitrite is an intravenous infusion. Risks associated with the use of these agents include potent vasodilatation and hypotension and an inappropriate induction of methemoglobinemia. This may result when a fire victim is already carbon monoxide poisoned and has a high level of carboxyhemoglobin present. The addition of a second "abnormal" hemoglobin, methemoglobin, may further compromise the patient's oxygen-carrying capacity.

The third agent in this kit is **sodium thiosulfate** and is by far the most important. Remember that the body naturally is exposed to very small amounts of cyanide regularly and detoxifies this by binding thiosulfate to cyanide via an enzyme called rodanese (see figure below). This forms a much less toxic compound, thiocyanate, that is eliminated in the urine. Infusing sodium thiosulfate exploits this enzyme by providing it significant

CYANIDE TREATMENT

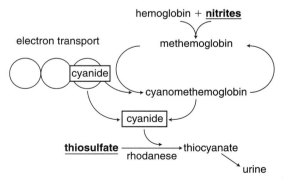

hemoglobin + **nitrites**
electron transport
cyanide
methemoglobin
cyanomethemoglobin
cyanide
thiosulfate → thiocyanate
rhodanese
→ urine

Cyanide treatment. Nitrites create methemoglobin from hemoglobin. This has a much higher affinity to cynanide and "attracts" it from the electron transport chain, forming cyanomethemoglobin. Thiosulfate is bound to cyanide by rhodanese enzyme, which produces the much less toxic and renally eliminated thiocyanate.

substrate and greatly increasing its ability to remove cyanide. Sodium thiosulfate has limited toxicity, and it's reasonable to administer this part of the kit alone in patients for whom the history or presentation is not clear, or in fire victims when the risk of concomitant carboxyhemoglobin will not allow patients to tolerate an induced methemoglobinemia. Instructions for administration of these agents and their dosing is on the inside of the kit lid, so do not discard the lid upon opening the kit.

The present patient was treated with sodium thiosulfate and good supportive care. Over the next few hours, she became more and more alert and awake. She confessed to eating one peanut-sized crystal of potassium cyanide she had removed from the laboratory where she worked in a suicide attempt. She fully recovered.

Clinical Pearls

1. Rapid onset of loss of consciousness or coma and a large lactic acidosis strongly suggest a cellular asphyxiant like cyanide.

2. Once you identify a wide anion gap metabolic acidosis, be sure to carefully consider the differential diagnosis through targeted history and laboratory study.

3. Clues from the history related to specific occupations, such as the jewelry or electroplating industries or work in a research laboratory, strongly support cyanide poisoning in the proper clinical setting.

4. Aggressive resuscitation, oxygenation, and supportive care remain the mainstay of treatment for cyanide-poisoned patients.

5. Antidotal treatment includes inducing a methemoglobinemia with nitrites to attract cyanide from the oxygen transport chain, and then providing thiosulfate to be bound to cyanide by an enzyme rhodanese, forming the relatively nontoxic thiocyanate.

REFERENCES

1. Kirk MA, Gerace R, Kulig KW: Cyanide and methemoglobin kinetics in smoke inhalation victims treated with the cyanide antidote kit. Ann Emerg Med 22(9):1413-1418, 1993.
2. Johnson WS, Hall AH, Rumack BH: Cyanide poisoning successfully treated without "therapeutic methemoglobin levels." Am J Emerg Med 7(4):437-440, 1989.
3. Hall AH, Rumack BH: Clinical toxicity of cyanide. Ann Emerg Med 15(9):1067-1073, 1986.
4. Graham DL, Laman D, Theodore J, et al: Acute cyanide poisoning complicated by lactic acidosis and pulmonary edema. Arch Intern Med 137(8):1051-1055, 1977.
5. Oh MS, Carroll HJ: The anion gap. N Engl J Med 297(15):814-817, 1977.
6. Chen KK, Rose CL: Nitrite and thiosulfate therapy in cyanide poisoning. JAMA 149(2):113-115, 1952.

PATIENT 10

A 2½-year-old boy who drank drain opener

A previously healthy 2½-year-old boy explored the bathroom cabinets at his home and drank some drain opener. He is now drooling and crying.

Physical Examination: Temperature 37.4° C, pulse 140/min, respirations 24/min, blood pressure 105/62 mmHg. General: alert, anxious and uncomfortable. HEENT: red and swollen lips, drooling, no corneal defects. Chest: mild stridor with agitation. Cardiovascular: well-perfused. Abdomen: soft. Skin: erythema of the chin.

Laboratory Findings: Chest radiograph: normal. Lateral neck radiograph: edema of the epiglottis (see figure).

Question: What intervention is indicated emergently?

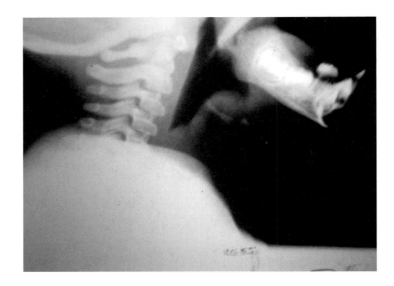

Diagnosis and Treatment: Caustic epiglottitis is an emergent threat to the boy's airway, and endotracheal intubation should be performed.

Discussion: Household drain openers are typically strong acids such as sulfuric acid, or, as in this case, strong alkali such as sodium hydroxide. Tens of thousands of acid and alkali exposures are reported to American Poison Control Centers annually, and these reports include several deaths. The degree of injury that occurs after caustic ingestion depends upon the pH of the product, its concentration, and its duration of contact with tissues. The duration of contact is, in turn, dependent upon the mode of exposure, the volume of exposure, and the viscosity of the product.

Initial evaluation of an alkali ingestion should focus on the airway, breathing, and circulation of the patient. In the present patient, laryngeal and glottic burns may become immediately life-threatening. Pneumonitis, esophageal or gastric perforation, metabolic acidosis, and shock may also occur. Care should be taken to decontaminate exposed skin and eyes with copious amounts of water or other suitable irrigation fluid. Neutralization of alkali injuries with weak acids is discouraged, as the chemical reaction produces heat.

Delayed complications of esophageal or gastric alkali injury include esophageal strictures, impaired gastric function, and pyloric obstruction. The presence of oropharyngeal burns and symptoms in the present patient suggests likely esophageal injury. An absence of signs or symptoms would suggest that esophageal injuries are unlikely, but the negative predictive value is not 100%. Early endoscopy to define the extent of the injury, to define prognosis, and to direct pharmacological and surgical therapy is probably warranted after any suicidal or large-volume alkali ingestion, after ingestion of a concentrated alkali of high pH, or when the patient is vomiting or significantly symptomatic.

First-degree alkali-burns of the esophagus typically heal uneventfully, and circumferential third-degree burns will uniformly scar with stricture. The role of **corticosteroid therapy** to reduce stricture formation after circumferential second-degree alkali-burns remains controversial. Some recommend methylprednisolone plus prophylactic antibiotics in instances where circumferential second-degree esophageal burns are confirmed within 24 hours of exposure.

The present patient was mechanically ventilated and received steroids for several days while his glottic edema resolved. Endoscopy demonstrated extensive circumferential second-degree burns of the esophagus. Esophageal stricture resulted, as demonstrated with a barium-swallow radiograph (see figure). The boy suffered from years of feeding difficulties, and was treated with repeated esophageal dilatations. It is estimated that patients with caustic esophageal injury have a 1000-fold increased incidence of esophageal carcinoma, with a mean latency period of nearly 40 years.

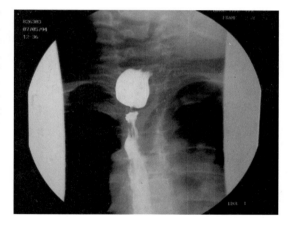

Clinical Pearls

1. Families often do not appreciate the dangerous nature of drain cleaners and gun-bluing agents, and this is an important anticipatory guidance message.

2. Airway compromise is the most immediate danger to life after caustic ingestion.

3. The role of corticosteroid therapy in the prevention of alkali-induced esophageal strictures is controversial, but some evidence exists to suggest a possible benefit among patients with circumferential second-degree esophageal burns.

REFERENCES
1. Howel J, Dalsey W, Hartsell F, et al: Steroids for the treatment of corrosive esophageal injury: a statistical analysis of past studies. Am J Emerg Med 1992; 10:421-425.
2. Rao RB, Hoffman RS: Caustics and batteries. In Goldfrank LR, Flomenbaum NE, Lewin NA, et al. (eds): Goldfrank's Toxicologic Emergencies, 7th ed. New York, McGraw Hill, 2002, 1323-1345.

Paul Ishimine, MD
Kevin C. Osterhoudt, MD

PATIENT 11

A 2-year-old girl with status epilepticus

A 2-year-old, previously healthy girl develops seizures. Diazepam stopped her initial seizure, but she subsequently has three more seizures in the emergency department that are stopped with lorazepam. A phenytoin infusion is started, but she continues to have seizures and undergoes endotracheal intubation. She has no history of fever, trauma, or previous seizures. She lives with her grandmother, who is taking medicine for "lung problems."

Physical Examination: Temperature 38.1° C, pulse 137/min, blood pressure 87/58 mmHg. General: obtunded. HEENT: pupils 4 mm, equal and reactive; moist mucous membranes. Chest: clear to auscultation. Cardiovascular: normal heart rhythm with good perfusion. Abdomen: normal. Extremities: normal. Skin: normal. Neuromuscular: cranial nerve function intact, opens eyes and moves extremities to painful stimuli.

Laboratory Findings: Hemogram: WBC 15,800/μL (78% segmented neutrophils; 4% band forms), otherwise normal. Serum chemistries: sodium 137 mEq/L, potassium 4.2 mEq/L, chloride 102 mEq/L, HCO_3^- 8 mEq/L; blood urea nitrogen 12 mEq/L; creatinine 0.4 mEq/L, glucose 143 mg/dL, lactate 17 mEq/L. Serum osmolarity: 298. Arterial blood gas (100% Fio_2 immediately after intubation): pH 7.02, $Paco_2$ 28 mmHg, Pao_2 393 mmHg, HCo_3^- 6 mmHg. Salicylate, acetaminophen, and ethanol levels: non-detectable. Urine immunoassay for drugs of abuse: negative. Electrocardiogram: sinus tachycardia with normal intervals. Chest x-ray: normal, endotracheal tube in good position. Head CT: normal.

Question: In the face of unexpected status epilepticus refractory to standard anticonvulsant therapy, and with salicylate intoxication excluded, what empiric pharmacological therapy should be considered next?

Discussion: Status epilepticus can result from many different etiologies. These causes include metabolic derangements, such as hyponatremia and hypoglycemia; infections (the most common cause of status epilepticus in children is prolonged febrile seizures); central nervous system lesions; and subtherapeutic levels of anticonvulsant agents used to treat patients with known seizure disorders. However, poisoning should be considered in the differential diagnosis of any child with the abrupt onset of unexplained status epilepticus. While many toxic exposures can lead to seizures, some toxins are more frequently associated with status epilepticus than others (see table). In addition to her status epilepticus, this patient also has a significant metabolic acidosis with an elevated anion gap:

$$\text{anion gap} = Na^+ - (Cl^- + HCO_3^-);$$
$$\text{normal range } 7 \pm 4 \text{ mEq/L.}$$

An elevated anion gap can be caused by either a decrease in unmeasured cations or by an increase in unmeasured anions within the serum. The wide-anion-gap metabolic acidosis provides a further clue to this child's malady.

Both isoniazid and theophylline are medications that can cause status epilepticus and metabolic acidosis; they are both used to treat pulmonary diseases. A family member was sent to retrieve the grandmother's pill bottles, and a serum theophylline level was measured. The family member returned with an empty bottle for isoniazid, and the serum theophylline level was undetectable.

Isoniazid (INH, isonicotinic hydrazide) is an antibiotic widely used for the treatment of tuberculosis. Isoniazid interferes with mycolic acid synthesis, which is an essential component of the mycobacterial cell wall. INH produces its toxic effects in the setting of acute overdose by causing a functional depletion of pyridoxine (vitamin B_6).

This occurs through several mechanisms. INH inhibits pyridoxine phosphokinase, the enzyme that coverts pyridoxine to its active form, pyridoxine-5-phosphate. Additionally, INH directly interferes with cellular pyridoxine and pyridoxine-5-phosphate, resulting in the inactivation of pyridoxine activity. Pyridoxine is a coenzyme for L-glutamic acid decarboxylase, an enzyme required for the synthesis of gamma aminobutyric acid (GABA), the primary inhibitory neurotransmitter in the brain. The decrease in GABA production is thought to cause the seizures seen in INH toxicity.

The therapeutic dosage of INH is typically 5–15 mg/kg. Seizures can be seen with doses as low as 20 mg/kg, but severe toxicity is most common after ingestion of 80–150 mg/kg. Symptoms of INH poisoning include slurred speech, ataxia, refractory seizures, and coma, and may be seen within 30 minutes of ingestion. Accumulation of lactate occurs during INH-induced seizures, leading to a wide-anion-gap metabolic acidosis.

Treatment for patients with isoniazid toxicity requires the usual initial attention to the airway, breathing, and circulation, neurological disability, and gastrointestinal decontamination. Benzodiazepines and other anticonvulsants may be used to attempt to control seizure activity, but seizures associated with INH toxicity are frequently difficult to control with standard anticonvulsants. Pyridoxine administration is the definitive antidote to isoniazid-induced seizures. If the amount of INH ingested is known, the same amount of pyridoxine should be given. If the amount of INH ingested is unknown, the recommended empiric dose 70 mg/kg up to 5 g.

The present patient was administered 70 mg/kg of pyridoxine and had no further seizure activity. Her metabolic acidosis subsequently subsided. She was discharged from the hospital 3 days later without any apparent neurological sequelae.

Drugs Commonly Associated with Seizures*

P	PCP, Pesticides, Propoxyphene
L	Lead, Lithium, Lindane, Local anesthetics
A	Antidepressants, Antipsychotics, Anticonvulsants, Antihistamines, Abstinence syndrome
S	Salicylates, Sympathomimetics, Strychnine, Solvents
T	Theophylline, Tricyclic antidepressants, Thallium, Tobacco (nicotine)
I	INH, Insulin (+ other hypoglycemic drugs), Insecticides, Inderal
C	Camphor, Cocaine, Cyanide, Chloroquine, Cicutoxin

*PLASTIC mnemonic adapted and modified from discussion developed by Dr. Jim Roberts at the Poison Control Center in Philadelphia, Pennsylvania.

Clinical Pearls

1. The combination of status epilepticus and an elevated-anion-gap metabolic acidosis should suggest isoniazid toxicity.

2. Theophylline and isonicotinic hydrazide (INH) may produce similar seizure syndromes. Since both medications are used to treat pulmonary diseases, theophylline toxicity may be confused with isoniazid toxicity.

3. Seizures caused by INH toxicity may be refractory to standard anticonvulsants, but administration of pyridoxine often results in rapid termination of seizure activity.

REFERENCES

1. Boyer EW: Antituberculous agents. In Goldfrank LR, Flomenbaum NE, Lewin NA, et al (eds): Goldfrank's Toxicologic Emergencies, 7th ed. New York, McGraw-Hill, 2002, pp 655-666.
2. Santucci KA, Shah BR, Linakis JG: Acute isoniazid exposures and antidote availability. Pediatr Emerg Care 15:99-101, 1999.
3. Shah BR, Santucci K, Sinert R, Steiner P: Acute isoniazid neurotoxicity in an urban hospital. Pediatrics 95:700-704, 1995.
4. Alvarez FG, Guntupalli KK: Isoniazid overdose: Four case reports and review of the literature. Intensive Care Med 21: 641-644, 1995.
5. Wason S, Lacouture PG, Lovejoy FH: Single high-dose pyridoxine treatment for isoniazid overdose. JAMA 246:1102-1104, 1981.

Sara Abbruzzi, DO
Jeanmarie Perrone, MD

PATIENT 12

A 40-year-old woman with hypoglycemia and lactic acidosis

A 40-year-old woman with a history of severe depression, hypothyroidism, and diabetes is brought to the emergency department by ambulance following a polysubstance overdose. Upon arrival, the patient is confused but awake, and exhibits slow speech. Within 8 hours of arrival, the patient vomits multiple times and has two episodes of hypoglycemia.

Physical Examination: Afebrile, pulse 79/min, respirations 14/min, blood pressure 126/49 mmHg. General: awake but confused. HEENT: pupils 3 mm, equal and reactive; conjunctiva pink, mucous membranes moist. Neck: supple, no jugular venous distention, no thyromegaly, no masses. Chest: decreased respiratory effort, clear to auscultation. Cardiovascular: regular rhythm without murmurs, rubs, or gallops. Abdomen: soft, obese, nontender, nondistended, no palpable masses. Extremities: no clubbing, cyanosis, or edema. Skin: warm and dry, no rashes. Neuromuscular: oriented to person and place only, normal reflexes, no focal deficits.

Laboratory Findings: **On admission**—Hemogram: WBC 15,400/μL, hemoglobin 15.4 g/dL, platelets 339,000/μL. Serum chemistries: sodium 135 mEq/L, potassium 3.8 mEq/L, chloride 98 mEq/L, HCO_3^- 25 mEq/L, BUN 8 mg/dL, creatinine 1.0 mg/dL, glucose 257mg/dL, anion gap 12, salicylate < 4 mg/dL, acetaminophen 33 μg/ml, lithium 0.38 mEq/L. **8 hours later**—Sodium 141 mEq/L, potassium 4.3 mEq/L, chloride 104 mEq/L, HCO_3^- 13 mEq/L, BUN 10 mg/dL, creatinine 2.3 mg/dL, glucose 58 mg/dL, anion gap 24, lactic acid 21 mmol/L. Arterial blood gas: pH 6.95, $Paco_2$ 26. EKG: sinus tachycardia. Chest radiograph: normal.

Question: What drug might this woman have been prescribed that could produce hypoglycemia as well as profound lactic acidosis in overdose?

Diagnosis: Additional history confirms that this patient has been prescribed a combination agent of metformin and glyburide (Glucovance) for diabetes.

Discussion: Metformin overdose was suspected when this diabetic patient developed a profound **lactic acidosis** and a blood pH of 6.95. While the differential diagnosis for a wide anion gap metabolic acidosis is quite broad (see table, *top*), attention in this case could be narrowed to those toxins known to cause lactic acidosis (see table, *bottom*). Serum testing excluded salicylate poisoning. Isoniazid ingestion causes a lactic acidosis by promoting status epilepticus that leads to lactate production. Isoniazid poisoning was excluded in this case since initial laboratory data was normal and no seizures occurred after hospitalization. Iron poisoning was exluded because gastrointestinal distress was not massive. Cyanide poisoning was also excluded because it causes rapid demise after ingestion. Since the patient was diabetic, metformin overdose was the most likely possibility. The patient also had recurrent episodes of hypoglycemia that did not stabilize with intravenous dextrose therapy. Refractory hypoglycemia is not characteristic of metformin poisoning; therefore, the hypoglycemia was an important clue suggesting co-ingestion of a sulfonylurea in a **new combined formulation**. Several combined formulations have become available in the past several years including Metaglip (glipizide and metformin) and Glucovance (glyburide and metformin).

Metformin is prescribed for diabetes because it enhances insulin sensitivity, increases glycogen formation and decreases insulin resistance. Metformin decreases hyperglycemia primarily by decreasing hepatic gluconeogenesis. Lactate, alanine, and pyruvate utilization decrease, and a lactic acidosis may occur. The specific mechanism is not clearly elucidated.

Lactic acidosis was a relatively common adverse effect of phenformin, a related drug. Phenformin caused lactic acidosis by binding to mitochondrial enzymes and inhibiting lactate utilization. This occasionally (approximately 64 cases per 100,000 patient-years) resulted in profound toxicity, including death, and was removed from the U.S. market in 1976. Occasional cases still occur among U.S. immigrants and visitors, who may be taking the drug prescribed abroad.

The incidence of lactic acidosis with metformin is much lower than with phenformin (approximately three cases per 100,000 patient-years). However, the risk is increased among patients with renal insufficiency or among patients with dehydration, congestive heart failure, and alcohol abuse. There are few published cases of intentional overdose with metformin. The observed toxicity has been variable; however, lactic acidosis has occurred in some cases. Lactic acidosis is managed with sodium bicarbonate therapy, and sometimes with hemodialysis to correct acid base disturbances and to remove metformin.

The present patient was emergently dialyzed and was given aggressive fluid resuscitation in combination with vasopressor support for circulatory collapse, supplemental bicarbonate therapy for profound acidemia, and dextrose and octreotide for the refractory hypoglycemia. Within 24 hours of admission, she became progressively more lethargic and profoundly hypotensive, and developed a worsening anion gap acidosis that was refractory to bicarbonate therapy. The patient ultimately died. A metformin level was obtained to ascertain and confirm the suspected diagnosis. The metformin level from admission was later reported to be 150 µg/mL (therapeutic 1–2 µg/mL). This case illustrates the potential for severe lactic acidosis and death with metformin poisoning.

Mnemonic for the Differential Diagnosis of Wide Anion Gap Metabolic Acidosis

M Methanol, metformin
U Uremia
D Diabetic ketoacidosis (and other ketoacidoses)
P Phenformin, paraldehyde
I Isoniazid, iron, inborn errors of metabolism
L Lactic acidosis
E Ethylene glycol
S Salicylates, solvents, strychnine

Drugs Associated with the Production of Lactic Acidosis

Cyanide
Iron
Isoniazid
Metformin
Phenformin
Salicylates

Clinical Pearls

1. The accumulation of lactate is an important finding in the evaluation of a patient with a wide anion gap metabolic acidosis.

2. Metformin or phenformin poisoning may produce severe lactic acidosis.

3. Hypoglycemia does not typically occur with isolated metformin or phenformin overdose, but may occur if another diabetes medication (such as a sulfonylurea) is co-ingested.

4. Metformin poisoning should be treated with large doses of sodium bicarbonate to buffer severe acidosis. Hemodialysis may be useful for correction of severe acidosis and to help eliminate metformin.

REFERENCES

1. Barrueto F, Meggs WJ, Barchman MJ: Clearance of metformin by hemofiltration in overdose. J Toxicol Clin Toxicol 40: 177-180, 2002.
2. McLaughlin SA, Crandall CS, McKinney PE: Octreotide: An antidote for sulfonylurea-induced hypoglycemia. Ann Emerg Med 36:133-138, 2000.
3. Spiller HA: Management of antidiabetic medications in overdose. Drug Saf 19:411-24, 1998.
4. Teale KF, Devine A, Stewart H, Harper NJ: The management of metformin overdose. Anaesthesia 53:698-701, 1998.

Esther H. Chen, MD
Jeanmarie Perrone, MD

PATIENT 13

An agitated youth from Jamaica

An 18-year-old woman is brought by customs officials from the international airport to the emergency department. She had just arrived from Jamaica and was apprehended by customs officials on arrival to the United States and suspected of drug smuggling. She adamantly denies any ingestion of drug or drug packets.

Physical Examination: Temperature 37.2° C, blood pressure 135/70 mmHg, pulse 88/min, respirations 20/min, pulse oximetry 98% in room air. General: alert, oriented, and anxious. HEENT: pupils mid-position and reactive. Chest: clear to auscultation. Cardiovascular: regular rhythm. Abdomen: soft, normal bowel sounds, non-tender, non-distended. Extremities: well-perfused. Neuromuscular: mild resting tremor in upper extremities, otherwise non-focal.

Laboratory Findings: Hemogram: normal. Serum chemistries: normal. Urinalysis: normal. EKG: sinus tachycardia, QRS duration 0.08 seconds, no ventricular ectopy. Chest x-ray: normal, no free air. Abdominal x-ray: small, round densities seen best in rectum, no dilated loops of bowel (see figure on left). Abdominal CT scan: (see figure on right).

Questions: What is the next step in the management of this patient? How might you obtain additional information if the patient is uncooperative?

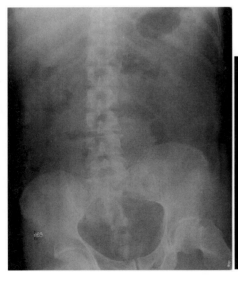
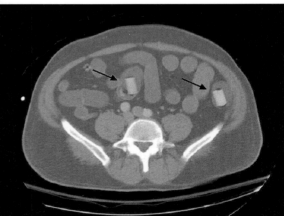

Answers: Although the patient denies any ingestion, the abdominal radiograph shows uniform foreign bodies in her abdomen, consistent with a diagnosis of body packing. Several factors may help clarify the contents of the packets, including country of origin, toxic signs or symptoms in the patient, or a urine drug screen. Most often patients are asymptomatic because the packets are still intact.

Discussion: Body *"packers"* ingest professionally wrapped packets of drugs, usually cocaine or heroin, for the purposes of smuggling. In contrast, *body "stuffers"* ingest poorly wrapped packets, usually in an effort to avoid police apprehension. Body stuffers also are more likely to be exposed to co-ingestants. Patients may present acutely ill with signs and symptoms consistent with the type of drug ingested, secondary to drug absorption from poorly wrapped packets, or they may prematurely pass packets while in transit. The diagnosis is made by history or direct visualization of the packets, i.e., on abdominal x-ray, as in this patient.

Radiographic imaging is a useful adjunct in the diagnosis and management of body packers. Proper imaging in body stuffers is more difficult because ingested containers are small and inconsistently apparent. An emergency bedside ultrasound may show hyperechogenic linear or round foreign bodies with dorsal echo extinction, but has limited resolution to distinguish the exact number. A flat-plate abdominal radiograph may help delineate quantities, but a detailed history of ingestion also should be obtained. Follow-up radiography after clearing the bowel is most important to verify that the packets are removed; however, the most sensitive imaging study for this purpose is still controversial.

Depending on the type of packing, the abdominal radiograph may show circular or tubular, hyperdense, radiolucent foreign bodies outlined by bowel gas ("halo sign") throughout the abdomen (see figure). However, they may be confused with stool or gas within the intestine ("pseudocondoms"). The sensitivity of abdominal radiography for detecting body packers ranges from 71% to 92%, with less reliability in body stuffers. In one series of body stuffers, the abdominal radiograph was falsely negative in all patients who were imaged. Alternatively, the use of oral-contrast plain radiography with complete bowel follow-through, after surgical or non-surgical bowel decontamination, may have merit.

Another commonly used modality is computed tomography (CT) without contrast, which shows packets as radio-opaque densities. Although typically not used as the initial screening modality, CT may be helpful in locating retained packets in persistently symptomatic patients. CT is about 60% sensitive at identifying healthy volunteers who have swallowed small packets of rock sugar to mimic body stuffers. However, there have been multiple case reports of false-negative CT scans and even false-negative laparotomies.

Asymptomatic body packers are managed with a dose of activated charcoal, followed by whole bowel irrigation with polyethylene glycol (PEG-ELS) at 2 liters/hour until all containers are passed. Serial oral-contrast plain radiographs with small bowel follow-through, or CT scan, may be helpful to detect retained packets if the history is unreliable as to the numbers of packets ingested. Patients with signs of toxicity after leakage of cocaine-containing body packets should be managed with surgical removal of the retained packets, since supportive care is often inadequate in the setting of massive cocaine exposure. Benzodiazepines should be used in the interim to ameliorate toxicity and prevent seizures. Leakage from heroin-containing packets can be managed with naloxone as needed, and continued whole bowel irrigation. Supportive care often is sufficient for heroin exposure. Small-bowel obstructions or ileus are common and may mandate surgical intervention.

The present patient was given 3.5 liters of Go-Lytely via a nasogastric tube, and she passed 18 packets. A single abdominal radiograph with barium, performed after decontamination, showed no remaining packets and no evidence of obstruction. She was observed, then discharged to police custody.

Clinical Pearls

1. Body *stuffers* hastily ingest poorly wrapped containers of smaller quantities of drugs and may frequently present with mild toxicity.

2. Body *packers* carry massive, life-threatening quantities of drug in their gut. The drug is carefully packaged.

3. Activated charcoal and whole bowel irrigation are commonly used together in an effort to safely purge containers from the gut of body packers.

4. Contrast imaging studies are important adjuncts used to confirm that the gut has been cleared of all drug packages. Estimates from patients tend to be inaccurate.

REFERENCES

1. Olmedo R, Nelson L, Chu J, Hoffman R: Is surgical decontamination definitive treatment of "body-packers"? Am J Emerg Med 19:593-596, 2001.
2. Hibbard R, Wahl M, Kirshenbaum M, Nellamattiathil G: Spiral CT imaging of ingested foreign bodies wrapped in plastic: A pilot study designed to mimic cocaine body stuffers. J Toxicol Clin Toxicol 37:644, 1999.
3. Sporer K, Firestone J: Clinical course of crack cocaine body stuffers. Ann Emerg Med 29:596-601, 1997.
4. Hierholzer J, Cordes M, Tantow H, et al: Drug smuggling by ingested cocaine-filled packages: Conventional x-ray and ultrasound. Abdom Imaging 20:333-338, 1995.
5. McCarron M, Wood J: The cocaine 'body packer' syndrome. JAMA 250:1417-1420, 1983.

Nancy Vinca, MD
Jeanmarie Perrone, MD

PATIENT 14

A 28-year-old man with a tremor and a seizure

A 28-year-old software salesman was traveling home from a 4-day business trip. While in an airport he had a generalized seizure, but he refused transport to the hospital. He subsequently had a second brief seizure while on the airplane. The plane landed, and paramedics were summoned again to assess the patient. Although he attempted to refuse transport a second time, he was mildly confused and very tachycardic with a pulse of 160/minute. He was transported to the emergency department (ED) against his wishes.

In the ED he is agitated, anxious, and tremulous and adamantly refuses further evaluation. His medical history is unremarkable. He denies a history of prior seizures or thyroid disease. He denies use of cocaine, amphetamines, diet drugs, herbal remedies, caffeine, steroids, or excess alcohol.

Physical Examination: Temperature 37° C, pulse 138/min, respirations 20/min, blood pressure 180/90 mmHg, oxygen saturation 96% in room air. General: tremulous, anxious, warm skin with diaphoresis, robust and healthy appearing. HEENT: pupils 5 mm and equally reactive. Chest: clear. Cardiovascular: tachycardic, no murmurs or rubs. Abdomen: normal bowel sounds, soft, non-tender. Extremities: well-perfused. Skin: diaphoretic, no rash. Neuromuscular: marked resting tremor which increases with intention, lower extremity clonus, otherwise non-focal.

Laboratory Findings: Hemogram: WBC 14,300/μL, hemoglobin 15.9 g/dL, platelets 122,000/μL, mean corpuscular volume (MCV) 97 μm^3. Coagulation profile: INR 1.6. Serum chemistries: glucose 238 mg/dL, GGT 199 IU/L, AST 88 IU/L, ALT 91 IU/L, CPK 421 IU/L, troponin negative; otherwise normal. Thyroid function tests: normal. Urinalysis: small blood, otherwise negative. Urine toxicology screen: negative. Electrocardiogram: tachycardia and 1.0- to 1.5-mm lateral ST depression (see figure). Chest radiograph: normal.

Questions: What could be causing the noted agitation, tachycardia, and hypertension following two brief seizures? Which laboratory clues help to confirm the diagnosis?

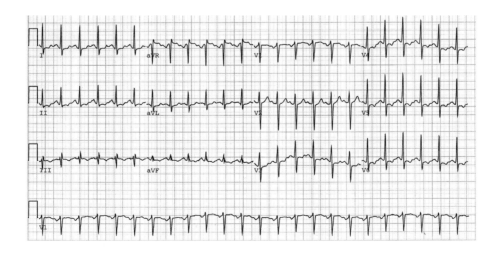

Diagnosis: Ethanol withdrawal was suspected because of the history of seizures and the sympathetic findings of tachycardia, hypertension, diaphoresis, and agitation. The high MCV of 98 μm^3 suggests folate deficiency and macrocytosis, presumably from heavy ethanol consumption. His relatively low platelet count may also indicate bone marrow toxicity from alcohol use. Elevated serum GGT can be a surrogate (but nonspecific) marker of alcohol consumption.

Discussion: An elaborate list of possible diagnoses can be ruled out by much of the data already obtained. On initial presentation the patient's symptoms and exam were most consistent with a sympathomimetic toxidrome, with seizures, tremors, diaphoresis, dilated and reactive pupils, and tachycardia. Also considered were thyrotoxicosis, pheochromocytoma, steroid use, and possible adrenal insufficiency. However, normal thyroid studies exclude thyrotoxicosis, and negative urine drug screening makes use of the more common stimulant drugs unlikely.

After observing and treating the patient in the ED and obtaining laboratory data, ethanol withdrawal became the more likely diagnosis. Sympathetic findings, seizures, and tremors are common in ethanol withdrawal. Although he did not readily admit to excess drinking, he was quite defensive when questioned about his alcohol use. In addition, his improvement after administration of lorazepam supported a diagnosis of alcohol withdrawal. EKG findings of ST depression appear to have been rate related and resolved with rate control.

Alcohol exerts its effects at the gamma aminobutyric acid (GABA) and *N*-methyl-D-aspartate (NMDA) type glutamate receptors. Its greatest effect is inhibition/depression of neurotransmitter release and of neuronal excitability. During a period of abstinence from alcohol there is reduced GABA activity and increased GABA-A sensitivity, causing a net decrease in neuronal inhibition. Thus, when faced with cessation of alcohol use, there is a resultant state of autonomic excitability, causing withdrawal symptoms. Signs and symptoms include two or more of the following: autonomic hyperactivity (tachycardia, hypertension, diaphoresis), tremor, insomnia, transient hallucinations, nausea/vomiting, anxiety/agitation, and seizures. Typically, symptoms start 5 to 10 hours after the last alcohol ingestion, peak at 48 to 72 hours, and subside by day 5 to 7.

Alcohol withdrawal includes a spectrum of clinical manifestations. It is important to realize that *alcohol withdrawal can begin even in the presence of an elevated ethanol level.* Seizures occur in 3–10% of patients in alcohol withdrawal. Alcohol withdrawal seizures or hallucinosis occur early after alcohol cessation. Untreated, either can progress to delirium tremens, characterized by fulminant agitation (delirium) and autonomic hyperactivity, including fever. The most important consideration in the diagnosis of alcohol withdrawal is to **determine why the patient stopped drinking**. Among chronic alcoholics, alcohol withdrawal is often precipitated by infection, which prevents the patient from being able to drink. By the time the patient presents to the ED with alcohol withdrawal, the underlying infectious process may be difficult to diagnose as fever may be ascribed to the withdrawal process. Failure to diagnose and treat the underlying pneumonia or meningitis often results in the greatest morbidity associated with ethanol withdrawal.

Any parenteral benzodiazepine will be efficacious in alcohol withdrawal, although lorazepam has been studied in alcohol withdrawal complicated by seizures. Either lorazepam or diazepam are most commonly used and titrated toward quelling the central nervous system (CNS) hyperexcitability and resolving any vital sign abnormalities. Barbiturates or propofol can be used for refractory cases; however, such treated patients often are supported with endotracheal intubation due to profound CNS and respiratory depression with these agents. Sympatholytics, such as beta receptor antagonists or clonidine, should not be used as monotherapy. They can decrease autonomic manifestations and, as a result, provide *a false sense of security* to the physician. Beta receptor antagonists should be used in conjunction with benzodiazepines only in cases of angina or marked anxiety. Clonidine may be used in the setting of severe hypertension or combined opioid/alcohol withdrawal. Thiamine therapy may prevent Wernicke's encephalopathy; magnesium, folate, and multivitamins help reverse nutritional deficiency. The goal of treatment is to prevent seizures, delirium tremens, and medical or psychiatric complications and, ideally, to bridge the patient to a stable state of abstinence. In the outpatient setting, disulfiram and naltrexone may be used for alcohol dependence as adjuncts to abstinence maintenance therapy.

Over a period of 4 days in the hospital the present patient improved greatly. He was initially treated with parenteral lorazepam as needed, and then switched to maintenance oxazepam every 4 hours by mouth. The EKG findings of lateral ST depression resolved, and he did not seize while in the hospital. Also, his tremor and anxiety decreased. His course was complicated by rhabdomyolysis (up to a total CPK of 7000 IU/L), which quickly resolved with intravenous fluid administration. He was aware of his problem with alcohol addiction and was open to seeking therapy on discharge.

Clinical Pearls

1. Seizures followed by tachycardia, hypertension, and tremor should prompt consideration of ethanol withdrawal as the etiology of the seizures.

2. A mean corpuscular volume greater than 97 μm^3 is unusual in an otherwise healthy, robust 28-year-old, and suggests nutritional deficiency such as that observed during chronic alcohol use.

3. Alcohol withdrawal can begin even in the presence of an elevated ethanol level, since the patient may be used to a much higher level.

REFERENCES

1. Chang P, Steinberg MB: Alcohol withdrawal. Med Clin North Am 85:1191-1209, 2001.
2. D'Onofrio G, Rathlev NK, Ulrich AS, et al: Lorazepam for the prevention of recurrent seizures related to alcohol. N Engl J Med 340:915-919, 1999.
3. Hall W, Zador D: The alcohol withdrawal syndrome. Lancet 349:1897-1900, 1997.
4. Saitz R, O'Malley, SS: Pharmacotherapy for alcohol abuse. Med Clin North Am 81:881-902, 1997.

Thomas Joseph Lydon, MD, PhD
Jeanmarie Perrone, MD

PATIENT 15

A 38-year-old woman with bizarre behavior on the job

A 38-year-old woman was found alone in the basement at her job. She was awake, but not speaking or acting normally. According to her colleagues, the patient had arrived on time that morning, met with clients, and subsequently ate lunch with several co-workers. She was not seen for approximately 1 hour prior to being discovered in the basement. No other co-workers in the building were ill.

On arrival in the emergency department, the patient is able to give her name but is unable to recall her birth date, the day, the year, or describe any of the events of the afternoon. She denies headache, nausea, vomiting, shortness of breath, chest pain, or abdominal pain.

Physical Examination: Temperature 37.4° C, pulse 116/min, respirations 18/min, blood pressure 114/79 mmHg. General: alert, oriented to self only; cooperative, but giving incorrect and inconsistent answers (she responded that the year was "1890," then later "1999," and then "1990"). HEENT: no obvious trauma; clear tympanic membranes bilaterally; pupils 4 mm, equal and reactive; no lacerations on the tongue or inner cheeks; no meningismus. Chest: clear. Cardiovascular: tachycardic but without murmur, rub, or gallop. Abdomen: soft, non-tender, non-distended. Genitourinary: no bruising, no urinary incontinence, no diarrhea. Extremities: no cyanosis, no edema. Skin: no rashes, warm and dry. Neuromuscular: cranial nerves intact, 2+ reflexes bilaterally, 5/5 strength in upper and lower extremities, uncooperative with gait exam; tolerant of arterial blood gas sampling from her right wrist without signs of discomfort.

Laboratory Findings: Hemogram: WBC 7100/μL, hemoglobin 13g/dL, platelets 238,000/μL. Coagulation profile: normal (INR = 0.9). Serum chemistries: Na^+ 140 mEq/L, K^+ 4.4 mEq/L, Cl^- 106 mEq/L, HCO_3^- 22 mEq/L, BUN 10 mg/dL, creatinine 0.7 mg/dL, glucose 93 mg/dL, anion gap 12, calcium 8.5 mg/dL, magnesium 1.9 mg/dL. Serum osmolality: 346 mOsm/L, osmolal gap 51 mOsm (normal range −7 to +10 mOsm). Cardiac profile: CPK 124 U/L, troponin-I <0.3 ng/mL. Arterial blood gas (32% Fio_2): pH 7.50, $Paco_2$ 34 mmHg, Pao_2 150 mmHg; carboxyhemoglobin 0.7%. Urinalysis: large ketones. Urine pregnancy: negative. Urine immunoassay for drugs of abuse: (+) ethanol. Serum toxicology: ethanol 27 mg/dL, salicylate 5.0 mg/dL, acetaminophen <10 mg/L. Electrocardiogram: rate 106, otherwise normal. Chest radiograph: normal. CT head: normal.

Question: What toxicological cause of altered mentation is notable for ketosis and an elevated osmolal gap in the *absence* of an increased anion gap acidosis?

Diagnosis: Isopropyl alcohol ingestion. The low ethanol level is not consistent with altered mental status. In contrast, isopropyl alcohol causes more profound central nervous system (CNS) effects and is metabolized to acetone, causing a ketosis and an elevated osmolal gap. However, unlike methanol and ethylene glycol, it does not cause a metabolic acidosis.

Discussion: Isopropyl alcohol (commonly known as rubbing alcohol) is a readily available and occasionally abused inexpensive substitute for ethanol. Although more intoxicating than ethanol, it induces significant gastric irritation and metabolic disturbances. Isopropyl alcohol is metabolized by alcohol dehydrogenase to acetone (see figure), which is then excreted renally. Isopropranol and the metabolite acetone are both CNS depressants. While the terminology "toxic alcohols" commonly refers to isopropyl alcohol, methanol, and ethylene glycol, only the latter two lead to morbidity-producing metabolic acidosis. Massive ingestion of isopropranol (concentrations >300 mg/dL) can result in hemorrhagic gastritis and tracheobronchitis in addition to extreme CNS depression. Such patients may benefit from endotracheal intubation, gastritis therapy, and possibly hemodialysis.

To confirm clinical suspicion of toxic alcohol ingestion, serum levels of toxic alcohols can be obtained in the laboratory. However, many hospitals are not equipped to run these levels on a "stat" basis, and thus surrogate markers for the presence of an unmeasured osmotically active substance are used to detect the possibility of a toxic alcohol ingestion. The **osmolal gap** represents the difference between the measured serum osmolality and the calculated serum osmolarity utilizing the values for sodium, BUN, and glucose obtained in the laboratory:

Osmol gap = Measured serum osmolality – calculated serum osmolarity.

Measured serum osmolality in the laboratory was 343 mosm/L, while the calculated osmolarity:

$$\text{Calculated osmolarity} = 2\,(Na^+\ mEq/L) + (\text{glucose mg/dL})/18 + (\text{BUN mg/dL})/2.8 + (\text{ethanol mg/dL})/4.6$$

was 295 mOsm. Thus, the osmol gap is 51 mOsm. An osmol gap of 51 is significantly elevated and is adequate to confirm suspicion of a toxic alcohol ingestion. While this number could represent severely elevated methanol and ethylene glycol levels, the absence of any elevation in the anion gap or significant decrease in the serum bicarbonate is not consistent with these toxic alcohols and this time course. In addition, the presence of serum ketones suggests that serum acetone is elevated, as it might be if resulting from isopropyl metabolism. The combination of depressed mental status, ketonuria, ketonemia, the large osmolal gap and the lack of an anion gap acidosis suggests isopropyl alcohol ingestion. Finally, the clinical and laboratory conclusions were confirmed by a serum isopropyl concentration of 198 mg/dL, serum methanol level of 0, and serum acetone level of 58 mg/dL.

The present patient was treated with intravenous fluids, zantac, thiamine, folate, and magnesium. After 4 hours in the emergency department, she was more alert and oriented and was admitted to the medical intensive care unit. The patient's belongings were examined for clues to her presentation. While no narcotics or medications were discovered, the name and address of her physician were found. The primary care provider stated that the patient had a history of alcohol abuse and had been through a rehabilitation program approximately 6 months ago. The physician provided the phone number of the emergency contact, her mother, who lived in another state. The mother reported that the patient had visited her on the previous weekend and seemed sad, but did not demonstrate any unusual behavior. On further questioning, the mother noted that she had found a bottle of rubbing alcohol in her bathroom closet. Although she kept rubbing alcohol in her home, she noted the discovery because the brand name on the bottle was not available in her area.

The patient improved in the ICU, and her altered mental status gradually resolved. Prior to discharge, the patient stated that she had tried rubbing alcohol (70% isopropranol) as a substitute for ethanol while staying with her mother on the previous weekend. On the morning of the day of admission, the patient had several glasses of wine before work (which explained the slightly elevated ethanol level) and then consumed the rubbing alcohol prior to lunch. The last thing she could remember was lunch with her co-workers, and she had no recollection of the events in the emergency department. The patient denied any attempt to harm herself, was seen and evaluated by psychiatry but refused any treatment.

ISOPROPANOL METABOLISM

Isopropanol

Acetone

Clinical Pearls

1. Isopropranol ingestion should be suspected in any patient presenting with a change in mental status, ketonuria and ketonemia, and a normal acid-base status.

2. Isopropranol ingestion is common in alcoholics because isopropranol is inexpensive and readily available in the home.

3. While the intoxicating effects of isopropranol can be severe, treatment is usually supportive, and deaths are rare.

4. Isopropyl alcohol is a notable "toxic" alcohol in that it does not typically cause a metabolic acidosis.

REFERENCES

1. Sharma AN: Toxic alcohols. In Goldfrank LR, Flomenbaum NE, Lewin NA, et al (eds): Goldfrank's Toxicologic Emergencies, 7th ed. New York, McGraw-Hill, 2002, pp 980-990.
2. Zaman F, Pervez A, Abreo K: Isopropyl alcohol intoxication: A diagnostic challenge. Am J Kidney Dis 40:E12, 2002.
3. Church AS, Witting MD: Laboratory testing in ethanol, methanol, ethylene glycol, and isopropanol toxicities. J Emerg Med 15:687-692, 1997.
4. Lacouture PG, Wason S, Abrams A, Lovejoy FH Jr: Acute isopropyl alcohol intoxication. Diagnosis and management. Am J Med 75:680-686, 1983.

Nancy N. Sun, MD
Francis DeRoos, MD

PATIENT 16

A 46-year-old man with auditory hallucinations

A 46-year-old man expresses the feeling that his housemates are "out to get him" and that they are trying to poison him. On review of systems, he notes a few days of increasing difficulty with breathing and inability to walk up a flight of stairs without stopping to rest. He admits to auditory hallucinations, but denies suicidal or homicidal ideations. His past medical history is significant for schizophrenia, bipolar disorder, and depression. His current medications consist of lithium and quetiapine.

Physical Examination: Temperature 36.1° C, pulse 101/min, respirations 32/min, blood pressure 114/78 mmHg. Pulse oximetry 100% in room air. General: pleasant, disheveled, in mild respiratory distress, having difficulty concentrating on questions; appears to be responding to internal stimuli. HEENT: normal; pupils 3 mm, round, reactive to light and accommodation. Chest: hyperpnea, bilateral basilar crackles. Cardiovascular: regular rate and rhythm without gallops or murmurs. Abdomen: normal. Extremities: no cyanosis or edema. Neuromuscular: awake and oriented to person, place, and time; normal muscle strength and reflexes.

Laboratory Findings: Hemogram: WBC 6300/μL, hemoglobin 15.2 g/dL, platelets 210,000/μL. Serum chemistries: sodium 138 mEq/L, potassium 3.6 mEq/L, chloride 105 mEq/L, bicarbonate 13 mEq/L, BUN 23 mg/dL, creatinine 2.3 mg/dL, glucose 116 mg/dL. Serum drug levels: lithium 0.6 mEq/L; acetaminophen <5 μg/mL. Urinalysis: pH 5, otherwise negative. Chest radiograph (see figure): bilateral lower lobe fluffy infiltrates consistent with pulmonary edema.

Questions: What additional information would you want to obtain from the patient? What additional tests might you consider and why?

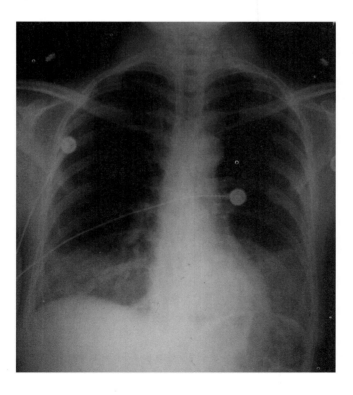

Diagnosis: Hyperpnea, wide-anion gap metabolic acidosis, and non-cardiogenic pulmonary edema (PE) should provoke suspicion for salicylate intoxication. Arterial blood gas (ABG) analysis and a serum salicylate level are warranted.

Discussion: Derived from willow bark, salicylates have been used for hundreds of years for their anti-inflammatory, analgesic, and antipyretic properties. Due to widespread availability, a significant number of accidental and intentional salicylate poisonings occur each year. Fatal overdoses can occur with single acute ingestions of 10–30 g in adults, and as little as 3 g in children.

The signs and symptoms of salicylism are numerous and can be surprisingly subtle. Minor symptoms may include nausea, vomiting, tinnitus, and vertigo. Major symptoms may include shortness of breath, lethargy, altered mental status, and seizures. Serious sequelae of salicylate poisoning include dehydration, metabolic acidosis, non-cardiogenic pulmonary edema, cerebral edema, and death. At toxic levels, salicylate uncouples oxidative phosphorylation and impairs normal Krebs cycle activity. This results in a wide-anion gap metabolic acidosis, ketosis, hyperpyrexia, and cellular dysfunction in multiple organs. Therefore, assessment of acid base status with serum electrolytes and blood gases is a critical part of managing salicylate poisoning. Classically, early in salicylate poisoning patients may have a pure respiratory alkalosis due to salicylate's ability to directly stimulate the brain's respiratory center. As the poisoning continues, metabolic acidosis develops, often resulting in a mixed disorder with a primary respiratory alkalosis and primary metabolic acidosis. When poisoning is severe, or if the patient also ingests any sedating drugs, such as ethanol or benzodiazapines, a pure metabolic acidosis may be detected. In the present patient, an ABG revealed a mixed disorder with a pH of 7.52 and a CO_2 of 16 mEq/L (previously measured serum bicarbonate 13 mEq/L).

There is much confusion pertaining to the interpretation of serum salicylate levels. Therapeutic serum levels range from 10 to 30 mg/dL. Symptoms of toxicity typically develop as serum levels rise above 40 mg/dL. Although the most critically ill patients typically have the highest levels, do not use serum salicylate levels alone to determine treatment. Serum salicylate concentration is dependent upon pH-dependent tissue distribution. Also, chronically poisoned patients may manifest significant toxicity at salicylate levels approaching only 50 or 60 mg/dL. While acutely poisoned patients typically present with a clear ingestion history, chronically poisoned patients often present with a constellation of clinical signs and symptoms (see table). These patients frequently are initially misdiagnosed as having sepsis, encephalopathy, worsening mental illness, dementia, alcoholic ketoacidosis, congestive heart failure, or even acute pulmonary edema. The longer a patient remains undiagnosed, the poorer the prognosis. It is imperative to consider and rule out salicylism in any patient with unexplained change in mental status, wide-anion gap metabolic acidosis, or new non-cardiogenic pulmonary edema.

In addition to supportive care, treatment options include oral activated charcoal, intravenous sodium bicarbonate and potassium infusion to alkalinize the urine, and hemodialysis. Raising the urine pH via **intravenous sodium bicarbonate** will "trap" salicylic acid within the renal tubules, resulting in increased renal excretion. Hydrogen ion gradients are necessary for this process to occur, but require adequate serum potassium so potassium supplementation is typically needed. One method of creating an effective intravenous solution is to place approximately 150 mEq of $NaHCO_3$ (three adult ampules found in most resuscitation carts) and 20–40 mEq KCl into a 1000 mL bag of D5W. This will result in essentially D5 normal bicarbonate with KCl. This infusion may be run at about two or three times maintenance rates (~ 250 mL/hr for an adult). In addition to serial salicylate and acid base assessments, also regularly check the urine pH to make certain it is being alkalinized successfully.

Hemodialysis is a potentially life-saving intervention because it not only removes salicylate from the serum, but also rapidly corrects acid-base disturbances. Hemodialysis should be used in clinically severely poisoned patients, such as those with altered mental status, seizures, intolerance of the significant fluid load (e.g., those with non-cardiogenic pulmonary edema or renal

Signs and Symptoms of Chronic Salicylate Poisoning

Nausea, vomiting
Dizziness, hearing loss
Fever
Shortness of breath, tachypnea
Palpitations, tachycardia
Hallucinations
Confusion
Agitation
Seizures

failure), or severe acid-base disturbances. Because of the significant salicylate burden and end-organ dysfunction, patients with levels greater than 100 mg/dL should also strongly be considered for hemodialysis.

Being an acid, salicylate's movements in the body are determined largely by changes in pH; the more acidic the environment, the less ionized the salicylate is and the easier it can move across membranes. As salicylate poisoning and acidosis develop, both the primary and compensatory respiratory alkalosis help maintain an alkalemic or normal pH. As the poisoning worsens, however, and the patient becomes lethargic and somnolent, respiratory function is depressed, which allows the metabolic acidosis to go unchecked, drops the serum pH, and promotes salicylate to move into tissues (e.g., the central nervous system). This vicious cycle often results in the patient's rapid deterioration and sometimes death, and because of the sedation and paralytic agents used during rapid sequence induction, the cycle can be acutely precipitated by emergent orotracheal intu-bation. Therefore, even though aspirin-poisoned patients often appear to have dramatic respiratory distress, exercise caution when considering mechanical ventilation of the alert, hyperventi-lating patient with clinical salicylism. When employed, endotracheal intubation should be accompanied by bicarbonate administration and subsequent hyperventilation.

Although the present patient presented with symptoms of persecutory thoughts and auditory hallucinations, initially thought to be an exacerba-tion of his underlying psychiatric illness, careful evaluation led to the suspicion of aspirin poison-ing. Indeed, upon further questioning, the patient admitted to self-treatment of a toothache with the ingestion of 9 or 10 tablets of aspirin each day for the past 3 weeks. His serum salicylate level was 64.4 mg/dL. Due to the significant non-cardiogenic pulmonary edema, the patient was unable to tolerate significant bicarbonate infusion, so hemodialysis was performed. Over the next 48 hours his paranoia significantly diminished, and his metabolic and respiratory status improved.

Clinical Pearls

1. The key to diagnosing salicylism in chronically poisoned patients is to have a high index of suspicion in those with unexplained hyperpnea or non-cardiogenic pulmonary edema, altered mental status, or wide-anion gap metabolic acidosis.

2. Shortness of breath and hyperventilation are commonly seen in aspirin poisoning. Patients with psychiatric illness may only present with mania or psychosis, or an appar-ent exacerbation of their illness.

3. Alkalinization of urine via sodium bicarbonate must be accompanied by potas-sium repletion for adequate excretion of ionized salicylate.

4. Endotracheal intubation of the salicylate-poisoned patient should be approached with caution. Intubated patients require aggressive hyperventilation to prevent against potentially fatal drug redistribution that may accompany acidemia.

REFERENCES
1. Greenberg, M: Deleterious effects of endotracheal intubation in salicylate poisoning. Ann Emerg Med 41:583-584, 2003.
2. Yip Dart RC, Gabow PA: Concepts and controversies in salicylate toxicity. Emerg Med Clin North Am 12:351-364, 1994.
3. Walters JS, Woodring JH, Stelling CB, et al: Salicylate-induced pulmonary edema. Radiology 146:289-293, 1983.
4. Gabow PA, Anderson RJ, Potts DE, Schrier RW: Acid-base disturbances in the salicylate poisoning in adults. Arch Intern Med 138:1481-1484, 1978.
5. Anderson RJ, Potts DE, Gabow PA, et al: Unrecognized adult salicylate intoxication. Ann Intern Med 85:745-748, 1976.
6. Hill JB: Experimental salicylate poisoning: Observations on the effects of altering blood pH on tissue and plasma salicylate concentrations. Pediatrics 47:658-665, 1971.

PATIENT 17

A toddler in status epilepticus

A 3-year-old boy is taken to the ED by a rescue squad for a prolonged seizure. He had been well until 3 days before, when he developed symptoms of a cold; over the next 2 days he began vomiting and became less playful. On the day of admission, he vomited several times and became drowsy. That evening he was noted to develop seizure activity, which prompted the rescue squad call.

Medical history is notable for developmental delay, especially in the language and personal/social spheres. There is no history of recent head trauma or ingestion, but his mother does recall that 3 weeks previously she had to remove paint chips from the boy's mouth.

Soon after arrival, the child has another seizure. He is treated with intravenous diazepam but respiratory depression develops, and he undergoes endotracheal intubation.

Physical Examination: Temperature 38.3° C, pulse 120/min, respirations 25/min (manually ventilated), blood pressure 84/50 mmHg. General: no evidence of external trauma. HEENT, cardiac, pulmonary, and abdominal exams: normal. Neurological: obtunded, intermittent withdrawal to pain; periodic extensor posturing; pupils 3 mm and sluggishly reactive; fundi normal; deep tendon reflexes 3+ to 4+ on the left and 2+ to 3+ on right lower extremities; bilateral sustained ankle clonus; plantar extension present on left, equivocal on right.

Laboratory Findings: Hemogram: WBC 11,300/μL, hemoglobin 6.6 g/dL, mean corpuscular volume 50 μm^3, platelet count 473,000/μl, peripheral blood smear positive for RBC basophilic stippling. Serum chemistries: sodium 139 mEq/L, potassium 4.3 mEq/L, chloride 105 mEq/L, bicarbonate 22 mEq/L, blood urea nitrogen 15 mg/dL, creatinine 0.3 mg/dL, glucose 170 mg/dL, calcium 9.4 mg/dL, magnesium 1.9 mg/dL, ammonia 44 μmol/L. CSF: opening pressure 46 cm H_2O, 3 WBC/μL, 0 RBC/μL, protein 96 mg/dL, glucose 108 mg/dL. Urinalysis: 4+ glucose, 5–10 WBC/hpf, 0–5 RBC/hpf, 1+ protein. CT scan of head: diffuse cerebral edema and loss of gray-white matter differentiation (see figure). Radiographs: abdomen negative for foreign bodies; wrist positive for dense metaphyseal bands.

Questions: What is the etiology of this unfortunate child's severe encephalopathy? What are the immediate management considerations?

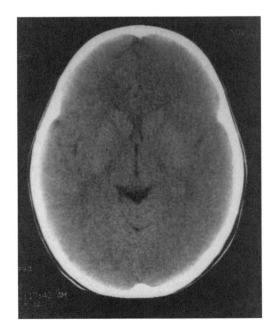

Diagnosis: Lead encephalopathy. Blood lead was 220 µg/dL, and erythrocyte protoporphyrin was 649 µg/dL.

Discussion: Lead encephalopathy is the most severe manifestation of childhood lead poisoning and, though rare nowadays, may still challenge pediatricians and emergency medicine physicians. This child presented in 1994, not the Dark Ages! This discussion will focus on symptomatic lead poisoning (plumbism) in childhood. A much more common problem, of course, is the large number of asymptomatic children who have mildly elevated blood lead levels, about whom much concern has been raised regarding potential subtle neurocognitive dysfunction, including decreased intelligence, poor school performance, and findings similar to attention deficit disorder. The prevention and management of asymptomatic childhood lead exposure has been reviewed extensively (see References). Adult lead poisoning, usually a consequence of occupational exposure, is also an important problem (see Patient 31). In the U.S., pediatric plumbism is usually the result of hand-to-mouth activity in children living in lead paint-dust contaminated homes. Other pediatric sources occasionally include drinking from improperly glazed ceramics, the use of contaminated water to prepare infant formula, exposure to some lead-containing folk remedies or cosmetics, and ingested metallic lead foreign bodies.

Lead exposure is generally via the gastrointestinal (GI) route in children. After absorption, it is distributed to bone, soft tissues (the brain being of particular concern), and blood. Excretion is very slow, primarily through urine, feces, and sweat. Children are at particular risk for ingested lead, because they have more efficient intestinal absorption, compartmentalize more into soft tissues, and have more immature brains, which are therefore especially susceptible to the chronic sequelae of lead toxicity. Lead is believed to exert its toxic effects at the cellular level via two general mechanisms: by being "mistaken" for calcium at many subcellular sites and thus interfering with normal calcium function; and by binding with sulfhydryl groups on proteins and thus inhibiting critical enzymes. In children, these effects are most manifest by injury to the brain and inhibition of the heme synthesis pathway. Lead neurotoxicity involves disorganized brain microanatomy in young children, along with interference to neurotransmitter and protein kinase function. As neurotoxicity progresses to encephalopathy, the brain microvasculature (blood-brain barrier) is injured, with leakage of proteinacious fluid exudates resulting in brain edema and increased intracranial pressure.

Lead toxicity often begins with vague and non-specific signs and symptoms, as demonstrated by this patient. Unfortunately, these may often overlap with the "picky eating" and "terrible twos" that many parents complain about in regard to their otherwise perfectly healthy toddlers, or with common, self-limited illnesses such as viral gastroenteritis. Initially, GI symptoms such as anorexia, colicky abdominal pain, vomiting, and constipation predominate. The child may then appear slightly less playful, or "fussier" than usual. With onset of encephalopathy, persistent vomiting, lethargy, and ataxia develop. As encephalopathy worsens, coma and seizures occur. Even with appropriate therapy, children who survive lead encephalopathy have a 25–30% incidence of residual brain injury, including mental retardation, seizure disorder, blindness, and hemiparesis. Peripheral neuropathy is very uncommon in children, but may be observed in children who also have sickle cell disease. Other organ systems damaged by lead include the kidneys (tubular nephropathy with aminoaciduria, glycosuria, and phosphaturia, i.e. Fanconi syndrome) and the bone marrow, with microcytic anemia resulting from defective heme synthesis (often compounded by concomitant iron deficiency).

Symptomatic lead poisoning may be recognized by a combination of characteristic clinical findings and laboratory results (see table). Children in the pica-prone age range (1–5 years) with a prodrome of persistent vomiting, listlessness and/or irritability, clumsiness, or ataxia who progress to seizures and coma should be highly suspect, especially if they live in deteriorated housing or older homes recently renovated. Contributory laboratory findings include microcytic anemia, elevated erythrocyte protoporphyrin, basophilic stippling of RBCs on smear, abnormal urinalysis, and radiopaque flecks on abdominal radiographs or dense metaphyseal bands on x-rays of knees and wrists ("lead lines," see figure next page). CSF examination may reveal increased pressure, lymphocytic pleocytosis, and elevated protein, but is not necessary to confirm diagnosis, and lumbar puncture may be hazardous if there is markedly increased intracranial pressure. Blood lead level is diagnostic, but unfortunately is not typically available on a stat basis. The combination of nonspecific clinical and laboratory findings noted above might constitute sufficient evidence to initiate specific therapy if suspicion is strong and there are no compelling alternative diagnoses.

Major Clinical Findings of Symptomatic Lead Poisoning in Children

Clinical Severity	Usual Range of Blood Lead
Mild to Moderate	50–70 µg/dL
GI: anorexia, abdominal pain, vomiting, constipation	
CNS: irritability, lethargy, less playful, "terrible two"	
Severe	>70 (usually >100) µg/dL
GI: persistent vomiting	
Heme: pallor (microcytic amenia)	
CNS: encephalopathy (apathy, ataxia, loss of milestones, coma, seizures, papilledema, cranial nerve palsies, increased intracranial pressure)	

Adapted from Henretig FM: Lead. In Goldfrank LR, Flomenbaum NE, Lewin et al (eds): Goldfrank's Toxicologic Emergencies, 7th ed. New York, McGraw-Hill, 2002, pp 1200-1238.

The treatment of symptomatic lead poisoning is three-part, including removal of the child from further lead exposure, specific antidotal (chelation) therapy, and appropriate supportive care, including pediatric intensive care for patients with encephalopathy (see table next page). The specific chelating drugs for lead poisoning are calcium disodium edathamil (CaEDTA), 2,4-dimercaptopropanol (British Anti-Lewisite or

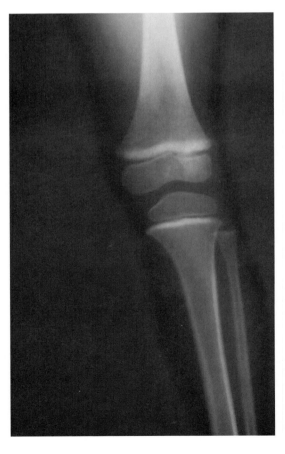

BAL), and dimercaptosuccinic acid (DMSA or succimer). The latter can be administered orally and is frequently used in the outpatient therapy of asymptomatic children with significantly elevated blood lead, but experience with its use in symptomatic patients is limited. Side effects of CaEDTA include local reactions at injection sites, hypercalcemia, fever, and renal dysfunction (at high doses—rarely seen with current regimens). BAL may cause nausea and vomiting (exacerbated if used with concurrent iron therapy), hemolysis in patients with G6PD deficiency, liver dysfunction, and transient hypertension.

The concomitant intensive care for children with lead encephalopathy should be designed to minimize intracranial pressure exacerbations and maintain adequate urine flow to enhance chelation efficacy. Generally, fluid provision that supplies basal water requirements is appropriate, with the goal of maintaining urine output at 0.35 to 0.5 mL/kcal/day. Treat seizures aggressively. Recent advances in the management of elevated intracranial pressure have not been evaluated critically in this context, but it seems reasonable that relatively noninvasive measures in addition to judicious fluid administration—such as modest hyperventilation, mannitol or glycerol osmotic therapy, and high-dose steroids—might have a salutary effect.

The present patient experienced intermittent seizure activity for several days despite aggressive chelation therapy, phenobarbital loading, midazolam infusion, and subsequent high-dose pentobarbital. He was hospitalized for 23 days and required further rehabilitative care. His neurological status prior to transfer was notable for choreoathetosis and hypotonia, inability to localize auditory or visual stimuli, and non-purposeful movements of his extremities. An MRI exam on the 22nd hospital day revealed cerebral and cerebellar atrophy and multiple areas of infarction in the frontal and parietal lobes.

Clinical Status/ BLL	Medication and Dose	Route, Regimen
Encephalopathy	BAL 450 mg/m^2/d[a] CaNa$_2$EDTA 1500 mg/m^2/d[a]	75 mg/m^2 IM every 4 h for 5 d Continuous infusion, or 2–4 divided IV doses, for 5 d (start 4 h after BAL)
Symptomatic, or >70	BAL 300–450 mg/m^2/d[a] CaNa$_2$EDTA 1000–1500 mg/m^2/d[a]	50–75 mg/m^2 IM every 4 h for 3–5 d Continuous infusion, or 2–4 divided IV doses, for 5 d (start 4 h after BAL). Base dose total on BLL, severity of symptoms
Asymptomatic, 45–69	Succimer 700–1050 mg/m^2/d or CaNa$_2$EDTA 1000 mg/m^2/d[a]	350 mg/m^2 tid for 5 d, then bid for 14 d Continuous infusion, or 2–4 divided IV doses, for 5 d
20–44	Generally not indicated	If succimer used, same regimen as per BLL 45–69 (above)
<20	Chelation not indicated. Attempt exposure reduction.	

[a]Doses expressed as mg/kg: BAL 450 mg/m^2 (24 mg/kg); 300 mg/m^2 (18 mg/kg). CaNa$_2$EDTA 1000 mg/m^2 (25–50 mg/kg); 1500 mg/m^2 (50–75 mg/kg) adult maximum 2–3 g/d. Succimer 350 mg/m^2 (10 mg/kg).
Subsequent treatment regimens based on postchelation BLL and clinical symptoms.
BLL = blood lead level (μg/dL); IM = intramuscular; IV = intravenous.
Adapted from Henretig FM: Lead. In Goldfrank LR, Flomenbaum NE, Lewin NA et al (eds): Goldfrank's Toxicologic Emergencies, 7th ed. New York, McGraw-Hill, 2002, pp 1200-1238.

Clinical Pearls

1. Symptomatic pediatric lead poisoning is uncommon today but may still occur; prompt recognition and treatment are crucial for optimal outcome and mitigation of neurological sequelae.

2. Early prodromal gastrointestinal and neurological symptoms are vague, nonspecific, and overlap with common parental complaints about otherwise well toddlers!

3. Suspect lead encephalopathy especially in critically ill 1- to 5-year-old children with a history of characteristic prodrome, progression to coma, seizures and/or focal neurological signs; environmental risk factors such as an older home with peeling paint and/or recent home remodeling; and nonspecific laboratory abnormalities including microcytic anemia, increased erythrocyte protoporphyrin, abnormal urinalysis, and positive abdominal or long-bone radiographs.

4. Order blood lead level before instituting chelation therapy, but consider such treatment presumptively if there is strong clinical and corollary laboratory evidence.

5. Combination chelation therapy and pediatric intensive care is mandatory for any child with lead encephalopathy.

REFERENCES

1. Henretig FM: Lead. In Goldfrank LR, Flomenbaum NE, Lewin NA et al (eds): Goldfrank's Toxicologic Emergencies, 7th ed. New York, McGraw-Hill, 2002, pp 1200-1238.
2. Campbell C, Osterhoudt KC: Prevention of childhood lead poisoning. Curr Opin Pediatr 12:428-437, 2000.
3. Wiley J, Henretig F, Foster R: Status epilepticus and severe neurologic impairment from lead encephalopathy. [abstract]. J Toxicol Clin Toxicol 33:529-530, 1995.

PATIENT 18

A 52-year-old man with a swollen tongue

A 52-year-old man with a history of hypertension presents with a concern of tongue swelling. He reports that his tongue began to swell 4 hours ago and has progressively worsened. He has never had an allergic reaction and reports no recent illness, dental work, or fever. He has no family or personal history of similar swelling. His antihypertensive medications are hydrochlorothiazide and captopril.

Physical Examination: Temperature 36.8° C, pulse 126/min, respirations 24/min, blood pressure 142/82 mmHg. Oxygen saturation 96% in room air. General: alert, anxious, with garbled but comprehensible speech and drooling. HEENT: non-pitting homogenous edema of tongue, lips, and submandibular region (see figure); no subcutaneous masses, erythema or warmth; no lymphadenopathy. Chest: normal. Cardiovascular: normal. Abdomen: normal. Skin: no rashes or urticaria.

Laboratory Findings: Hemogram: normal. Serum chemistries: normal. Electrocardiogram: sinus tachycardia, LVH, no ischemic changes. Arterial blood gas (room air): pH 7.48, $Paco_2$ 30 mmHg, PaO_2 90 mmHg.

Question: What is the cause of this swelling?

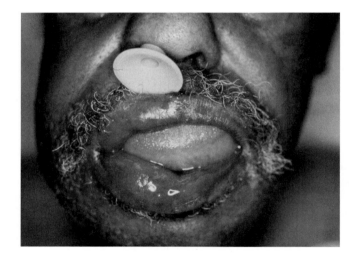

Diagnosis: A definitive diagnosis may be difficult in the acute setting. However, acute facial or oral edema that is soft and nontender in a patient with hypertension makes angiotensin-converting enzyme inhibitor (ACEI)–induced angioedema a likely diagnosis.

Discussion: The approach to this patient begins with the evaluation of his airway and a rapid assessment of the potential need for an artificial oral, nasal, or surgical airway. Although the patient is adequately ventilating and oxygenating currently, ACEI-induced angioedema can progress rapidly and completely obstruct the upper airway within minutes. Anticipation of this progression and early airway intervention is critical to avert acute airway obstruction.

Decisions regarding the best method by which to perform **endotracheal intubation** are not easy. The swelling of the tongue and sublingual tissue may hamper orotracheal or blind nasotracheal intubation. Use of pharmacologic adjuncts such as sedation or rapid sequence induction may become problematic if orotracheal intubation is unsuccessful, because the now relaxed and swollen tongue may fall back and prohibit either placement of a rescue airway device such as a laryngeal mask airway or even adequate bag valve mask ventilation. Awake fiberoptic intubation should be considered early, and additional physicians knowledgeable in advanced airway techniques—including anesthesiologists, otolaryngologists, general surgeons, and/or emergency medicine physicians—should be mobilized. Emergent surgical airway equipment should be available at the bedside at all times until a definitive airway has been obtained. If imminent airway obstruction is not anticipated, vigilant observation and serial assessments are mandatory.

ACEI-induced angioedema is a non-pitting edema of the skin and mucous membranes that most commonly affects the face and orophayrnx. The swelling may range from slight edema of the lip to massive lingual and pharyngeal edema causing complete upper airway obstruction. Although the majority of these reactions occur within in the first few weeks to months of ACEI therapy, they can occur at any time and have been reported in patients who have been taking these medications for years. ACEIs have been implicated in 38% to 79% of all reported cases of angioedema.

The mechanism by which ACEIs produce angioedema is thought to be a side effect of their primary antihypertensive effect of inhibition of angiotensin-converting enzyme. Blockade of this enzyme not only decreases conversion of angiotensin I to angiotensin II, a potent vasoconstrictor, it also results in the undesired reduced breakdown of bradykinin, a vasodilator. These elevated bradykinin levels are thought to induce the angioedema. This is the same mechanism by which cough, another common but under-recognized side effect of ACEIs, is produced. However, this theory recently has been questioned, after an angiotenin II receptor blocker, losartan, which does *not* inhibit the degradation of bradykinins, was reported to induce angioedema. Other possible mechanisms include alteration of the level or activity of C1 esterase.

Prospective analysis of treatment modalities has never been performed, and therapy is based on angioedema's physical similarities to allergy-induced swelling, including therapy with intravenous antihistamines and corticosteroids. Warm, humidified oxygen and racemic or subcutaneous epinephrine have been used as well, but oxygen masks may exacerbate the anxiety and choking sensation that patients with oropharyngeal edema may experience. As emphasized earlier, early airway intervention with awake fiberoptic intubation should be strongly considered.

The present patient began captopril therapy 4 months prior to the tongue swelling event to improve his blood pressure control. He was managed with 100% humidified oxygen with nebulized racemic epinephrine, intravenous diphenhydramine, dexamethasone, and famotidine while an airway team with fiberoptic intubating equipment was mobilized. His trachea was successfully intubated in the emergency department in a controlled manner. Therapy with diphenhydramine, dexamethasone and famotidine was continued. The swelling resolved over 24 hours, and the patient was extubated. He was discharged with instructions to consider this a life-threatening reaction to ACEI and given a list of all the ACEIs to avoid.

Clinical Pearls

1. ACE inhibitor–induced angioedema may occur at any time during ACE inhibitor therapy.

2. Pharmacological therapy for ACEI-induced angioedema may include intravenous antihistamines, corticosteroids, and subcutaneous or nebulized catecholamines, although systematic clinical trials have not been performed.

3. Patients who develop ACEI-induced angioedema should be instructed that this reaction may occur with any of the ACEI antihypertensives.

4. Early airway intervention, such as awake fiberoptic intubation, should be considered in all patients with ACEI-induced airway edema, particularly those with severe or rapidly progressive swelling.

REFERENCES

1. Chiu AG, Krowiak EJ, Deeb ZE: Angioedema associated with angiotensin II receptor antagonists: Challenging our knowledge of angioedema and its etiology. Laryngoscope 111:1729-1731, 2001.
2. Chiu AG, Newkirk KA, Davidson BJ, et al: Angiotensin-converting enzyme inhibitor–induced angioedema: A multicenter review and an algorithm for airway management. Ann Otol Rhinol Laryngol 110:834-840, 2001.
3. Agostoni A, Cicardi M: Drug-induced angioedema without urticaria. Drug Safety 24:599-606, 2001.
4. Agostoni A, Cicardi M, Cugno M, et al: Angioedema due to angiotensin-converting enzyme inhibitors. Immunopharmacology 44:21-25, 1999.
5. Nadel ES, Brown DF: Angioedema. J Emerg Med 16:477-479, 1998.
6. Kyrmizakis DE, Papadakis CE, Fountoulakis EJ, et al: Tongue angioedema after long-term use of ACE inhibitors. Amer J Otolaryngol 19:394-396, 1998.
7. Megerian CA, Arnold JE, Berger M: Angioedema: 5 years' experience, with a review of the disorder's presentation and treatment. Laryngoscope 102:256-260, 1992.

Ronald Perry, MD
Francis DeRoos, MD

PATIENT 19

A 58-year-old man with a large anion gap metabolic acidosis

A 58-year-old man fell down a flight of stairs. He admits to being despondent over the loss of his lifetime job several months earlier and states he has been "drinking." The man is otherwise without complaints and denies any suicide attempt. However, his suspicious neck and wrist wounds and admitted depression led the paramedics to consider a possible suicide attempt and to search the premises. They found two bloodied antifreeze bottles in a room near the top of the stairs.

Physical Examination: Temperature 34.5° C (tympanic), pulse 77/min, respirations 26/min, blood pressure 112/74 mmHg. General: lethargic with slightly slurred speech. HEENT: abrasion over bridge of nose; pupils equal and reactive, nystagmus bilaterally, which extinguishes; orophayrnx without lesions. Neck: nontender; two right-sided linear abrasions approximately 8 cm long each, no active bleeding. Chest: lungs clear. Cardiovascular: normal. Abdomen: normal. Extremities: multiple transverse linear abrasions. Neuromuscular: lethargic but appropriate and moving all extremities well; symmetric reflexes.

Laboratory Findings: Hemogram: mild leukocytosis, otherwise normal. Serum chemistries: sodium 137 mEq/L, potassium 4.0 mEq/L, chloride 104 mEq/L, bicarbonate 7 mEq/L, BUN 5 mg/dL, creatinine 0.9 mg/dL, calcium 8.2 mEq/L, phosphorus 5.1 mEq/L, anion gap 26 mEq/L, glucose 96 mg/dL. Arterial blood gas (100% Fio_2): pH 7.23, Pco_2 16 mmHg, Po_2 423 mmHg. Chest and c-spine radiographs: negative. Head CT: negative.

Question: What is the next reasonable plan of action?

Diagnosis: Armed with the history and after detecting a significant anion gap metabolic acidosis, the next step is to block any further metabolism of ethylene glycol into its toxic metabolites, with either ethanol or fomepizole, and to contact a nephrologist for possible hemodialysis.

Discussion: Ethylene glycol is a saturated alcohol used commercially for its effect in lowering the freezing point of water. It is best known as automobile antifreeze but is also a common industrial solvent. It is a colorless and odorless liquid with a slightly sweet taste. The fluorescent green or blue coloration associated with many automotive antifreeze products is from added dyes that allow for easier identification of radiator leaks. Ethylene glycol is metabolized in the liver by NAD-dependant sequential oxidation, initially by alcohol dehydrogenase and then by aldehyde dehydrogenase. Subsequent metabolism produces a wide variety of acids, including glycolic acid, glyoxylic acid, oxalic acid, formic acid, and alpha-hydroxy beta-ketoadipate. The first enzyme, alcohol dehydrogenase, is the target of antidotal therapy with ethanol or fomepizole to block ethylene glycol metabolism and subsequent development of significant toxicity.

The clinical effects of ethylene glycol poisoning initially resemble ethanol intoxication. This is a potential pitfall because alcoholics are uniquely at risk of self-poisoning with ethylene glycol and methanol, and their altered sensorium may be attributed to routine ethanol intoxication instead. Over the next several hours the ethylene glycol undergoes metabolism into the numerous toxic acids, particularly formic acid, and a potentially lethal anion gap metabolic acidosis develops. This manifests clinically in 8 to 36 hours with increased respiratory rate in compensation for the metabolic acidosis, tachycardia, and, if severe, cardiovascular collapse. During this phase patients may manifest a wide variety of clinical findings, including visual changes, confusion, agitation, seizures, pulmonary edema, or coma. After 48 hours a patient enters a phase that is characterized by azotemia and acute renal failure secondary to acute tubular necrosis from renal deposition of calcium oxalate crystals. Rarely, patients may manifest cranial nerve dysfunction several days after the initial ingestion, possibly due to precipitating calcium oxalate crystals.

The laboratory abnormalities associated with ethylene glycol poisoning are noteworthy and can aid in the diagnosis. As previously discussed, a **severe wide anion gap metabolic acidosis** is the predominant toxicity induced by ethylene glycol. While other etiologies for an anion gap metabolic acidosis exist, this in combination with an **elevated osmolar gap** strongly suggests a toxic alcohol like ethylene glycol or methanol. An osmolal gap is the difference between the measured or actual serum osmolality and the calculated or "estimated" osmolarity. Since the osmolality is almost completely accounted for by the sodium, BUN, glucose, and any alcohols present, the following formula is used: calculated serum osmolality = (2 Na + BUN/2.8 + serum glucose/18 + serum ethanol/4.6). In our patient the measured serum osmolality was 342 mOsm/kg, and the calculated was 281 mOsm/kg ([2 × 137 + 5/2.8 + 96/18 + 0/4.6] = [274 + 1.8 + 5.3 + 0] = 281) producing an osmolal gap of 61 mOsm/kg. In the setting of garage product ingestion or measured wide anion gap metabolic acidosis, this strongly suggests ethylene glycol or methanol poisoning and is an indication for initiating ethanol or fomepizole blockade and hemodialysis. However, remember that even if the osmolal gap is normal (<10 mOsm/kg), the patient can still be severely poisoned and may require hemodialysis.

One rapid analytical study that may be helpful is a **urinalysis**. Calcium oxalate crystals are formed in ethylene glycol–poisoned patients and can be seen in the urine under microscopy. The crystals are either needle-shaped (monohydrates) or envelope-shaped (dehydrates) (see figure). If these crystals are not present in initial urinalysis, they often develop later in the clinical course. Also, examination of the urine sample in a plastic (not glass) container with a Wood's lamp may detect fluorescence, and this identifies ingestion of flourescein-containing antifreeze. This test is not sensitive so, if absent, poisoning is still very possible. As a result of the precipitating calcium oxalate crystals throughout the body (most notably in the renal system as well as the CNS), hypocalcemia often develops. The present patient's calcium dropped to 7.0 mEq/L during the first 36 hours of care.

Ethylene glycol levels are obviously diagnostic; however, in many hospitals the turn-around time for these may be several hours. An ethylene glycol level >25 mg/dL can cause significant injury, and the patient requires treatment.

Initial evaluation and management of the patient starts with attention to the basics of airway, breathing, and circulation. All patients with any significant ingestion will present with a degree of CNS depression. Concomitant ethanol ingestion is present in a large portion of these patients, so protection of the airway by endotracheal intubation must be considered early. In addition, if using ethanol as therapy, patients may develop hypotension or progressive CNS depres-

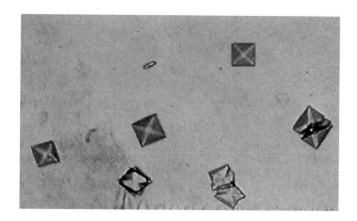

sion during therapy, necessitating intubation. All patients should have two large-bore intravenous lines in anticipation of infusion of fluids, bicarbonate, and antidotes. Patients who present with severe acidosis (pH <7.0) should receive bicarbonate to support their pH. Pertinent laboratory studies should include electrolytes, glucose, BUN, creatinine, alcohol levels (including ethanol, methanol, isopropanol, and ethylene glycol), serum osmolarity, and an arterial blood gas. The urine should be examined for crystals, and for fluorescence with a Wood's lamp.

After the initial evaluation, stabilization, and resuscitation, the treatment of ethylene glycol poisoning involves limiting the formation of toxic metabolite and eliminating the ethylene glycol. In this case, the patient was initially hemodynamically and cognitively stable, but during his almost immediate ethanol infusion he became more lethargic and hypotensive, leading to intubation prior to hemodialysis. Ethanol levels were maintained throughout the dialysis by tripling the ethanol infusion rate. This was because during hemodialysis the ethanol, as well as the ethylene glycol, is removed. Since the affinity of alcohol dehydrogenase is 100 times greater for ethanol than for ethylene glycol, in most cases an ethanol level of 100 mg/dL effectively blocks significant ethylene glycol metabolism. Monitor ethanol levels every few hours before and after dialysis, and hourly during dialysis.

Alternatively, there is a newer, more specific, and equally effective agent called fomepizole (Antizol) that is being used to treat ethylene glycol and methanol poisoned patients. Fomepizole, a direct inhibitor of alcohol dehydrogenase, is safer but more expensive. The advantages of fomepizole are more predictable pharmacokinetics, ease of administration, longer half-life, and no CNS depression. It is dosed at 15 mg/kg followed by 10 mg/kg every 12 hours for four doses. Then after the first five doses it is dosed at 15

mg/kg every 12 hours, until ethylene glycol levels are undetectable and the patient is asymptomatic with normal anion gap and pH. Dosing changes are required for hemodialysis, but a constant infusion is not necessary as it is for ethanol. Patients with less toxic levels, say 25–50 mg/dL, may be effectively treated with fomepizole alone without hemodialysis. The ethylene glycol metabolism is blocked via alcohol dehydrogenase, but it still can be eliminated via the kidneys and possibly other metabolic pathways.

Even after successfully preventing the further development of acidosis by blocking additional metabolism of ethylene glycol, hemodialysis may still be required to remove the remaining ethylene glycol as well as any acids already formed (see table). Some patients with extremely elevated levels may benefit from a second session of hemodialysis; therefore, it is important to continue antidotal therapy even after hemodialysis has been performed until a level <20 mg/dL returns. Alternatively, a continued treatment with fomepizole may be equally efficacious in preventing toxicity while allowing the body to clear the ethylene glycol. Administration of thiamine (100 mg/day), pyridoxine (100 mg), and magnesium theoretically facilitates metabolism into nontoxic metabolites such as alpha-hydroxy beta-ketoadipate, although no animal or human research has explored this.

Indications for Hemodialysis in the Setting of Suspected Ethylene Glycol Poisoning

Suspicion of exposure high
Unexplained anion gap metabolic acidosis
Unexplained osmolal gap
Severe metabolic acidosis
End organ dysfunction
Ethylene glycol level >50 mg/dL

The present patient's post-dialysis course was complicated by aspiration pneumonia and ethanol withdrawal. Nevertheless, he regained normal neurological and cognitive function and was admitted to an inpatient psychiatric facility for treatment of his depression.

Clinical Pearls

1. Patients who present with signs of self-inflicted injuries are at high risk for ingestions, even if they deny it.

2. Patients who have a large anion gap metabolic acidosis should have an osmolal gap calculated to help determine if a toxic alcohol is the causative agent. However, a normal osmolal gap does not eliminate the possibility of toxic alcohol poisoning.

3. Early inhibition of ethanol dehydrogenase by either ethanol or fomepizole is essential in preventing further metabolism of ethylene glycol into its toxic and acidosis-producing metabolites.

4. Hemodialysis is the main treatment for any significant ethylene glycol or methanol ingestion, as it removes these chemicals from the serum and improves the profound acid base disturbances that their metabolism produces.

REFERENCES

1. Brent J, McMartin KE, Philips S, et al: Fomepizole for the treatment of ethylene glycol poisoning: Methylpyrazole Toxic Alcohols Study Group. N Engl J Med 344(6):832-837, 1999.
2. Jacobsen D, Hewlett TP, Webb R, et al: Ethylene glycol intoxication: Evaluation of kinetics and crystalluria. Am J Med 84(1): 145-150, 1988.
3. Gabow PA, Clay K, Sullivan JB, Lepoff R: Organic acids in ethylene glycol intoxication. Ann Intern Med 105(1):16-20, 1986.
4. Gennari FJ: Serum osmolarity: Uses and limitations. N Engl J Med 310(2):102-105, 1984.
5. Peterson CD, Collins AJ, Himes JM, et al: Ethylene glycol poisoning: Pharmacokinetics during therapy with ethanol and hemodialysis. N Engl J Med 304(1):21-23, 1981.
6. Cadnapaphornchai P, Taher S, Bhathena D, McDonald FD: Ethylene glycol poisoning: Diagnosis based on high osmolal and anion gaps and crystalluria. Ann Emerg Med 10(2):94-97, 1981.

Susan A. O'Malley, MD
Jeanmarie Perrone, MD

PATIENT 20

A 35-year-old man with chest pain

A 35-year-old man is brought by ambulance to the emergency department (ED) with a chief concern of chest pain. He reports that the pain started 8 hours prior, was of sudden onset, and began approximately 1 hour after snorting cocaine. He describes the pain as a dull pressure, "7" on a severity scale to 10, that is exacerbated by exertion and improves with rest. He denies associated nausea, vomiting, sweating, or dyspnea. He reports that the pain is similar to prior episodes of chest pain associated with his cocaine use. His last ED visit for chest pain was 2 years ago. His medial history is significant for tobacco, cocaine, and alcohol abuse: he smokes two packs of cigarettes per day, drinks beer daily, and snorts cocaine a few times a month. He is employed as a carpenter. His father died at age 65 from an acute myocardial infarction, and his mother has a history of hypertension.

Physical Examination: Temperature 38.3° C, pulse 86/min, respirations 22/min, blood pressure 160/96 mmHg. General: well-developed, well-nourished, slightly agitated. HEENT: pupils 7 mm, equally round, reactive bilaterally; sclera non-icteric; dry mucous membranes. Chest: clear. Cardiovascular: regular rate, no murmurs, rubs or gallops, no S3 or S4. Abdomen: normal. Extremities: no edema. Skin: pale, warm, dry. Neuromuscular: alert and oriented, 5/5 strength, sensation intact, no gross deficits.

Laboratory Findings: Hemogram: WBC 12,000/µL, hemoglobin 14 g/dL, platelets 140,000/µL. Serum chemistries: Na^+ 140 mEq/L, K^+ 4.2 mEq/L, Cl^- 110 mEq/L, CO_2^- 20 mEq/L, BUN 20 mg/dL, creatinine 0.8 mg/dL, glucose 100 mg/dL. Cardiac panel: CPK 854 IU/L, troponin <0.04 ng/mL. Urinalysis: pH 6.0, trace protein, trace heme, no RBCs microscopically. Electrocardiogram (EKG) : sinus rhythm, ST elevation >2 mm II, III, aVF; ST depression I, aVL; no Q waves, normal intervals (see figure). Chest radiograph: mild cardiomegaly.

Questions: Why is this patient having chest pain? What therapy should be considered?

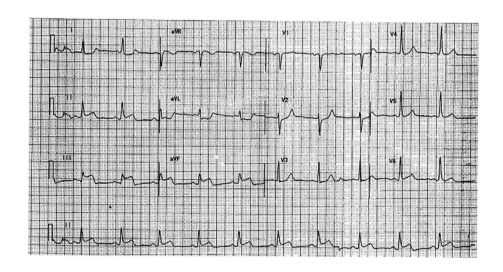

Diagnosis and Treatment: This patient is having an acute coronary syndrome likely secondary to coronary artery vasoconstriction induced by his cocaine use. Although he meets criteria for thrombolytic therapy, it may be prudent to first try more conventional methods for the treatment of cocaine-associated chest pain.

Discussion: The approach to the cocaine-intoxicated patient is multi-faceted, as cocaine is a unique compound with numerous physiological effects. Proarrhythmic effects result from antagonism of fast sodium channels in the heart. Sympathomimetic effects including hypertension and tachycardia result from cocaine-induced catecholamine release. Cocaine causes increased synaptic levels of norepinephrine, dopamine, and serotonin secondary to blockade of neuronal reuptake of these neurotransmitters as well as release of epinephrine from the adrenal axis.

Cocaine users are at increased risk for stroke and numerous other cerebrovascular events including, but not limited to, subarachnoid hemorrhage, seizure, transient ischemic attack, and migraine headaches. Cocaine also has disastrous effects on the cardiovascular system. Myocardial infarction (MI) occurs in approximately 6% of patients with cocaine-induced chest pain. The risk in the first 60 minutes is 24-fold. Acutely, cocaine may induce coronary vasoconstriction with resultant ischemia and hypertension. It also increases the permeability of endothelial cells to low-density lipoproteins, causing accelerated atherosclerosis in chronic users. Chronic users also develop dilated cardiomyopathy and left ventricular hypertrophy.

Another cause of cocaine-induced morbidity and mortality is **hyperthermia**. Cocaine is known to cause hyperthermia via multiple mechanisms: increased psychomotor activity causing increased heat production and peripheral vasoconstriction leading to decreased heat dissipation. Experimental evidence involving animal models showed that therapeutic modalities that decreased hyperthermia increased survival. In New York City, deaths related to cocaine are noted to increase with increased ambient temperatures.

Concerns with the present patient are multiple. He is slightly agitated, with an elevated temperature and blood pressure, and he is having chest pain. The agitation will improve with a parenteral benzodiazepine. Due to the direct pharmacological and toxicological relationship between the neuropsychiatric and cardiovascular systems, parenteral benzodiazepines (lorazepam 2–4 mg IV or diazepam 5–10 mg IV per dose) may be considered first-line therapy for his chest pain. The goal should be to dampen the adrenergic syndrome associated with cocaine use. Frequently, when the neuropsychiatric component has been treated, the cardiovascular component begins to recede.

Prudent therapeutic interventions for this patient might include administration of aspirin, a benzodiazepine, and sublingual nitroglycerin.

Following treatment of agitation and chest pain, temperature should be closely monitored. In patients with significantly elevated temperatures, cooling techniques (mist and fan or ice baths, depending on severity) are warranted until the temperature normalizes. Blood pressure should improve with the benzodiazepine therapy. However, if more aggressive therapy were indicated, beta blockers should be avoided. Cocaine-induced vasoconstriction is induced by an alpha-adrenergic mechanism. Beta blockade, even with short-acting agents such as esmolol, may lead to unopposed alpha effects. Labetalol should also be avoided. Although it has mixed alpha- and beta-adrenergic antagonist effects, it has a much larger beta-adrenergic antagonist effect. Vasodilating agents, such as sodium nitroprusside and nitroglycerin, are first-line therapy in treating cocaine-associated hypertension. Phentolamine, an alpha antagonist, can also be considered if hypertension is refractory to nitrates.

There are several case reports of poor outcomes with thrombolytic therapy among patients with cocaine-induced chest pain. A significant proportion of cocaine-induced chest pain patients will meet EKG criteria for thrombolysis, but will have negative cardiac markers. One approach to thrombolytic therapy among patients with cocaine-associated chest pain is to administer it only to those patients who are at low risk for cerebrovascular bleeding, have received vasodilator therapy without effect, have a contraindication for percutaneous intervention, and are definitely having an acute MI.

Although this patient has an elevated CPK, his troponin is normal 8 hours after his chest pain started. Analysis of his urine revealed heme without red cells on microscopy. Rhabdomyolysis is a reasonable explanation for his elevated serum CPK. His serum electrolytes also reveal a component of dehydration. Intravenous fluid hydration may prevent renal toxicity related to his elevated CPK. However, his chest radiograph does reveal cardiomegaly; thus fluid administration should be cautious, and he should be monitored for signs of volume overload. This patient warrants inpatient observation and monitoring of potential cardiac ischemia. The EKG is very concerning as is his history of chronic cocaine use, which puts him at risk for a thrombotic event.

The present patient was admitted to a chest pain observation unit. His repeat cardiac panel revealed a normal troponin 16 hours after his initial onset and a mildly elevated CPK of 986 IU/L. His EKG remained unchanged. An echocardiogram revealed no wall motion abnormalities. Social work was consulted, and the patient was given referral to substance abuse centers. He was discharged home 10 hours after his admission, advised to follow-up for substance abuse and to see his primary care physician within 24 hours.

Clinical Pearls

1. Thrombolytics should be used cautiously among patients with cocaine-induced chest pain.

2. Benzodiazepines may be considered first-line agents for cocaine-induced chest pain.

3. Treatment of the CNS effects of cocaine will often resolve the cardiovascular effects.

4. Beta-blocker therapy should be avoided in patients with cocaine intoxication.

REFERENCES

1. Hollander JE, Hoffman RS: Cocaine. In Goldfrank LR, Flomenbaum NE, Lewin NA, et al (eds): Goldfrank's Toxicologic Emergencies. New York, McGraw-Hill, 2002, pp 980-990.
2. Baumann BM, Perrone J, Hornig SE, et al: Randomized controlled, double-blind, placebo controlled trial of diazepam, nitroglycerin or both for treatment of patients with potential cocaine associated acute coronary syndromes. Acad Emerg Med 7:878-885, 2000.
3. Hollander JE, Burstein JL, Shih RD, et al: Cocaine associated myocardial infarction: Clinical safety of thrombolytic therapy. Chest 107:1237-1241, 1995.
4. Hollander JE, Hoffman RS, Gennis P, et al: Prospective multicenter evaluation of cocaine associated chest pain. Acad Emerg Med 1:330-339, 1994.
5. Lange RA, Cigarroa RG, Flores ED, et al: Potentiation of cocaine-induced coronary vasoconstriction by beta adrenergic blockade. Ann Intern Med 112:897-903, 1990.

PATIENT 21

An 11-day-old boy with cyanosis

An 11-day-old baby boy, born full-term from an uncomplicated pregnancy and delivery, developed lethargy and cyanosis. He was solely breast fed and had been well upon circumcision 24 hours earlier. There is no history of fever, vomiting, diarrhea, congestion, or oral medication use.

Physical Examination: Temperature 37.0° C, pulse 182/min, respirations 34/min, blood pressure 88/58 mmHg; oxygen saturation 85% in room air and in 40% oxygen. General: somnolent but non-distressed, well-nourished. HEENT: nomal. Chest: no retractions, clear to auscultion with good aeration of all lung fields. Cardiovascular: normal S1 and S2, no murmur, equal blood pressures in all four extremities. Abdomen: normal. Extremities: well-perfused. Skin: cyanotic. Neuromuscular: good startle and suck, moves all extremities, good tone.

Laboratory Findings: Hemogram: normal. Serum chemistries: normal. Urinalysis: normal. Arterial blood gas (40% FiO_2): pH 7.44, $PaCO_2$ 36 mmHg, PaO_2 190 mmHg. Electrocardiogram (EKG): sinus tachycardia. Chest radiograph: normal heart size, no pulmonary infiltrates.

Question: What test will best confirm the cause of this infant's cyanosis?

Diagnosis: Cyanosis unresponsive to oxygen, despite normal arterial oxygen tension, is the hallmark of methemoglobinemia. Co-oximetric measurement of methemoglobin should confirm the diagnosis.

Discussion: Although the differential diagnosis of cyanosis is broad (see table), the acute onset of cyanosis within the first 2 weeks of life must raise the concern of a ductus-dependent congenital heart abnormality. The failure of supplemental oxygen administration to raise the oxygen saturation measured by pulse-oximetry, and the normal lung exam, makes pulmonary disease unlikely in this infant. Even though the baby has a normal cardiac exam and EKG, it might be tempting to administer prostaglandin and obtain an echocardiogram to evaluate his heart. However, the results of the arterial blood gas deserve closer inspection.

Cyanotic heart disease occurs through shunting of deoxygenated blood from the right heart to the left. In this situation, administration of supplemental oxygen should not greatly affect the arterial oxygen tension. Note that although the baby's oxygen saturation measured by pulse oximetry did not rise above 85%, he was not hypoxemic as demonstrated by a PaO_2 of 190 mmHg. A "saturation gap" between the measured oxygen saturation of the blood and the oxygen saturation calculated by blood gas analysis suggests the presence of an abnormal hemoglobin such as **methemoglobin**. Methemoglobin absorbs light at different wavelengths than oxyhemoglobin and deoxyhemoglobin, resulting in aberrant oxygen saturation measurement by the pulse-oximeter. Methemoglobin can be quantified using multiple-wavelength co-oximetry, typically available in a hospital's blood gas laboratory.

Methemoglobin is a form of hemoglobin unable to transport oxygen, created when deoxygenated heme iron within the red blood cell is oxidized from the ferrous to ferric state. Cyanosis will become clinically apparent in the presence of 1.5 g/dL of methemoglobin within the blood. In healthy individuals, symptoms of hypoxia often become notable with methemoglobin concentrations above 30%, and levels above 50% may be acutely threatening.

There are both congenital and acquired causes of methemoglobinemia. Methemoglobinemia may be found in as many as two thirds of infants under 6 months of age with severe diarrheal illness, as well as in occasional infants with dietary intolerance or infection. In addition, many oxidant medications, chemicals, and pollutants can cause methemoglobinemia (see table on next page). The principles of treatment are to provide supplemental oxygen, to remove or treat the cause of the oxidant stress, and to consider antidotal therapy with 1 to 2 mg/kg of **methylene blue** in a 1% solution. Methylene blue serves as a co-factor stimulating an otherwise dormant NADPH-dependent methemoglobin reductase system.

Methemoglobinemia was not initially considered in the present patient, and an echocardiogram and sepsis evaluation were performed. Ultimately, the methemoglobin concentration was found to be 39%. The methemoglobinemia resolved with administration of methylene blue. Further investigation discovered that the baby's father, a physician, had been applying a lidocaine/prilocaine (known inducers of methemoglobinemia) cream to the baby's circumcision site every 2 to 3 hours.

Differential Diagnosis of Cyanosis

Low Oxygen Tension
  Environmental hypoxia
  Pulmonary disorders
    Airway compromise
    Oxygen diffusion barrier
    Mismatch of ventilation and perfusion
    Vascular shunting
  Cardiovascular disorders
    Right-to-left shunting
    Congestive heart failure
    Shock
    Vasoconstriction
Abnormal Hemoglobin Variants
  Methemoglobinemia
  Sulfhemoglobinemia
Factitious
  Discoloration of skin or blood by dyes

Medications and Chemicals Implicated in Producing Methemoglobinemia

Acetanilid
Aminophenones
Aniline dyes
Antipyrine
Arsine
Bismuth subnitrate
Chlorates
Chloroquine
Chromates
Cobalt
Copper
Dapsone
Flutamide
Hydrazines

Hydroquinones
Hydrogen peroxide
Hydroxylamines
Local anesthetics
Methylene blue
Metoclopramide
Naphthalene
Nitrates
Nitrites
Nitroalkanes
Nitrobenzenes
Nitroglycerin
Nitroprusside
Petroleum octane booster

Phenacetin
Phenazopyridine
Phenetidin
Phenylenediamines
Potassium permanganate
Primaquine
Propanol
Quinones
Resorcinol
Rifampin
Toluidine
Trinitrotoluene
Sulfonamides
Vitamin K_3 (menadione)

Clinical Pearls

1. Cyanosis unresponsive to oxygen, despite normal arterial oxygen tension, should suggest methemoglobinemia.
2. Iatrogenic induction of methemoglobinemia is a relatively common occurrence.
3. Clinical interpretation of methemoglobin percentages must take into account the total hemoglobin value.
4. In the setting of glucose-6-phosphate dehydrogenase deficiency there may be insufficient NADPH available for methylene blue to reduce methemoglobin.

REFERENCES
1. Wright RO, Lewander WJ, Woolf AD: Methemoglobinemia: Etiology, pharmacology, and clinical management. Ann Emerg Med 34:646-656, 1999.
2. Avner JR, Henretig FM, McAneney CM: Acquired methemoglobinemia—The relationship of cause to course of illness. Am J Dis Child 144:1229-1230, 1990.

Charlene H. An, MD
Francis DeRoos, MD

PATIENT 22

A 34-year-old man with palpitations

A 34-year-old man without any significant medical history has been bothered by palpitations and lightheadedness since this morning. The patient denies other symptoms and has been feeling well otherwise. Interestingly, the patient has begun a new fitness regimen over the past few weeks that includes daily exercise combining running and weight training and an herbal supplement marketed to enhance weight reduction.

Physical Examination: Temperature 37.1° C, pulse 136/min and irregular, respirations 20/min, blood pressure 126/66 mmHg. Pulse oximetry 99% in room air. General: well developed, well nourished, slightly anxious. Chest: normal. Cardiovascular: tachycardic and irregularly, irregular rhythm. Extremities: no edema

Laboratory Findings: Serum chemistries: unremarkable. Urine drug screen (GC/mass spec): + for caffeine. EKG (see figure): atrial fibrillation at a rate of 130, no ischemic ST/T-wave changes. Chest radiograph: normal.

Questions: What are the concerns with the use of herbal supplements? Are any herbals associated with cardiac dysrythmias?

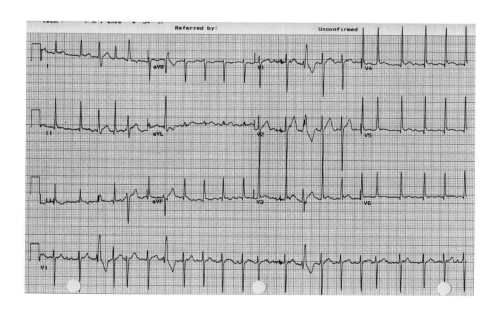

Diagnosis and Treatment: Herbal supplements should be considered medicinals with real, but poorly controlled therapeutic and toxic pharmacological effects. In this case, the herbal supplement included ma huang (ephedra 20 mg) and guarana (caffeine 200 mg) per tablet. Both of these chemicals are associated with atrial fibrillation.

Discussion: In the U.S., complementary alternative medicines, especially "natural" or herbal medications, are becoming increasingly popular. While many have been demonstrated to have significant, yet poorly understood, physiological effects similar to pharmaceutically manufactured drugs, under current Federal Drug Administration (FDA) policies they are not subject to the same manufacturing standards and checks as synthetic or purified medicines. Herbal medicines are categorized as dietary supplements and fall under the **Dietary Supplement Health and Education Act of 1994**. Under these sets of regulations, the manufacturing company is responsible for the safety and quality control of the product and for accurate product labeling. Therefore, any herb use is fraught with potential problems, including inconsistencies in "doses" of active ingredients, potential impurities and contaminants within the product (such as heavy metals or pharmaceuticals), lack of demonstrated efficacy for the prescribed malady, and unknown side effects or dose effects. Dietary supplements registered as such prior to 1994 are not even required to register with the FDA before the product is sold. However, the law allows the FDA to restrict sales after market if the product poses a "significant risk for injury."

Ephedra is the active ingredient derived from the plant ma huang. Other aliases are Mormon tea, yellow horse, desert tea, and "herbal ecstasy." The similar chemical compounds ephedrine and pseudoephedrine are found in common, over-the-counter drugs (e.g., Primatene Mist, Sudafed). In Traditional Chinese medicine, ma huang has been used to treat asthma, nasal congestion, and weight control and is considered a general health promoter. More recently in the U. S., it has been used extensively as a sports performance enhancer, energy booster, and dietary pill for weight loss. Ephedra is a mixed-action adrenergic agent, meaning it stimulates the release of stored norepinephrine as well as acts directly on alpha and beta receptors. In addition, it is *not* inactivated by monoamine oxidase (MAO), resulting in a longer duration of action than endogenous sympathomimetic chemicals. Ephedra is a sympathetic central nervous system stimulant producing vasoconstriction, bronchodilation, and cardiac stimulation. It increases the metabolic rate by promoting thermogenesis and may increase contractile strength of muscle fibers.

Symptoms of overdose include palpitations, nervousness, headache, insomnia, and delirium. Like other sympathomimetics, strokes, myocardial ischemia, seizures, and sudden death have all been associated with ephedra use in otherwise healthy adults. Concurrent use with caffeine, decongestants, beta-agonists (inhalers), or antidepressant-like MAO inhibitors can increase the chance of adverse affects, such as cardiac arrhythmia, hyperactivity, insomnia, tremors, headaches, and nausea. Recently the FDA issued a caution regarding use of dietary supplements containing ephedra, especially among athletes and those doing strenuous workouts. In the present patient the combination of this potent sympathomimetic agent and caffeine likely precipitated his atrial fibrillation. Within 1 hour of arrival to medical attention the patient spontaneously converted into normal sinus rhythm. He received continuous cardiac monitoring for a few more hours, remained well, and was encouraged to discontinue herbal supplement use.

Two other commonly used herbals that may have significant pharmacological toxicity include *Ginko biloba* and St. John's wort. **Ginkgo biloba** has been used in Traditional Chinese medicine for thousands of years. The different parts of the tree (e.g., seeds, leaves, and nut) are used to treat specific ailments including urinary incontinence, poor short-term memory, asthma, dysmenorrhea, cardiovascular disease, and sexual dysfunction. The active ingredients in the *Ginkgo biloba* extract are collectively called ginkgolides and can be separated into two major types—ginkgolide B and bilobalide. Their biological activity is just beginning to be understood, but ranges from antioxidant effects to antagonizing platelet-activating factor to vasodilatation. Some clinical data suggest this herb may stabilize or delay the progression of dementia. Ginkgo may also be useful in improving the symptoms of intermittent claudication and chronic tinnitus. Complications can include bleeding (antiplatelet activating effect) and possibly seizures. Several case reports of spontaneous intracranial or intraocular hemorrhages have been reported in patients already using other anticoagulants, including aspirin and warfarin.

St. John's wort (*Hypericum perforatum*) contains two main active compounds, hypericum and hyperforin. These agents inhibit the reuptake of serotonin, dopamine, and norepinephrine at respective presynaptic sites. St. John's wort has been used for centuries and is currently employed as an antidepressant in patients with mild depression. Cases exist of the **serotonin syndrome** developing in patients who are taking St. John's wort plus other serotonergic antidepressants, such as selective serotonin reuptake inhibitors. Serotonin syndrome is a clinical syndrome that consists classically of rigidity, autonomic instability, agitation, and delirium, but most patients present with symptoms of anxiety, agitation, insomnia, and lower extremity muscle stiffness.

St. John's wort also induces activation of the hepatic enzyme cytochrome P450 and may decrease the plasma levels and effectiveness of some pharmaceuticals, including warfarin, estrogen, theophylline, digoxin, cyclosporin, and the HIV protease inhibitor indinavir. Several countries are now warning against the use of St. John's wort with HIV-protease inhibitors. Patients on oral contraceptives should be counseled about using alternative forms of birth control.

Clinical Pearls

1. Herbal supplements or medications, while not regulated to the same extent as pharmaceuticals by the FDA, still have significant and potentially toxic physiological effects.

2. In general, treatment of herbal ingestions should be supportive and directed toward the symptoms and signs.

3. Ma huang, an herbal commonly found in many dietary supplements, weight reduction therapies, and performance enhancers, contains ephedra, a potent sympathomimetic agent. Ma huang has been associated with dysrhythmias, seizures, and sudden death in otherwise healthy people.

4. Because of the under-regulated processing and minimal scrutiny of herbal preparations, the risk of impurities, contaminants, and variable dosing of active ingredients increase the possibility for adverse events in patients using these products.

REFERENCES

1. Palmer MD: Adverse events associated with dietary supplements: An observational study. Lancet 361:101-107, 2003.
2. Tesch BJ: Herbs commonly used by women: An evidence-based review. Am J Obst Gyn 188:44-55, 2003.
3. Ernst E: The risk-benefit profile of commonly used herbal therapies: Ginkgo, St. John's wort, ginseng, echinacea, saw palmetto, and kava. Ann Intern Med 136:42-53, 2002.
4. Haller CA, Anderson IB, Kim SY, Blanc PD: An evaluation of selected herbal reference texts and comparison to published reports of adverse herbal events. Adv Drug React Toxicol Rev 21:143-150, 2002.
5. Hung OL, Lewin NA, Howland MA: Herbal preparations. In Goldfrank LR, Flomenbaum NE, Lewin NA, et al (eds): Goldfrank's Toxicologic Emergencies, 7th ed. New York, McGraw-Hill, 2002, pp 1129-1148.
6. Jacobs KM, Hirsch KA: Psychiatric complications of ma-huang. Psychosomatics 41:58-62, 2000.
7. Mills K: Serotonin syndrome: A clinical update. Crit Care Clin 13:763-783, 1997.

PATIENT 23

A 4-year-old girl with a cough after drinking from a soda bottle

A 4-year-old girl drank from a cola bottle in the garage of her home. She choked and coughed after sipping the noxious liquid within the bottle. The girl's father realized that he had stored lamp oil within the bottle, phoned the regional poison control center, and was referred for hospital evaluation. The girl continues to cough and breathe fast.

Physical Examination: Temperature 37.7° C, pulse 118/min, respirations 38/min, blood pressure 106/66 mmHg, pulse oximetry 95% breathing room air. General: alert, slightly anxious. HEENT: petroleum odor to breath, no oral lesions. Chest: tachypnea and diffuse rhonchi. Cardiovascular: normal. Abdomen: soft. Extremities: well perfused. Neuromuscular: normal.

Laboratory Findings: Chest radiograph: see figure.

Question: What physical properties of lamp oil are responsible for its propensity to cause aspiration pneumonitis?

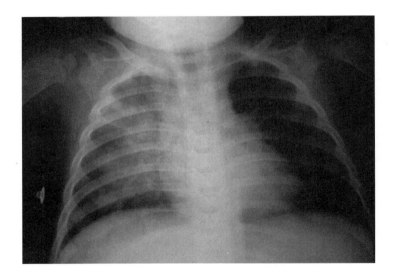

Answer: Low viscosity and low surface tension

Discussion: Hydrocarbons are aptly named organic compounds comprised primarily of hydrogen and carbon atoms and are typically derived from plants or through distillation of petroleum. Aliphatic, or "straight chain," petroleum-based hydrocarbons pose danger to children primarily via pulmonary aspiration. Hydrocarbon compounds extracted from plants (e.g., pine oil), with aromatic rings (e.g., benzene) or with halogen-atom side groups (e.g., carbon tetrachloride), have additional inherent toxicities. Aliphatic hydrocarbons (gasoline, kerosene, mineral seal oil, and lamp oil) are common household chemicals that place exploring children at risk when not properly stored. In the present case, lamp oil had been improperly stored in an attractive cola bottle within easy reach of a curious child.

Hydrocarbon chemicals cause lung injury on contact with pulmonary surfactant and cellular structures. The potential for pulmonary aspiration is influenced by a hydrocarbon's physical properties of viscosity and surface tension. *Viscosity* is a liquid's ability to resist flow. *Surface tension* is a measure of the adherence of a liquid to a surface. Hydrocarbons with low viscosity and low surface tension are most likely to spread into the lungs during drinking, swallowing, or vomiting.

Medical evaluation is recommended for any child developing symptoms after hydrocarbon ingestion. Children suffering from hydrocarbon aspiration will typically cough, gasp, or choke within 30 minutes of ingestion, although they frequently appear well on initial medical evaluation. The majority of such asymptomatic children will remain well, but some will develop progressive pneumonitis. Among children who develop clinically significant pneumonitis, the majority will have abnormal chest radiographs within 4 hours of ingestion, and almost all will have radiographic findings within 12 hours. Children without symptoms and with normal radiographs after a 4- to 6-hour period of observation may be candidates for close outpatient observation. Hospitalization is recommended for symptomatic patients.

Lamp oil is poorly bound by activated charcoal and less toxic in the stomach than in the lungs, thus gastric emptying is rarely advisable. Respiratory support remains the mainstay of therapy after lamp oil ingestion. Radiographic lung injury often progresses over several days to a week, then slowly resolves. Volume- and pressure-limited mechanical ventilation, high-frequency oscillatory mechanical ("jet") ventilation, and extracorporeal membrane oxygenation (ECMO) have all been employed in the treatment of fulminant hydrocarbon pneumonitis. Current data do not support the routine use of corticosteroids, and surfactant replacement therapy remains experimental.

The present patient's chest radiograph demonstrated diffuse patchy infiltrates of the right lung consistent with pneumonitis. She subsequently experienced rapid clinical deterioration and radiographic opacification. Standard mechanical ventilation and jet ventilation failed to provide adequate oxygenation, and the girl was treated with ECMO. Slow clinical improvement was noticed on the 9th day, and she was discharged to home after several weeks of hospitalization. Fortunately, she seems neurologically well on follow-up; however, pulmonary function testing demonstrates chronic restrictive lung disease.

Clinical Pearls

1. Never store drugs or chemicals in anything other than original, or specially designated, containers.

2. Families may be unaware of the hazard posed by several common household hydrocarbon products.

3. Hydrocarbon pneumonitis may develop in the absence of vomiting and may be delayed in presentation.

REFERENCES

1. Lewander WJ, Aleguas A Jr: Petroleum distillates and turpentine. In Haddad LM, Shannon MW, Winchester JF (eds): Clinical Management of Poisoning and Drug Overdose. Philadelphia, WB Saunders, 1998, pp 913-918.
2. Chyka PA: Benefits of extracorporeal membrane oxygenation for hydrocarbon pneumonitis. J Toxicol Clin Toxicol 34:357-363, 1996.
3. Truemper E, De La Rocha SR, Atkinson SD: Clinical characteristics, pathophysiology, and management of hydrocarbon ingestion: Case report and review of the literature. Pediatr Emerg Care 3:187-193, 1987.

Otilia Capellan, MD
Jeanmarie Perrone, MD

PATIENT 24

A 20-year-old pregnant woman 20 hours after acetaminophen overdose

One day prior to admission, a 20-year-old woman went to see her doctor to obtain emergency contraception. Upon evaluation she was found to have a positive urine pregnancy test and was advised that she could not be given the prescription. Based upon the dates of her last menstrual period she was 6 weeks pregnant. The patient became distraught and ingested twenty "extra strength" 500-mg tablets of acetaminophen. She vomited twice and eventually called her doctor and was instructed to come to the emergency department for evaluation. She denies any other ingestions or complaints.

Physical Examination: Temperature 36.5° C, pulse 93/min, respirations 16/min, blood pressure 116/71 mmHg. General: well-developed, well-nourished, no acute distress. HEENT: pupils equally round and reactive; sclera anicteric; oropharynx clear. Chest: normal. Cardiovascular: normal. Abdomen: soft, non-distended, normal bowel sounds; right upper quadrant tenderness to palpation, especially at liver edge; no hepatomegaly. Extremities: normal capillary refill. Skin: normal. Neuromuscular: awake, alert, oriented; no motor weakness, normal coordination and gait.

Laboratory Findings: Hemogram: WBC 7300/μL, hemoglobin 12 g/dL, platelets 325,000/μL. Serum chemistries: sodium 138 mEq/L, potassium 3.9 mEq/L, chloride 101 mEq/L, CO_2 22 mEq/L, BUN 8 mg/dL, creatinine 0.7 mg/dL, total bilirubin 0.8 mg/dL, alanine aminotransferase 32 U/L, aspartate aminotransferase 20 U/L, alkaline phosphatase 61 U/L. Human chorionic gonadotropin level: 5750 mIU/mL Acetaminophen level: 17.1 mcg/mL. Salicylate level: 1.4 mg/dL

Question: If the time of ingestion was 20 hours ago, how should the "therapeutic" acetaminophen level of 17.1 mcg/mL be interpreted?

Diagnosis and Treatment: According to the Rumack-Matthew nomogram, an acetaminophen level of 17.1 mcg/mL at 20 hours after ingestion is considered toxic (see figure). Patients taking single acute acetaminophen overdoses, with serum levels determined by the nomogram to be potentially toxic, should be considered candidates for *N*-acetylcysteine (NAC) therapy. *Early* therapy (NAC starting within 8 hours after overdose) is very effective. Risk of hepatic injury increases with every hour of treatment delay after 8 hours postingestion.

Discussion: Acetaminophen is the most common analgesic medication used during pregnancy. In therapeutic doses it is safe for both mother and fetus. However, in large amounts it can cause lethal hepatic necrosis in both.

Acetaminophen is primarily metabolized by the liver through sulfation and glucuronidation. Less than 5% undergoes direct renal elimination. The remaining fraction (up to 15%) is oxidized by the cytochrome P-450 system to a toxic metabolite (*N*-acetyl-*p*-benzoquinoneimine: NAPQI). NAPQI is quickly detoxified by conjugation with glutathione to a nontoxic cysteine or mercapturic acid conjugate that is readily excreted by the kidneys.

After overdose, saturation of metabolic pathways leads to increased NAPQI production; hepatic stores of glutathione quickly diminish; and hepatic toxicity ensues. NAPQI readily binds to sulfur-containing enzymes and proteins in the liver, resulting in the characteristic hepatic centrilobular necrosis. The antidote NAC, when metabolized to cysteine, provides a glutathione precursor capable of conjugating excess toxic metabolites and preventing further liver damage.

Acetaminophen is known to cross the placenta. Metabolism of acetaminophen by the fetal liver microsomes and isolated fetal liver cells is limited. Fetal microsomal activity is minimal in the first trimester (12 weeks or less) and increases with gestational age (18–23 weeks). The cytochrome P-450 system responsible for the production of the toxic acetaminophen metabolites is present in the 16-week-old fetus.

It is unclear if NAC crosses the human placenta. Animal studies have been conflicting; however, the fetus is probably best protected by early maternal NAC therapy. Several human cases of acetaminophen overdose in pregnancy have been reported, with variable outcomes. In some cases, fetal demise with histological evidence of fetal hepatotoxicity was noted. However, other cases revealed good outcome following NAC therapy. The largest study of poisoned pregnant patients describes 60 women with acetaminophen overdoses at different stages in pregnancy. This confirmed that there is a *statistically significant correlation between the time that NAC therapy is started and pregnancy outcome*, with an increase in spontaneous abortions and fetal demise when NAC treatment was started late (16–24 hours).

The present patient was administered antiemetics, and the first dose of NAC was given via nasogastric tube. The remainder of the NAC therapy was administered orally. Liver function tests remained normal during the hospitalization. Symptoms (i.e., abdominal pain, nausea, and vomiting) resolved, and she continued to receive NAC therapy × 17 doses. She subsequently had a therapeutic abortion. In light of the information available on pregnancy and acetaminophen overdose, it is appropriate to start immediate NAC therapy in a pregnant patient who has ingested a potentially toxic amount of acetaminophen.

SINGLE ACUTE ACETAMINOPHEN OVERDOSE NOMOGRAM

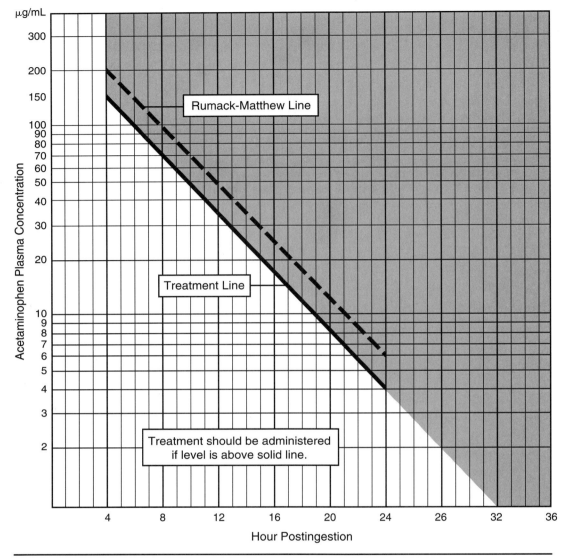

Nomogram: acetaminophen plasma concentration vs time after acetaminophen ingestion (adapted from Rumack and Matthew, 1975, with permission).

The nomogram has been developed to estimate the probability of whether a plasma acetaminophen concentration in relation to the interval postingestion will result in hepatoxicity and, therefore, whether acetylcysteine therapy should be administered.

CAUTIONS FOR USE OF THIS CHART:
1. Time coordinates refer to time postingestion.
2. Graph relates only to plasma concentrations following a single, acute overdose ingestion.
3. The Treatment Line is plotted 25% below the Rumack-Matthew Line to allow for potential errors in plasma acetaminophen assays and estimated time from ingestion of an overdose.

Clinical Pearls

1. In pregnant women with an acetaminophen overdose and a potentially toxic serum level, *N*-acetylcysteine (NAC) therapy showed be started as soon as possible.

2. Serum acetaminophen levels can be interpreted using the Rumack-Matthew nomogram within the first 4–24 hours postingestion.

3. When in doubt, start NAC therapy as early as possible postingestion. Therapy can be discontinued if not necessary.

4. Although NAC therapy IS NOT CLEARLY hepatoprotective in the fetus, fetal outcome depends on the mother's survival. Thus, the mother should be treated aggressively to prevent complications from the ingestion.

REFERENCES

1. Fine J: Reproductive and perinatal principles. In Goldfrank LR, Flomenbaum NE, Lewin NA, et al (eds): Goldfrank's Toxicologic Emergencies, 7th ed. New York, McGraw-Hill, 2002, pp 1606-1628.
2. Horowitz RS, Dart RC, Jarvie DR, et al: Placental transfer of N-acetylcysteine following human maternal acetaminophen toxicity. J Toxicol Clin Toxicol 35:447-451, 1997.
3. Selden BS, Curry SC, Clark RF, et al: Transplacental transport of N-acetylcysteine in an ovine model. Ann Emerg Med 20:1069-1072, 1991.
4. Riggs BS, Bronstein AC, Kulig K, et al: Acute acetaminophen overdose during pregnancy. Obstet Gynecol 74:247-253, 1989.
5. Wang LH, Rudolph AM, Benet LZ: Pharmacokinetic studies of the disposition of acetaminophen in the sheep maternal-placental-fetal unit. J Phamacol Exp Ther 238:198-205, 1986.
6. Robertson RG, Van Cleave BL, Collins JJ: Acetaminophen overdose in the second trimester of pregnancy. J Fam Pract 23:267-268, 1986.
7. Ludmir J, Main DM, Landon MB, Gabbe SG: Maternal acetaminophen overdose at 15 weeks gestation. Obset Gynecol 67:750-751, 1986.
8. Hairbach H, Akhter JE, Muscato MS, et al: Acetaminophen overdose with fetal demise. Am J Clin Pathol 82:240-242, 1983.
9. Byer AJ, Traylo TR, Semmer JR: Acetaminophen overrdose in the third trimester of pregnancy. JAMA 247:3114-3115, 1982.

Aaron J. Donoghue, MD

PATIENT 25

A 2½-year-old boy with a verapamil ingestion

A 2½-year-old boy with no significant medical history presents to the emergency department approximately 30 minutes after ingesting a handful of pills from a vial left unattended on the living-room table. The medication belonged to his aunt, who knows for certain that a total of 12 pills are now unaccounted for. The tablets are sustained-release verapamil, 240 mg per tablet. The boy is completely asymptomatic.

Physical Examination: Temperature 37° C, pulse 147/min, respirations 24/min, blood pressure 108/64 mmHg. General: crying but consolable. HEENT: mucous membranes moist. Chest: clear to auscultation bilaterally. Cardiovascular: tachycardic, no murmur. Abdomen: soft, nontender. Genitourinary: normal male genitalia. Extremities: warm, pulses normal. Skin: warm and dry. Neuromuscular: nonfocal.

Laboratory Findings: A complete blood count, electrolytes, coagulation profile: normal. Electrocardiogram: sinus tachycardia, PR interval 110 ms, QRS interval 50 ms.

Question: What should be the medical disposition for this well-appearing child?

Treatment: Admission to a tertiary-care hospital intensive care unit (ICU) with capacity for maximal cardiac support.

Discussion: Verapamil is a calcium channel blocker (CCB) widely prescribed to adults for dysrhythmias, coronary artery disease, hypertension, and congestive heart failure. Its therapeutic use in children is rare, and adverse events from exploratory ingestions among children have been well described. Verapamil has been characterized as one of several medications that could be fatal to toddlers in a single dose. However, the clinical severity of CCB exposures varies widely, and the majority of toddlers with a known or suspected single-dose CCB ingestion do not suffer major morbidity or death. Clearly, a history of ingestion of a "handful" of pills portends a dangerous situation.

The cardiovascular effects of verapamil and other CCBs occur through multiple pathophysiological mechanisms. Calcium influx responsible for sinoatrial (SA) and atrioventricular (AV) node depolarization is impaired by CCBs, with resultant depression of SA node discharge rate and slowed conduction through the AV node. Clinically, these effects result in bradycardia and heart block, and these effects have been noted to be particularly prominent for verapamil among the CCBs. Verapamil also affects the slow calcium channels responsible for the plateau of myocardial depolarization in systole; blockage of these channels by verapamil results in impaired contractility and depressed myocardial function. Additionally, verapamil and other CCBs inhibit calcium influx into vascular smooth muscle and consequently lower arteriolar vascular tone, producing significant reduction in blood pressure and systemic vascular resistance. The toxicity of verapamil and other CCBs, therefore, is an extension of these effects with bradycardia, poor myocardial function, heart block, and hypotension being features of overdoses in children.

Management of patients with verapamil overdoses, as always, begins with supportive attention to the airway, breathing, and circulation. It should be borne in mind that circulatory compromise in such patients can be severe, and preparation for central administration of cardiac medications and transcutaneous cardiac pacing is warranted. Decontamination measures for verapamil should be considered as with any other potentially toxic ingestion, and general agreement suggests that activated charcoal should be administered as early as possible. Gastric lavage is more controversial, but may be indicated in patients presenting within 30 to 60 minutes after high-dose ingestions, provided they are stable and asymptomatic at the time of presentation. Several sustained-release preparations of verapamil and other CCBs are in commonplace use; when such preparations are encountered, whole bowel irrigation may be strongly considered.

No specific antidotal therapy for verapamil exists. The use of calcium salts for reversal of cardiovascular side effects is supported by sound theory and several cases in the literature, but it should be noted that some patients fail to respond to calcium. Some clinician-researchers suggest that such failures simply represent under-dosing of calcium salts, but this remains unproven. Therapeutic agents that enhance inotropy and chronotropy via alternate pharmacological mechanisms, such as phosphodiesterase inhibitors and insulin/dextrose, have been reported to have some efficacy in experimental animal models, but clinical data on their utility are varied. A verapamil-specific immunoglobulin, analogous to the widely used preparation specific for digoxin, has been prepared and has been shown *in vitro* to attenuate myocardial impairment; however, clinical trials do not exist. Transcutaneous pacing has been successfully used to improve symptomatic bradycardia in CCB-poisoned patients, but effect upon overall hemodynamic status and blood pressure is varied. Intra-aortic balloon counterpulsation has been used successfully in adults, but is technically challenging in small children.

The successful use of extracorporeal life support for the poisoned patient has been documented in multiple case reports in children and adults after a variety of intoxications, including medications with specific cardiovascular toxicity such as flecainide and quinidine. However, the clinical experience pertaining to the use of extracorporeal membrane oxygenation (ECMO) in the treatment of poisoned patients remains very limited, and demonstration of improved patient outcomes when compared to other conventional means of critical care support has been difficult. A sound basis for its use in support of reversible causes of cardiovascular toxicity exists. More clinical experience with ECMO in the poisoned patient will likely be needed to better define its role, but it should be borne in mind as a viable option for poisonings with cardiovascular toxins.

The patient in this case had his stomach lavaged, which produced several pill fragments, and was given an initial dose of activated charcoal. He had a progressively worsening course over the first hospital day. Three to four hours after ingestion he began to have significant first-degree heart block (see figure) and hypotension despite fluids, calcium, and catecholamine infusions. He was transferred to the ICU of a tertiary

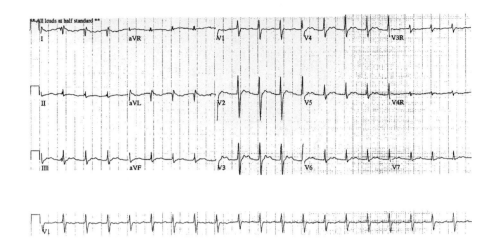

children's hospital, and shortly thereafter developed junctional bradycardia and subsequently suffered cardiac arrest. After approximately 10 minutes of cardiopulmonary resuscitation he was transcutaneously paced into a perfusing rhythm. He was subsequently placed onto venous-arterial ECMO. For his first 36 to 48 hours on ECMO, he remained in nearly complete cardiac electromechanical standstill, with a heart rate of 1 to 2 beats per minute. Cardiac function gradually returned (see figure below) with a normal sinus rhythm by day 4 post-ingestion, and he was taken off ECMO on hospital day 6. His remaining hospital course was marked by a gradual return to normal cardiac function, a tracheostomy for continued ventilatory support, and transfer to a rehabilitation facility for continued therapy. Long-term follow-up showed that he was converted back to a natural airway less than 1 year following his ECMO course and was neurologically intact.

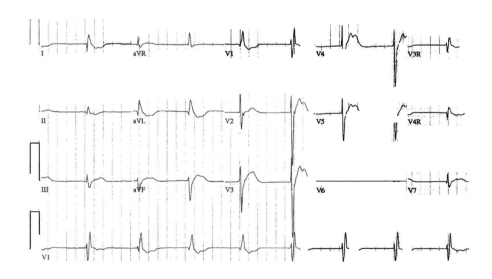

Clinical Pearls

1. Verapamil has no specific antidote.
2. Ingestions of sustained-release preparations of toxic medications may be amenable to decontamination via whole bowel irrigation.
3. Management of potentially toxic verapamil ingestions should occur in a critical care setting with capacity for aggressive cardiac support, possibly including extracorporeal life support.

REFERENCES

1. Hill RE, Heard K, Bogdan GM, et al: Attenuation verapamil-induced myocardial toxicity in an ex-vivo rat model using a verapamil-specific ovine immunoglobulin. AEM 8:950-956, 2001.
2. Osterhoudt KC: The toxic toddler: Drugs that can kill in small doses. Contemp Pediatr 17:73-89, 2000.
3. Belson MG, Gorman SE, Sullivan K, Geller RJ: Calcium channel blocker ingestions in children. Am J Emer Med 18: 581-586, 2000.
4. DeRoos F: Calcium channel blockers. In Goldfrank L. Flomenbaum N, Lewin N, et al (eds): Goldfrank's Toxicologic Emergencies, 7th ed. New York, McGraw-Hill, 1998, pp 762-774.
5. Banner W Jr: Risks of extracorporeal membrane oxygenation: Is there a role for use in the management of the acutely poisoned patient? J Toxicol Clin Toxicol 34:365-371, 1996.

Anthony P. Morocco, M.D.

PATIENT 26

A 45-year-old woman with a pale and painful fingertip

A 45-year-old woman complains of pain and numbness in her right index finger. She is a school nurse and inadvertently injected the finger while demonstrating the use of an epinephrine auto-injector. She denies chest pain, palpitations, or systemic complaints.

Physical Examination: Temperature 36.5° C, pulse 98/min, respirations 16/min, blood pressure 138/88 mmHg. General: no distress. Cardiovascular: normal. Extremities (see figure): puncture wound on volar aspect of right index fingertip; distal half of finger appears pale, and capillary refill is prolonged (>3 seconds); full range of motion (ROM) of finger, decreased light touch sensation in fingertip.

Question: What treatment, if any, is needed in this case?

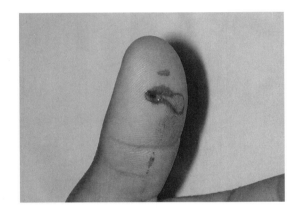

Diagnosis and Treatment: The patient has clinical signs of decreased blood flow to the fingertip due to the vasoconstrictive effect of the injected epinephrine. Treatment goals should be to assess the degree of ischemia, if any, and to attempt to restore perfusion.

Discussion: Epinephrine auto-injectors provide potentially lifesaving first aid to those suffering from severe allergic reactions to insect envenomation, food allergy, or other exposure. Anaphylaxis results from a foreign chemical or agent, the antigen, precipitating the degranulation of mast cells that release relatively large quantities of histamine and other inflammatory mediators. These substances induce a combination of clinical effects, including urticaria, wheezing, vasodilation, and increased vascular permeability. Epinephrine acts quickly to stop the release of these mediators from the mast cells. It also acts via alpha- and beta-adrenergic stimulation to increase cardiac contractility, cardiac output, vasomotor tone, and bronchodilation.

The epinephrine auto-injectors available in the United States are the EpiPen (see figure) and EpiPen Jr. The former yields a dose of 0.3 mg of epinephrine, the latter 0.15 mg. Each is designed to inject only 0.3 cc (epinephrine 1:1000 or 1:2000) of the 2 cc contained in the syringe, so a used injector appears to have only partially injected its contents. Both products are available in a kit that contains two auto-injectors, and a training device that contains no needle or medicine, so the patient can practice and become more comfortable with the device prior to requiring it in a true emergency. When properly used, the injector is first held tightly with the fist, the activator cap is then removed, and finally the unit is jabbed firmly into the anterolateral thigh to trigger the spring-loaded syringe. It is held in place for several seconds to deliver the full dose of epinephrine into the muscle before removal. Unfortunately, as many as 60% of patients and their physicians have difficulty using these devices properly. Improper use and careless handling of the auto-injectors have resulted in numerous cases of inadvertent discharge of epinephrine,

typically into fingers. The incidence of unintended injection has been estimated at 1 occurrence per 50,000 prescribed units. Upon injection, the alpha-adrenergic agonism of epinephrine results in vasoconstriction. In regions without collateral arterial circulation, such as fingers, toes, and nose, it is postulated that this may compromise vascular supply, resulting in irreversible ischemic injury.

Patients with an ischemic finger after epinephrine injection will complain of pain and numbness in the area. Examination may demonstrate pallor, delayed capillary refill, edema resulting in decreased ROM, and/or decreased sensation. The range of signs and symptoms depends on the degree and length of time of ischemia. If perfusion is not restored within 12 hours, the skin may begin to appear necrotic. Patients may also complain of systemic symptoms from the absorbed epinephrine, such as palpitations, rapid heart rate, tremor, and anxiety. The physical examination may reveal hypertension, tachycardia, tremor, and diaphoresis. Patients with underlying cardiovascular disease are at risk for cardiac ischemia and dysrhythmias.

The treatment for epinephrine auto-injector injury, and any iatrogenic alpha-adrenergic agent injection, depends on the degree of ischemia. Perfusion may be assessed by physical examination, particularly capillary refill and sensation. Pulse oximetry has also been utilized as a sensitive and readily available measure of perfusion in cases of epinephrine injection as well as traumatic injuries to the finger. In many cases, examination will reveal little or no evidence of decreased perfusion. These patients are often treated conservatively by soaking the finger in warm water or massaging the finger to encourage blood flow. Some patients have also been treated with topical nitroglycerin to the affected area to promote vasodilatation, but the efficacy of this treatment has not been rigorously tested. Patients with clear signs of ischemia can be treated with local injection of **phentolamine**. This drug is an alpha-adrenergic antagonist and reverses the epinephrine-induced vasoconstriction. Generally, 10 cc of a 1 mg/mL solution of phentolamine is prepared. Doses of 0.5 mg to 10 mg have been reported to be successful. Some authors advocate direct injection into the wound site and surrounding ischemic skin. However, given the limited volume that may be injected into a finger, particularly one that may already be edematous, it may be preferable to inject the phentolamine near the digital artery at

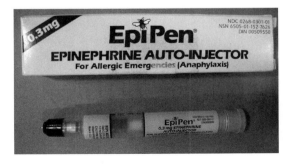

the base of the finger, in a manner similar to a digital nerve block. Lidocaine may be added to the phentolamine to relieve pain.

Local **terbutaline** injection has been employed as an alternative treatment, as phentolamine may not be readily available. Terbutaline is a beta2-adrenergic agonist, and stimulation of these receptors causes vasodilatation. A solution of 1 mg of the drug in 10 cc should be prepared and utilized in the same manner as described for phentolamine. Both agents may cause systemic effects, particularly if injected directly into a blood vessel. Phentolamine may cause hypotension, while terbutaline may cause tachycardia. Therefore it is important to have intravenous access prior to using these agents. Other vasodilators, such as amyl nitrate and sodium nitroprusside, have been used in the past but are not recommended due to limited efficacy and possibility of systemic hypotension. Finally, as with any wound, the patient's tetanus status and the degree of direct tissue trauma should be assessed.

This patient had evidence of significant ischemia to her fingertip with pain, pallor, and delayed capillary refill. She was treated with three injections of 0.5 mg phentolamine, one at the site of the injury and one at the base of each finger near the digital artery. Within 30 minutes, the fingertip appeared to be hyperemic with brisk capillary refill. The patient was subsequently discharged and had no sequelae on follow up.

Clinical Pearls

1. Inadvertent injection of epinephrine into the finger by auto-injector may cause vasoconstriction resulting in tissue ischemia.
2. Invasive therapy is generally unnecessary; suspected ischemia can be treated with injection of phentolamine or terbutaline.
3. The pulse oximeter may be useful in assessing perfusion of the affected finger.

REFERENCES

1. Mrvos R, Anderson BD, Krenzelok EP: Accidental injection of epinephrine from an autoinjector: invasive treatment not always required. South Med J 95:318-320, 2002.
2. Sicherer SH, Forman JA, Noone, SA: Use assessment of self-administered epinephrine among food-allergic children and pediatricians. Pediatrics 105:359-362, 2000.
3. Sellens C, Morrison L: Accidental injection of epinephrine by a child: A unique approach to treatment. CJEM 1:34-36, 1999.
4. Steir PA, Bogner MP, Webster K, et al: Use of subcutaneous terbutaline to reverse peripheral ischemia. Am J Emerg Med 17:91-94, 1999.
5. McCauley WA, Gerace RV, Scilley C: Treatment of accidental digital injection of epinephrine. Ann Emerg Med 20:665-668, 1991.

PATIENT 27

A 22-year-old man who has inhaled hair spray

A 22-year-old man presents to the emergency department (ED) via ambulance; he is unresponsive. According to his accompanying friends, the patient was inhaling hair spray that was released into a paper bag. Soon after taking three large inhalations the patient became very agitated, started screaming, and then collapsed. The paramedics were immediately called and the patient was rushed to the ED. The friends state that the patient has no medical history, has no drug allergies, and only abuses "inhalants" (see figure).

Physical Examination: No pulse and blood pressure are detected. The patient has no spontaneous respirations. HEENT: no gag reflex.

Laboratory Findings: Electrocardiogram: ventricular fibrillation.

Questions: What caused this patient's life-threatening dysrhythmia? What is the treatment?

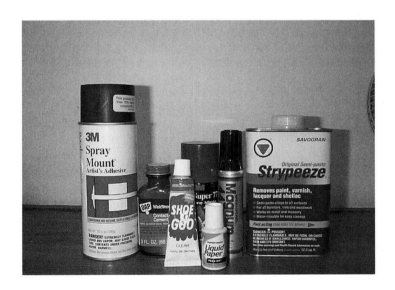

Diagnosis and Treatment: This patient is suffering from myocardial "sensitization" and subsequent ventricular fibrillation secondary to inhalant abuse. The treatment is standard cardiac defibrillation. If defibrillation is unsuccessful, then consider use of lidocaine or a beta-blocker.

Discussion: The inhaled substances of abuse are aromatic and short-chained volatile hydrocarbons that, upon inhalation, have a rapid onset of intoxicating effects. The volatilized inhalant used is well absorbed from the lungs and rapidly distributed to the central nervous system. One or two large inhalations of the inebriating substance intoxicates the user very quickly, and the effects can last for hours. It is very difficult to clinically differentiate inhalant-induced inebriation from ethanol-induced inebriation, although toxic inhalation inebriation is usually of shorter duration compared to alcohol.

Patients who abuse inhalants typically experience euphoria. However, the intentional abuse of inhalants is potentially dangerous, as patients can acutely die or suffer severe permanent organ damage. Organ systems that can be injured by inhalant abuse include the central and peripheral nervous systems, the hematological system, and the lungs, liver, kidneys, and heart.

There are several methods by which solvent abusers inhale the toxic fumes; "huffing" and "sniffing" are two of the more common methods. Huffing involves nasally inhaling the fumes from a solvent-saturated rag (e.g., glue, gasoline). Sniffing involves directly sniffing the fumes from the container or squeezing the toxic substance onto a rag and nasally sniffing the fumes from the rag. Another method involves transferring the toxic substance into a paper bag, placing this bag over the nose and mouth, and inhaling deeply (e.g., "bagging"). Some abusers transfer the toxic substance into a pan or other vessel, which is then heated; this results in a more rapid and concentrated vapor.

There are many reports of cardiovascular toxicity and death associated with inhalant abuse. During the late 1950s and 1960s, there was an epidemic of sudden deaths occurring among teenagers who recently inhaled volatile hydrocarbons. This scenario, termed **sudden sniffing death** (SSD), is believed to result from the volatile hydrocarbons sensitizing the myocardium to catecholamines, which subsequently produces lethal cardiac arrhythmias. A typical scenario of SSD postulated by many toxicologists occurs when teenagers are caught abusing inhalants by parents or police. After being caught, a rush of catecholamines occurs in these teenagers as they experience fear of parental punishment or they run to escape legal complications. The catecholamine rush then "excessively stimulates" the inhalant-sensitized myocardium, leading to lethal arrhythmias and death.

There are numerous other reports of human SSD associated with the recent abuse of inhalants. Some inhalants reported to cause lethal arrhythmias and SSD include freon, bromochlorodifluoromethane, butane, propane, 1,1,1-trichloroethane, gasoline, and trichloroethylene.

Patients who abuse inhalants and suffer cardiac sensitization may arrive to the ED suffering a life-threatening dysrhythmia. Standard cardiac pharmacological treatment and electrotherapy are reported to be unsuccessful. Beta-adrenergic blocking agents have been proposed as a treatment option for life-threatening arrhythmias induced by inhalants. Should conventional cardiac resuscitation fail, consider the use of beta-adrenergic blocking agents (e.g., esmolol, propanolol). Most patients who suffer cardiac consequences of inhalant abuse usually die at the scene or convert back to a normal rhythm prior to medical intervention.

The present patient was intubated in the ED, and cardiac pulmonary resuscitation (CPR) was provided. The patient was defibrillated with 200 joules, 300 joules, and finally with 360 joules. Following the third defibrillation, the patient became electrically asystolic. CPR was continued, and the patient was given several doses of atropine and epinephrine intravenously. After approximately 30 minutes of resuscitation the patient unfortunately remained asystolic. Eye examination revealed fixed and dilated pupils. The patient was then pronounced dead. The family did not request an autopsy.

Clinical Pearls

1. Acute inhalant abuse can sensitize the myocardium to catecholamine stimulation and subsequently produce lethal dysrhythmias (ventricular tachycardia, ventricular fibrillation).
2. Standard cardiac pharmacological treatment and electrotherapy may be unsuccessful in treating patients suffering lethal dysrhythmias induced by inhalant abuse.
3. Consider the use of beta-adrenergic blocking agents as a treatment option for life-threatening arrhythmias induced by inhalants should conventional cardiac resuscitation fail.

REFERENCES

1. LoVecchio F, Gerkin R: Inhalants of abuse. Top Emerg Med 19:4:44-52, 1997.
2. Linden CH: Volatile substances of abuse. Emerg Med Clin North Am 39:451-461, 1990.
3. Bass M: Sudden sniffing death. JAMA 219:1:33-37, 1972.

Chirag Patel, MD
Francis DeRoos, MD

PATIENT 28

A 52-year-old man with vomiting, diarrhea, sweating, and tremor

A 52-year-old man presents with several days of diarrhea followed by the sudden onset of confusion, frequent vomiting, loss of bowel and bladder control, rhinorrhea, cough, excessive tearing, and tremulousness. He had profuse sweating, but no fever or chills. The patient works at a chemical plant, and a few weeks prior to presentation he was seen by his family spraying for bees around his home.

Physical Examination: Temperature 35.6° C, pulse 94/min, respirations 18/min, blood pressure 144/82 mmHg. HEENT: mildly constricted pupils, increased tearing, copious saliva. Chest: scattered rhonchi. Cardiovascular: normal S1 and S2, no murmur or S3 or S4. Abdomen: normal. Extremities: well-perfused. Skin: diaphoretic. Neuromuscular: alert, oriented to person and place, diffuse weakness with tremor.

Laboratory Findings: Hemogram: WBC 21,800/μL, otherwise normal. Serum chemistries: normal. EKG: QTc 471 msec, otherwise normal. Chest x-ray: normal. Non contrast CT of the head: normal.

Question: What clinical presentation or toxidrome is this patient manifesting?

Diagnosis: The patient has a clinical presentation consistent with organophosphate or carbamate toxicity, termed the cholinergic toxidrome (see table). This is a constellation of signs and symptoms that most prominently consist of muscarinic effects, including increased GI motility, urinary incontinence, pupillary miosis, bronchospasm, bronchorrhea, lacrimation, and salivation.

Discussion: Organophosphates and carbamates are families of compounds that bind to carboxylic ester hydrolases including acetylcholinesterase (AChE), which is found on nerve terminals and within red blood cells, and pseudocholinesterase (BuChE), which is found in plasma. These chemicals are used most commonly as pesticides but have also been developed as chemical weapons. The Tokyo subway poisoning by the extremist group Aum Shinrikyo in fall of 1995 involved sarin, an organophosphate. The toxic effects of organophosphates and carbamates are primarily derived from their **anticholinesterase activity**, specifically against AChE. Toxicity is seen when the level of AChE activity is depressed to less than 20% of baseline. Generally, symptoms develop most rapidly with inhalational and parenteral exposures and more slowly with transdermal absorption; however, most patients display symptoms of poisoning within 6 to 12 hours of exposure. The exceptions to this pattern include a few highly fat-soluble compounds that first distribute into the body's vast fat stores and then slowly leech out into the systemic circulation manifesting toxicity only after several days or even weeks.

Organophosphates and carbamates bind at the active site of AChE, rendering it unable to hydrolyze acetylcholine into acetic acid and choline. Carbamates reversibly bind the AChE with an unstable bond lasting less than 24 hours. Organophosphates, on the other hand, form a much more stable bond with this enzyme that can be reversed only by a nucleophilic oxime such as the antidote pralidoxime (2-PAM). After 24 to 72 hours the organophosphate moiety irreversibly binds in a process called aging, making the enzyme forever useless. In order for normal physiological function to return, new AChE must be synthesized—a process that takes many weeks to a few months.

Acetylcholine is a neurotransmitter found at parasympathetic as well as sympathetic ganglia, terminals of postganglionic parasympathetic nerves, skeletal neuromuscular junctions, and some nerve endings within the central nervous system (CNS). Under physiological conditions, after acetylcholine is released from a nerve terminal into the synapse and activates the appropriate post-synaptic receptors, AChE rapidly breaks it down. However, when AChE is blocked or inactivated by a carbamate or organophosphate, acetylcholine accumulates within the synapse, causing greater than normal receptor stimulation. Therefore, the signs and symptoms of anticholinesterase toxicity manifest through activation of the parasympathetic nerves (muscarinic effects), activation of the sympathetic nervous system as well as somatic neuromuscular junction (nicotinic effects), and CNS effects. **CNS findings** can be varied and nonspecific and may include tremor, restlessness, insomnia, headache, dizziness, depression, and change in mental status including lethargy or obtundation. **Muscarinic effects** include increased GI motility, urinary incontinence, pupillary miosis, bradydysrhythmias, bronchospasm, bronchorrhea, lacrimation, and salivation. **Nicotinic effects** may include muscle fasiculations, weakness, and paralysis from overactivation of the neuromuscular junction, as well as mydriasis, bronchodilation, tachycardia, hypertension, and urinary retention from activation of the sympathetic nervous system. Because of the wide variety of physiological effects possible in the cholinergic toxidrome, most patients manifest a mixture of both muscarinic and sympathetic findings. Symptoms of anticholinesterase poisoning are very similar to more familiar conditions; bronchorrhea could be assumed to be pulmonary edema, and severe vomiting and diarrhea could be assumed to be gastroenteritis (see table next page).

Depressed cholinesterase activity is the gold standard to confirm the diagnosis of anticholinesterase toxicity. Red blood cell AChE activity closely correlates with neuronal activity in the first 5–7 days of symptoms and can be used as a marker for level of toxicity. Alternately but less reliably, because of less predictable correlation with neuronal activity, plasma pseudocholinesterase level also can be used. Unfortunately, both of these tests are not available emergently and treatment

DUMBBELS Mnemonic for the Cholinergic Toxidrome

Diarrhea
Urination
Miosis
Bronchorrhea
Bronchospasm
Emesis
Lacrimation
Salivation

Finding	Other Processes Substances Causing the Finding	Differentiating Findings
Miosis	Sedative-hypnotics, opioids, PCP, pontine hemorrhage	No muscarinic or nicotinic signs or symptoms
Muscarinic symptoms	Muscarine containing mushrooms, pilocarpine, bethanechol	No muscle weakness or fasciculations
Bronchorrhea, respiratory distress	Asthma, pulmonary edema, pulmonary embolism, salicylism	Should lack sialorrhea, diarrhea, cramping, myoclonus of fasciculations
Hypertension, seizures, tachycardia, mydriasis, tremor, clonus, diaphoresis	Sympathomimetic intoxication, sedative-hypnotic or alcohol withdrawal	Should lack "DUMBBELS" muscarinic findings; muscle activity should be coordinated

must be based upon both the exposure history and clinical presentation.

Treatment of anticholinesterase poisoning should focus on decontamination, reversing the muscarinic effects, and antidotal therapy to regenerate AChE. Because organophosphates and carbamates are found in various forms, decontamination often involves careful removal and disposal of all worn items and irrigation or washing of the patient's skin. Cases of healthcare providers manifesting cholinergic symptoms after decontaminating an organophosphate-poisoned patient underscore the importance of adequate self-protection, including impermeable gowns and gloves used for chemical exposure incidents. The earliest threat to life after cholinergic poisoning is from CNS toxicity and from respiratory failure and hypoxemia due to respiratory muscle failure and muscarinic effects. Therefore, the airway and ventilation should be controlled early with endotracheal intubation and mechanical ventilation in patients with significant weakness, patients unable to handle secretions, or obtunded patients. Remember that if succinylcholine is used as a paralytic agent, its duration of effect will be greatly prolonged and unpredictable because it is metabolized by AchE. The duration of effect of nondepolarizing paralytic agents is unaffected, because they are not metabolized by AchE.

Excess muscarinic activity should be controlled with **ACh antagonists** such as **atropine**. The initial dose is 1–2 mg IV in adults (0.05 mg/kg in children) and should be repeated every 2 to 3 minutes until the desirable clinical response is achieved, namely drying the tracheobronchial tree of its excessive secretions in order to enable oxygenation. This may require over 40 mg of atropine in *significantly* poisoned adults; *severely* poisoned patients have been administered over 1000 mg of atropine during the first 24 hours of their therapy. Initial tachycardia should not deter atropine administration and typically improves after significant doses of atropine. Nebulized itratropium or atropine may also be effective in treating bronchospasm and secretions. Significantly poisoned patients typically benefit from either repeat doses or a continuous infusion of atropine. The dose is highly variable and should be titrated to clinical effect. **Glycopyrrolate** (0.05 mg/kg IV) also can be used to treat the peripheral muscarinic effects without causing central effects. Remember that while atropine reverses the muscarinic effects of these agents, the nicotinic effects are unchanged. Therefore, patients must be continually monitored for progressive weakness and respiratory failure in an intensive care setting.

Lastly, antidotal therapy with a **nucleophilic oxime** such as **pralidoxime** (2-PAM) should be instituted as early as possible. Pralidoxime reverses the organophosphate-AChE bond and binds and inactivates free organophosphates in the body. Unfortunately, pralidoxime is unable to cleave aged organophosphate-AChE bonds, so the sooner it's administered, the more effective it will be. Note, however, that patients should receive pralidoxime even if they present up to 24 or 48 hours after exposure, because the rate of aging and redistribution from fat among organophosphates is quite variable. One suggested initial dose is 1–2 g intravenously over 10–15 minutes (25–50 mg/kg IV for children) followed by a constant infusion at 2–4 mg/kg/hr (5–10 mg/kg/hr in children). This infusion is also titrated to improvement in symptoms. There is some evidence to suggest that **benzodiazepines** such as **diazepam** may be neuroprotective in severe poisonings and should be strongly considered as a sedative agent.

If a patient remains asymptomatic 6 to 12 hours after exposure, he or she may be discharged home with close follow-up. Any symptomatic patient should be admitted for at least 24 hours. All patients who require atropine should also receive pralidoxime and be admitted to an intensive care unit.

Three neurological sequelae may result from organophosphate poisoning: cognitive deterioration, confusion, and personality changes. A poorly understood syndrome called the **intermediate syndrome**, characterized by respiratory failure and bulbar, nuchal, and proximal limb muscle weakness with slow recovery, also may occur. Finally, patients may develop a severe polyneuropathy.

This patient was stabilized with endotrachial intubation, mechanical ventilation, atropine, and pralidoxime. After 9 days of intensive care, he recovered without residual deficits after prolonged rehabilitation. Upon recovery, the man admitted to drinking a cup of an insecticide containing the organophosphate diazinon in an attempt to commit suicide.

Clinical Pearls

1. Organophosphate toxicity can present with mixed muscarinic ("DUMBBELS") and nicotinic (adrenergic stimulation and muscle weakness) findings. The constellation of suggestive symptoms and a high index of suspicion should prompt rapid therapy.

2. Early control of airway and muscarinic manifestations is essential to limiting morbidity and mortality.

3. Atropine is the treatment for significant organophosphate poisoning, and the dose should be titrated to improvement in muscarinic toxicity. Nicotinic effects, such as muscle weakness, are not improved with atropine.

4. Pralidoxime should be administered to all organophosphate-poisoned patients who receive significant atropine therapy and can be effective, depending upon the agent ingested, up to 48 hours after exposure.

REFERENCES

1. Clark RF: Insecticides: Organic phosphorous compounds and carbamates. In Goldfrank LR, Flomenbaum, NE, Lewin NA, et al (eds): Toxicologic Emergencies. New York, McGraw-Hill, 2002, pp 1346-1365.
2. Aaron CK: Organophosphates and carbamates. In Ford MD, Ling LJ, Delany KA (eds): Clinical Toxicology. Philadelphia, W. B. Saunders Company, 2001, pp 820-826.
3. DeBleecker J, Van Den Neucker K, Calardyn F: Intermediate syndrome in organophosphrus poisoning: A prospective study. Crit Care Med 21:1706-1711, 1993.
4. Karalliedde L, Senanayake N: Organophosphorus insecticide poisoning. Br J Anaesth 63:736-740, 1989.
5. Zwiener RJ, Ginsburg CM: Organophosphate and carbamate poisoning in infants and children. Pediatrics 81:121-126, 1988.

PATIENT 29

A 34-year-old man with gastroenteritis

A 34-year-old police officer with no previous relevant medical history suffers from crampy abdominal pain, intermittent nausea, occasional vomiting, and persistent diarrhea. These symptoms have been present for approximately 1 month, and this is his third emergency department visit for the evaluation of these problems since they began. His symptoms have reportedly worsened over the past month, and now he is also complaining of "pins and needles" sensations in both feet as well as some muscular weakness that began in his feet and has progressed to include his lower legs.

Physical Examination: Temperature 37° C, pulse 115/min, respirations 24/min, blood pressure 118/70 mmHg. Oxygen saturation: 97% in room air. HEENT: normal. Chest: no wheezes, rales, or rhonchi. Abdomen: soft, flat, diffusely tender, no rebound tenderness; increased bowel sounds; no organomegaly. Genitourinary: heme-positive stool. Neuromuscular: weak motor strength both lower extremities. Skin: exfoliative rash on palmer surface of both hands and plantar surfaces of both feet.

Laboratory Findings: Hemogram: WBC normal, hemoglobin 10 g/dL (normocytic, normochromic), platelets normal. Serum chemistries: normal.

Question: What is the cause of this man's apparent gastroenteritis?

Diagnosis: Gastrointestinal symptoms persisting for several weeks in conjunction with a palmar and plantar exfoliative rash are suggestive of acute arsenic intoxication.

Discussion: Acute arsenic poisoning can occur as a result of either ingestion or inhalation of arsenic-containing compounds. Since acute arsenic poisoning is a relatively uncommon event, diagnosing this problem can be challenging for any clinician. Equally challenging, at times, is determining the source of the arsenic exposure. Most cases of acute arsenic intoxication in the United States today result from either occupational exposures or exposures related to homicidal or suicidal intention.

Unremitting symptoms of gastrointestinal distress are the usual presenting symptoms associated with acute arsenic poisoning secondary to the ingestion of inorganic arsenic compounds. However, acute arsenic poisoning can manifest with multi-system abnormalities (see table).

Arsenic intoxication is best confirmed by the use of a 24-hour urine specimen for arsenic testing. However, note that general urine testing can be confounded by naturally occurring forms of organic arsenic, found in a variety of seafood. These forms can produce false-positive tests for urine arsenic for up to a week following ingestion. Thus, the appropriate test to order is a "**speciated urine arsenic level**." This test essentially separates the inorganic (potentially harmful) arsenic from organic (that derived from seafood, which is relatively harmless) and allows the clinician to obtain a true picture of the possibility of arsenic intoxication. Blood arsenic levels have limited utility since arsenic is cleared from the blood within hours.

The present patient was hospitalized for the treatment of dehydration due to "severe gastroenteritis." A neurological consultation was obtained when the patient began to complain of lower extremity weakness, and an astute neurologist ordered speciated urine arsenic levels. These levels were reported as positive for inorganic arsenic. It was later determined that the patient's wife had been adding small amounts of an arsenic-containing ant poison to the patient's evening meal for several weeks in an attempt to kill him. Once removed from exposure the patient recovered uneventfully and never required the use of chelation therapy or other treatment modalities beyond good supportive care.

Systems That May Be Affected by Arsenic and Related Clinical Manifestations

Central nervous system	Encephalopathy, seizures, coma, death
Peripheral nervous system	"Stocking-glove" neuropathies, painful paresthesias, fasciculations, foot/wrist drop
Cardiovascular system	QT prolongation, conduction blocks, ventricular tachycardia, torsades des pointes, ventricular fibrillation
Pulmonary system	Pulmonary edema, ARDS, respiratory failure, lung cancer
Gastrointestinal system	Abdominal pain, nausea, vomiting, bloody diarrhea, garlicky breath, metallic taste
Hematopoietic system	Hemolysis (associated with arsine gas exposure), pancytopenia, anemia,
Skin/nails	Exfoliative dermatitis, hyperpigmentation, Mees' lines, skin cancer

Clinical Pearls

1. Patients with unresolved symptoms of gastroenteritis should be evaluated for possible arsenic intoxication.

2. Any patient newly diagnosed with Guillain-Barré syndrome should be evaluated for possible arsenic intoxication.

3. Arsenic testing of 24-hour urine specimens should include speciation to account for the fact that ingested seafood may confound the test by causing a positive assay for a relatively harmless form of arsenic that exists in nature.

REFERENCES
1. Graeme KA, Pollack CV: Heavy metal toxicity. Part I: Arsenic and mercury. J Emerg Med 16:45-56, 1998.
2. Beckman KJ, Bauman JL, Pimental PA, et al: Arsenic-induced torsades des pointes. Crit Care Med 19:290-292, 1991.
3. Gorby MS: Arsenic poisoning. West J Med 149:308-315, 1988.
4. Donofrio PD, Wilbourn AJ, Algers JW, et al: Acute arsenic intoxication presenting as Guillain-Barré syndrome. Muscle Nerve 10:114-120, 1987.

PATIENT 30

Two men collapse in an area that smells of rotten eggs

A 27-year-old collapses while working in an empty tank at an oil refinery. A co-worker sees the man, descends into the tank to help him, and subsequently collapses. A third rescuer puts on a self-contained breathing apparatus and removes the men from the tank. The first man is dead at the scene. The second man is transported to the hospital. Multiple witnesses and other employees complain of a "rotten egg" smell.

Physical Examination: Temperature 36.8° C, pulse 125/min, respirations 28/min, blood pressure 130/90 mmHg, oxygen saturation by pulse-oximetry 100%. General: muscular, healthy; now groaning and more awake. HEENT: atraumatic, no signs of tongue biting. Chest: clear. Cardiovascular: tachycardic, regular rhythm, no murmurs. Abdomen: soft, nontender. Extremities: pale, faint distal pulses. Skin: warm and dry.

Laboratory Findings: Hemogram and coagulation profile: normal. Serum chemistries: normal. Arterial blood gas (40% Fio_2): pH 7.35, $Paco_2$ 32 mmHg, Pao_2 320 mmHg. Electrocardiogram (EKG): sinus tachycardia, no ischemia. Chest radiograph: see figure.

Question: When multiple serious casualties occur from a toxic inhalation, what should be suspected?

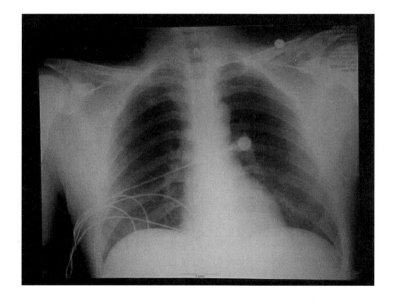

Diagnosis: Hydrogen sulfide gas inhalation

Discussion: When multiple people fall ill due to a toxic inhalant, the presence of a simple or chemical asphyxiant gas should be considered immediately. The scene should be evacuated and secured until the etiology and source of exposure is contained. If the industry where the exposure occurred is known, further clues as to the cause can be elucidated. Hydrogen sulfide gas is a common toxic byproduct of natural gas refining. At lower concentrations, it is notorious for a "rotten egg" sulfur odor. As concentrations increase, the odor becomes less reliable as olfactory fatigue may occur, and the victim may no longer be aware of ongoing risk. At high concentrations, there is a **"knockdown effect"** as cellular enzyme systems are poisoned and central nervous system and respiratory depression can occur quickly. Because it is rapid acting and very potent, multiple rescuers becoming victims is a common tale of hydrogen sulfide exposures. Both the industry where this accident occurred and the unfortunate severity of the illness prompt consideration of hydrogen sulfide gas. Another gas with similar knockdown effect is cyanide, but it is not used in oil refinery work. Treatment of hydrogen sulfide exposure is supplemental oxygen following immediate but safe removal from exposure.

Toxic inhalants can be grouped by mechanism for greater understanding (see table). **Simple asphyxiants**, gases such as nitrogen and carbon dioxide, replace oxygen in ambient air and can cause death (asphyxiation) when concentrations build in enclosed spaces. Other examples of asphyxiant gases include argon, helium, methane, and ethane. A second group of toxic inhalants is called **irritants**. These toxic inhalants, such as ammonia, cause noxious irritation to eyes, nose, and upper airways due to water solubility on exposed mucous membranes. The irritation is actually beneficial in that it prevents prolonged exposure. If exposure continues within an enclosed space, however irritant effects on the lower bronchi can lead to bronchospasm and pulmonary edema. Other toxic inhalants with low water solubility such as phosgene have greater potential for toxicity because there is minimal irritation to the upper airways and therefore exposure may not be associated with warning symptoms. Pulmonary edema may develop as exposure continues unknowingly. This is the premise of phosgene use as a chemical warfare agent. The most lethal group of toxic inhalants include the **chemical asphyxiants**, such as cyanide and hydrogen sulfide. These gases bind to cytochrome a-a$_3$ of the cytochrome oxidase pathway, disrupting oxidative phosphorylation in the electron transport chain and inhibiting oxygen utilization and cellular energy generation.

The present patient continued to improve in the hospital and returned to normal mentation within 15 minutes of arrival. The mild metabolic acidosis that was present on the initial arterial blood gas resolved on subsequent laboratory testing and probably represented a lactic acidosis secondary to the cellular asphyxiant effects of the hydrogen sulfide exposure. The chest radiograph was normal without evidence of pulmonary edema, ruling out irritant gases as the etiology of the sudden collapse. If the patient had not shown rapid signs of improvement, considerations for the use of the cyanide antidote kit would have been made, since the patient did have a metabolic acidosis and had collapsed suddenly.

An important clinical difference between cyanide and hydrogen sulfide poisoning is that cyanide-poisoned patients do *not* tend to improve just with removal from exposure and supportive care. Although cyanide binds to the same enzyme systems as hydrogen sulfide at the cellular level, cyanide does not "unbind" unless a specific antidote is utilized to release the cyanide bound to the cytochrome oxidase system. In cyanide poisoning, sodium nitrite is used to produce a methemoglobinemia to draw the cyanide from the cytochrome a-a$_3$ enzyme and form cyanomethemoglobin, thus liberating the cyanide from the

Toxic Inhalants

Simple Asphyxiants	Irritants	Chemical Asphyxiants
Carbon dioxide	Ammonia	Hydrogen sulfide
Nitrogen	Chloramine	Cyanide
Argon	Formaldehyde	Carbon monoxide
Helium	Ozone	Hydrazoic acid
Methane	Chlorine	
Ethane	Phosgene	

cytochrome and restoring the system's function. Conversely, hydrogen sulfide "unbinds" spontaneously after removal from exposure; thus, as in this case, if a hydrogen sulfide–poisoned patient is rescued and removed from exposure prior to sustaining anoxic injury, then he or she will improve with supplemental oxygen and supportive care alone.

Clinical Pearls

1. When multiple individuals collapse at an industrial workplace, suspect hydrogen sulfide poisoning. Subsequent rescue attempts should be performed with self-contained breathing apparatus in place.

2. Hydrogen sulfide is a cellular asphyxiant-like cyanide, but can be treated more simply by immediate removal of exposure and supplemental oxygenation and supportive care.

3. Although hydrogen sulfide has the notorious odor of rotten eggs, olfactory fatigue occurs rapidly, and thus detection and removal from exposure may be hindered.

REFERENCES

1. Nelson L: Simple asphyxiants and pulmonary irritants. In Gold-frank LR, Flomenbaum NE, Lewin NA, et al (eds): Goldfrank's Toxicologic Emergencies, 7th ed. New York, McGraw-Hill, 2002, pp 1453-1468.
2. Gabbay DS, De Roos F, Perrone J: Twenty-foot fall averts fatality from massive hydrogen sulfide exposure. J Emerg Med 20:141-144, 2001.
3. Fuller DC, Suruda AJ: Occupationally related hydrogen sulfide deaths in the United States from 1984 to 1994. J Occup Environ Med 42:939-942, 2000.
4. Milby TH, Baselt RC: Hydrogen sulfide poisoning: Clarification of some controversial issues. Am J Ind Med 35:192-195, 1999.
5. Snyder JW, Safir EF, Summerville GP, Middleberg RA: Occupational fatality and persistent neurological sequelae after mass exposure to hydrogen sulfide. Am J Emerg Med 13:199-203, 1995.

Fred M. Henretig. MD
Kevin C. Osterhoudt, MD

PATIENT 31

A 54-year-old man with muscle weakness
and altered mental status

A 54-year-old man experiences alteration in mental status over 1 to 2 weeks. Early symptoms included forgetfulness, losing track of time, and easily becoming lost. He has experienced anorexia and weight loss from 165 to 154 lb and has complained of pains in his elbows and knees and decreased muscle strength. In the day or two prior to admission he has become belligerent, confused, and agitated.

Physical Examination: Temperature 36.4° C, pulse 91/min, respirations 20/min, blood pressure 122/70 mmHg. General: confused and incoherent. Neurological: no focal signs. Remainder of exam normal.

Laboratory Findings: Hemogram: hemoglobin 10.4 g/dL. Serum chemistries: Na^+ 122 mEq/L, BUN 32 mg/dL, creatinine 1.4 mg/dL. Urinalysis: 2+ protein and trace glucose. EKG: normal. Computed tomography scan of brain: normal.

Questions: This patient presents with multisystem abnormalities occurring subacutely over several weeks, with recent exacerbation over 2 days. What general class of toxicants is classically responsible for such presentations? What specific exposure is most likely given CNS, peripheral nerve and/or muscle involvement, renal dysfunction, and anemia?

Diagnosis: Multisystem abnormalities are often seen in heavy metal toxicity. The combination of neurological, renal, and hematological findings is characteristic of lead poisoning (plumbism). The admission blood lead level (BLL) is 180 µg/dL.

Discussion: Further investigation and discussion with family members revealed that this patient had a fairly remarkable occupational history. For the preceding 7 years, he was self-employed as a salvager of bullets from several target-shooting ranges. He had made a routine of visiting each range one morning per week, working about 3 hours at each. He recovered pistol bullets from indoor ranges, and rifle bullets from outdoor ranges during the summer. Bullets were shoveled from the bullet tray of the indoor ranges or screened from the dirt backstops of the outdoor ranges, and loaded into 5-gallon pails to a weight of nearly 120 lb. In recent weeks, the patient had noted that he could only carry one pail at a time, rather than his usual one in each hand! This gentleman was clearly aware of his lead dust hazard, and had in fact been treated for lead poisoning 4 years earlier. He attempted to decrease his exposure by wearing inexpensive, disposable filter masks, work gloves, and coveralls, and by showering and changing clothes after work, though at home. He described graphically the sensation of breathing clouds of dust during his work (despite the mask), and noted that his clothes were covered with dust at the end of his shifts.

Most adults with lead poisoning are victims of respiratory exposure to lead dust and fumes in an occupational setting. Highest-risk exposures include those involved with welding, cutting, or burning lead-coated materials or metallic lead (shipbreakers, metal welders and cutters, lead smelter and refinery workers, storage battery industry workers, painters and construction workers involved in paint removal and/or demolition of lead-painted structures). Numerous other occupational (and recreational) exposures are described, including shooting range employees. Clinical findings in adults (see table below) overlap considerably with those in children (see Patient 17) but tend to be milder for a given range of BLLs. Adults tend to manifest more prominent peripheral (primarily motor) nerve involvement that generally results in extensor muscle weakness (foot and wrist "drop") and nephropathy (hypertension, decreased renal function, and gout).

Treatment issues were also detailed previously in the discussion of childhood plumbism (see Patient 17). For symptomatic adults, the same chelating drugs are used, at similar mg/m^2 doses, though the clinical indications for the various regimens differ slightly (see table next page). Asymptomatic adults with BLL <70 µg/dL are not routinely chelated but require prompt removal from exposure. Chelation therapy should never substitute for adherence to U.S. Occupational Safety and Health Association lead standards at the worksite and is not to be given prophylactically.

Over the next several weeks, the present patient was treated with two courses of parenteral BAL and CaNa$_2$EDTA chelation therapy, followed by oral succimer at the time of discharge. His mental status cleared completely, and his muscle strength seemed restored. He promised to look into alternative career paths!

Major Clinical Manifestations of Lead Poisoning in Adults

Clinical Severity	Typical Blood Lead Range (µg/dL)
Severe	100–150
CNS: encephalopathy	
PNS: foot and wrist drop	
GI: colicky abdominal pain	
Heme: pallor (anemia)	
Renal: hypertension, nephropathy, gout	
Moderate	80–100
CNS: headache, poor memory, insomnia	
GI: abdominal pain, anorexia, constipation	
Renal: nephropathy	
Misc: arthralgias, myalgias, muscle weakness, mild anemia	
Mild	40–80
CNS: tiredness, somnolence, irritability	
Misc: hypertension, mild psychometrics impairment	

CNS = central nervous system, GI = gastrointestinal, PNS = peripheral nervous system
Adapted from Henretig FM: Lead. In Goldfrank LR, Flomenbaum NE, Lewin NA, et al (eds): Goldfrank's Toxicologic Emergencies, 7th ed. New York, McGraw-Hill, 2002, pp 1200-1238.

Condition & Blood Lead (μg/dL)	Medication & Dose	Route & Regimen
Encephalopathy	BAL 450 mg/m^2/d* CaNa$_2$EDTA 1500 mg/m^2/d*	75 mg/m^2 IM every 4 h for 5 d Continuous infusion, or 2–4 divided IV doses, for 5 d (start 4 h after BAL)
Symptoms suggestive of encephalopathy or >100	BAL 300-450 mg/m^2/d* CaNa$_2$EDTA 1000-1500 mg/m^2/d*	50-75 mg/m^2 IM every 4 h for 3–5 d Continuous infusion, or 2–4 divided IV doses, for 5 d (start 4 h after BAL); base dose total on blood lead level, severity of symptoms
Mild Symptoms or 70-100	Succimer 700-1050 mg/m^2/d*	350 mg/m^2 tid for 5 d, then bid for 14 d
Asymptomatic and <70	Usually not indicated	Remove from exposure

*Doses expressed as mg/kg: BAL 450 mg/m^2 (24 mg/kg), 300 mg/m^2 (18 mg/kg). CaNa$_2$EDTA 1000 mg/m^2 (25-50 mg/kg), 1500 mg/m^2 (50-75 mg/kg) adult maximum 2–3 g/d. Succimer 350 mg/m^2 (10 mg/kg).
Subsequent treatment regimens based on postchelation BPb and clinical symptoms.
IM = intramuscular; IV = intravenous.
Adapted from Henretig FM: Lead. In Goldfrank LR, Flomenbaum NE, Lewin NA, et al (eds): goldfrank's Toxicologic Emergencies, 7th ed. New York, McGraw-Hill, 2002, pp 1200-1238.

Clinical Pearls

1. Take a careful occupational history in adult patients with multiorgan system abnormalities.
2. Treat symptomatic adults with chelation therapy as per their clinical severity.

REFERENCES

1. Henretig FM: Lead. In Goldfrank LR, Flomenbaum NE, Lewin NA, et al (eds): Goldfrank's Toxicologic Emergencies, 7th ed. New York, McGraw – Hill, 2002, pp 1200-1238.
2. Henretig F, Osterhoudt K, Greenberg M et al: Acute lead encephalopathy in a bullet salvager [abstract]. J Toxicol Clin Toxicol 35:525, 1997.
3. DeRoos FJ: Smelters and metal reclaimers. In Greenberg MI, Hamilton R, Phillips S (eds): Occupational, Industrial and Environmental Toxicology. St. Louis, Mosby-Year Book, 1997, pp 291-301.

PATIENT 32

A 20-year-old man with agitated delirium

A 20-year-old college student is brought to the emergency department (ED) by emergency medical services (EMS) after being found at the bottom of the steps in his dormitory. He is transported with cervical spine immobilization and is on a backboard. Per EMS personnel, the patient was found rambling, with confused, pressured speech. He has been very tachycardic en route, with a heart rate of 160 beats/min. A rapid bedside dextrose is 178 mg/dL. The patient history is limited; he is confused and disoriented but does mention that he takes lithium for his "moods." His roommate arrives and recalls seeing him a few hours prior to arrival. A plastic bag containing multiple soft blue gel caps was found with the patient.

Physical Examination: Temperature 36.6° C (orally), pulse 168/min, respirations 18/min, blood pressure 156/80 mmHg, oxygen saturation 99% in room air. General: well-developed, agitated, confused; attempting to climb off stretcher. HEENT: atraumatic; pupils dilated at 6 mm, symmetrical, not reactive to light (see figure); mucous membranes dry, oropharynx clear; tympanic membranes without hemotympanum; cervical collar in place. Chest: normal. Cardiovascular: tachycardic, normal S1 and S2, no murmurs, rubs, or gallops. Abdomen: soft, non distended, no bowel sounds auscultated. Extremities: warm, well-perfused, good pulses. Skin: flushed, with dry axillae and groin. Neuromuscular: agitated, confused, difficulty attending to exam, moves all extremities equally, follows simple commands, Glasgow Coma Scale score = 13. Foley catheter returns 1.5 L clear urine.

Laboratory Findings: Hemogram: normal. Serum chemistries: normal. Urinalysis: normal. Serum salicylate and acetaminophen: negative. Serum ethanol: negative. Serum lithium: 0.35 mmol/L (0.5–1.2 mmol/L.) CT head: no evidence of fracture, bleed, mass or midline shift. Cervical spine radiographic series: normal. Chest radiograph: normal. Electrocardiogram (EKG): sinus tachycardia (see figure on next page).

Questions: What is the most likely cause of this patient's delirium? Is antidotal therapy available to reverse such delirium?

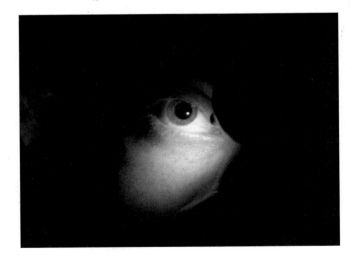

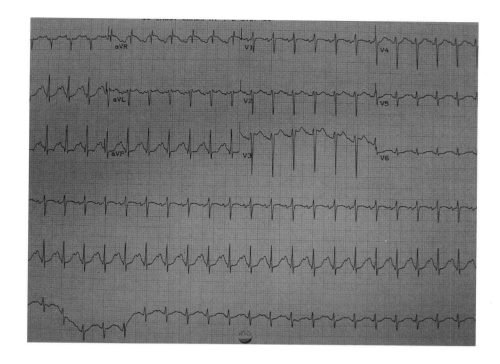

Diagnosis and Treatment: This patient demonstrates an anticholinergic toxidrome, in this case caused by diphenhydramine overdose. The cholinergic drug physostigmine can be used to reverse the patient's delirium.

Discussion: Although the differential diagnosis of altered mental status is broad, a careful history combined with a focused physical exam can help determine the etiology of this patient's distress. The causes of an agitated delirium include diverse etiological categories such as toxicological (sedative/hypnotic withdrawal, sympathomimetic intoxication, anticholinergic intoxication), metabolic (hypoglycemia), infectious (meningitis, encephalitis), neurological (tumor, subarachnoid hemorrhage), and/or psychiatric (schizophrenia, bipolar) illnesses, or a combination of any of the above. The patient's history of being found with a bag of pills, combined with the relatively rapid onset of his symptoms, make a toxicological etiology for this case more likely. Although other causes of this patient's mental status, such as trauma and infection, must still be excluded, the physical examination can lead us toward the answer.

The present patient exhibits features characteristic of the anticholinergic toxidrome. This toxidrome can be remembered with a mnemonic that identifies its salient features:

1. Blind as a Bat → mydriasis
2. Fast as a Hare → tachycardia
3. Mad as a Hatter → altered mental status, agitation
4. Dry as a Bone → dry mucous membranes
5. Red as a Beet → flushed skin
6. Hot as Hades → increased temperature (inability to sweat)
7. Full as a Tick → urinary retention, decreased GI motility

The anticholinergic toxidrome is, perhaps, more correctly referred to as the *anti-muscarinic* toxidrome. Its main manifestations are the result of blocking the effects of acetylcholine on the muscarinic subtype of the acetylcholine (or cholinergic) receptor. Muscarinic receptors are found in the CNS (brain), at postganglionic parasympathetic nerves and postganglionic sympathetic nerves (sweat glands.) The blockade of the central receptors leads to confusion, agitation, and other central effects. The peripheral manifestations lead to the muscarinic effects detailed above.

101

You must be able to differentiate the anticholinergic toxidrome from the sympathomimetic toxidrome, as is seen in intoxications with agents like cocaine. Both share many common features (e.g., tachycardia, increased temperature, altered mental status). There are a few physical exam findings that can be used to distinguish between these two. The first is the skin and mucous membrane exam. In the sympathomimetic toxidrome, patients are often diaphoretic, with moist axillae and groin. In the anticholinergic toxidrome, the axillae and groin are dry, as are the patient's mucous membranes ("dry as a bone.") One of the common descriptions of a patient with anticholinergic symptoms is a muffled, garbled, or "cotton mouth" voice, caused by the difficulty phonating from the very dry oropharynx and lack of saliva. A second differentiating physical finding is the pupil exam. Normally, pupillary dilation is mediated through sympathetic discharge, and pupillary constriction through the parasympathetic fibers. With sympathomimetic intoxication, pupils are dilated due to excess sympathetic stimulation of dilator fibers. The parasympathetic fibers are intact, so when a light is directed into the dilated pupil, they should still be able to constrict. In anticholinergic poisoning, the constrictor (parasympathetic) fibers are blocked. This leads to unopposed sympathetic tone and pupillary dilation. When a light is shone in the dilated pupil, it is unable to constrict (see initial figure). Also, in contrast to sympathomimetic toxicity, anticholinergic patients often have urinary retention, through inability to constrict the bladder and relax the urinary sphincter.

Common agents with anticholinergic properties are presented in the table. Note that anticholinergic toxicity is not usually the predominant manifestation of tricyclic antidepressant (TCA) poisoning, but can accompany the more concerning seizures and cardiavascular toxicity frequently noted after TCA overdose.

Common Toxic Agents with Anticholinergic Properties

Anticholinergic drugs, primary
  Atropine
  Glycopyrrolate
  Scopolamine
Antidepressants
Antihistimines
Antispasmodics
Phenothiazine antipsychotics
Plants
  Deadly nightshade
  Jimson weed
  Others

An effective antidote for the central and peripheral manifestations of anticholinergic poisoning is **physostigmine**. Physostigmine is a carbamate compound, derived from the Calabar bean, that reversibly inhibits central and peripheral cholinesterases. This leads to an accumulation of acetylcholine at the site of action, overcoming the blockade caused by the anticholinergic agent and reversing toxicity. The primary risk associated with physostigmine administration is the possibility of promoting a condition of cholinergic excess. It has been suggested that physostigmine may reduce the seizure threshold after certain poisonings. Additionally, there are several case reports of TCA-poisoned patients receiving physostigmine and subsequently experiencing asystolic arrest. Therefore, caution should be exercised when considering physostigmine administration to patients with a history of TCA ingestion, or among patients with cardiac conduction delay noted on EKG. Anticholinergic toxicity will typically abate with good supportive care.

Prudent physostigmine administration includes close cardiorespiratory monitoring and the presence of appropriate resuscitative equipment at the bedside. A dose of 0.5–2.0 mg may be given to adults intravenously over no less than 5 minutes (pediatric dosing may start at 0.02 mg/kg, not to exceed adult dosing). Rapid administration can lead to adverse effects of bradycardia, excessive secretions, and possibly seizures. Physostigmine has a relatively rapid onset of action, usually within minutes of administration. Clinical endpoints should include improvement of the anticholinergic state (presence of tearing, spontaneous voiding, improvement and clearing of mental status), without evidence of muscarinic effects. It can be re-dosed cautiously in 10–15 minutes if there has been a partial or inadequate response. Relative contraindications to the administration of physostigmine include patients with bronchospastic disease, intestinal or bladder outlet obstruction, and underlying cardiac conduction abnormalities.

The present patient was thoroughly evaluated for traumatic causes of his mental status. He remained agitated with anticholinergic signs, and a decision to administer physostigmine was made in consultation with a medical toxicologist. The patient received a total of 3 mg of physostigmine in two separate doses. After the initial 2-mg dose, he became much less agitated and more interactive. After the second dose of 1 mg, he was able to drink activated charcoal without assistance. He did not require additional doses of physostigmine overnight. The pills were identified as diphenhydramine, and this was correlated with serum toxicological analysis. The patient spent 1 day in the intensive care unit, and was subsequently admitted to inpatient psychiatry. Two days after his presentation, he was asymptomatic and able to relate the history of his ingestion and the events leading up to it.

Clinical Pearls

1. The unique toxicities of the large number of agents that can cause the anticholinergic toxidrome can help in determining the offending agent.

2. The anticholinergic toxidrome is characterized by hyperthermia, tachycardia, mydriasis, dry, flushed skin and dry mucous membranes, altered mental status, and urinary retention.

3. Physostigmine is an effective antidote in anticholinergic poisoning, but caution is warranted when considering its use among TCA-overdosed patients.

4. Physostigmine should be administered cautiously, with a clinical endpoint of resolution of altered mental status or development of muscarinic side effects.

REFERENCES

1. Howland MA: Antidotes in depth: Physostigmine. In Goldfrank LR, Flomenbaum NE, Lewin NA, et al (eds): Goldfrank's Toxicologic Emergencies, 7th ed. New York, McGraw-Hill, 2002, pp 544-547.
2. Weisman RS: Antihistamines and decongestants. In: Goldfrank's Toxicologic Emergencies, 7th ed. Goldfrank LR Flomenbaum NE, Lewin NA, Howland MA, Hoffman RS, Nelson LS (Eds): New York, NY, McGraw-Hill, 2002, pp 535-543.
3. Holger JS, Harris CR, Engebretsen KM: Physostigmine, sodium bicarbonate, or hypertonic saline to treat diphenhydramine toxicity. Vet Human Toxicol 44:1-4, 2002.
4. Leybishkis B, Fasseas P, Ryan K: Doxylamine overdose as a potential cause of rhabdomyolysis. Am J Med Sci 322:48-49, 2001.
5. Simons FER, Simons KJ: The pharmacology and use of H_1-receptor-antagonist drugs. N Engl J Med;330:1663-1670, 1994.
6. Clark RF, Vance MV: Massive diphenhydramine poisoning resulting in a wide-complex tachycardia: Successful treatment with sodium bicarbonate. Ann Emerg Med 1:318-321, 1992.
7. Köppel C, Tenczer J: Poisoning with over-the-counter doxylamine preparations: an evaluation of 109 cases. Human Toxicol 6:355-359, 1987.
8. Pentel P, Peterson CD: Asystole complicating physostigmine treatment of tricyclic antidepressant overdose. Ann Emerg Med 9:588-590, 1980.

PATIENT 33

An 82-year-old man with suicidal ingestion
of antidysrhythmia medication

An 82-year-old man with a medical history of atrial fibrillation and depression is brought by paramedics to the emergency department (ED). Approximately 20 minutes earlier, the patient ingested 30 200-mg quinidine (Quinidex) tablets. He confessed to his wife that he had stopped taking all his other medications 3 weeks ago and was saving his quinidine for this event. His wife called for emergency medical services immediately after the ingestion.

The man was awake with normal vital signs upon ambulance arrival to the home. An intravenous line was placed and the patient was rushed to the ED; the transport time was approximately 10 minutes. He was unresponsive upon arrival at the hospital.

Physical Examination: Pulse and blood pressure: none detected. Respirations: none spontaneous. HEENT: no gag reflex. Chest: no breath sounds heard. Cardiovascular: no heart sounds detected.

Laboratory Findings: Electrocardiogram (EKG): ventricular fibrillation.

Questions: What caused this patient's life-threatening dysrhythmia? What is the treatment?

Diagnosis and Treatment: Rapid cardiovascular toxicity is characteristic of quinidine poisoning. Alkalinization and sodium loading are important components of the treatment for poisoning by quinidine and other sodium-channel antagonists.

Discussion: Poisoning from quinidine and the other sodium-channel antagonists may feature four cardiotoxic events: intraventricular conduction defects, ventricular dysrhythmias, hypotension, and bradydysrhythmias. Intraventricular conduction defects occur secondary to a reduction in the slope of phase 0 of the non-pacemaker cell action potential resulting from sodium channel blockade, which in turn causes decrement in propagation of the myocardial action potential. Clinically, this is represented by a widening of the QRS complex or by bundle branch blockade. Severe blockade of phase 0 is accompanied by progressive QRS widening to the point of a "sine wave" or asystole. Ventricular dysrhythmias are thought to occur by slowing intraventricular conduction to the point that unidirectional block and re-entrant circuits develop. These re-entrant circuits can further degenerate into ventricular tachycardia and fibrillation. Rarely, poisoning by sodium-channel–blocking antiarrhythmics also produces polymorphic ventricular tachycardia (torsades de pointes). Hypotension following sodium channel blockade poisoning may result from decreased myocardial contractility, as sodium and calcium influx are coupled to the release of intracellular calcium stores. Hypotension may also occur secondary to reduced vascular smooth muscle contractility and resultant vasodilation. Large overdoses of these antidysrhythmics may depress pacemaker cell automaticity with resulting sinus bradycardia, junctional escape, or other ventricular arrhythmias, and even asystole.

Patients poisoned with immediate-release forms of antidysrhythmics that block sodium channels usually can be expected to become symptomatic within 6 hours after oral ingestion, and much sooner following parenteral overdoses. Patients poisoned with oral sustained-release antidysrhythmic preparations that block sodium channels may have delayed onset of symptoms. The diagnosis of sodium-channel blocking antidysrythmic poisoning is mainly clinical. In poisoned patients, intraventricular conduction defects often occur secondary to the block of phase 0 of the nonpacemaker cells (see figure). Clinically, these conduction defects are manifested by prolongation of the QRS greater than 100 milliseconds and typically develop within 6 hours of poisoning.

Primary treatment of quinidine poisoning and poisoning due to other sodium-channel blocking antidysrhythmics involves ensuring an adequate airway and proper ventilation. Place the patient on a cardiac monitor, and establish intravenous access. Hypotension can initially be treated with judicious crystalloid boluses, unless contraindicated (e.g., pulmonary edema). Because of the severe toxicity associated with overdose of these agents, gastrointestinal decontamination with either gastric lavage or activated charcoal may be considered if the patient presents within 1–2 hours after ingestion.

Hypertonic sodium bicarbonate is considered by many toxicologists as the treatment of choice for intraventricular conduction defects and ventricular dysrhythmias. Based on experience treating tricyclic antidepressant poisoning, it has become common practice to administer sodium bicarbonate boluses when QRS complex duration reaches or exceeds 120 milliseconds. Sodium

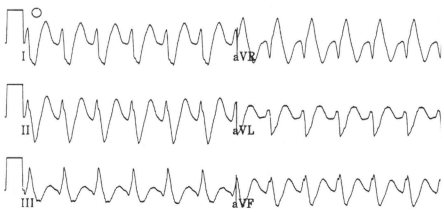

Significant tachycardia (rate ~ 150/minute) and profound QRS widening (190 ms), findings typically noted with poisoning due to sodium channel antagonist drugs.

bicarbonate is often administered as a 1- to 2-mEq/kg bolus initially and then titrated to an arterial pH in the range of 7.45–7.5. If life-threatening clinical manifestations are present (e.g., hypotension, ventricular arrhythmias), then the pH can be increased towards 7.55. Treatment options for intraventricular conduction defects and ventricular dysrhythmias resistant to sodium bicarbonate include lidocaine, bretylium, cardiac pacing, and cardiopulmonary bypass.

Hypotension that accompanies poisoning by quinidine and other sodium-channel antagonists usually responds to careful crystalloid challenges. Persistent hypotension unexplained by dysrhythmias most commonly results from myocardial depression and peripheral vasodilation. If hypotension is unresponsive to fluid boluses, norepinephrine is generally recommended for its inotropic effect and vasoconstrictive properties. In patients who require more than minimal doses of norepinephrine or who remain in shock, pulmonary artery cathetarization may be helpful. Intra-aortic balloon counterpulsation or even cardiopulmonary bypass may be life saving for patients in extremis.

Bradydysrhythmias are characteristic of severe sodium channel antiarrhythmic poisoning. In the face of severe bradycardia, a wide QRS complex, and hypotension, **epinephrine** may be considered if sodium bicarbonate therapy did not produce an immediate effect. Transcutaneous or transvenous cardiac pacing should be initiated if the hemodynamically significant bradydysrhythmia persists despite drug therapy. Although unclear, the mechanism for sodium-channel blockade–induced brady-dysrythmias is not believed to occur by depression of sinus node activity. Thus, avoid atropine when treating sodium-channel antagonist–induced bradydysrhythmias.

There are anecdotal reports of the successful treatment of ventricular arrhythmias, QRS widening, or hypotension that have been induced by sodium channel blockade poisoning, with **hypertonic saline** when initial hypertonic sodium bicarbonate therapy was unsuccessful. An accepted human dose of hypertonic saline has not been established, and careful attention is necessary to prevent the complications of hypernatremia.

The present patient was endotracheally intubated and given 2 ampules of sodium bicarbonate intravenously. Following the infusion of the sodium bicarbonate, the EKG revealed a wide complex rhythm with a rate of 140 beats per minute. The blood pressure was 90/50 mmHg. Sodium bicarbonate was then administered as a continuous infusion and titrated to keep his arterial pH at 7.5. An orogastric lavage tube was passed, and pill fragments were suctioned out of his stomach. One dose of activated charcoal was administered through the orogastric tube. The patient was then admitted to the intensive care unit. Over the next 48 hours his EKG returned to baseline; the sodium bicarbonate infusion was then discontinued, and the patient returned to his baseline health. Psychiatric evaluation prompted inpatient treatment for depression.

Clinical Pearls

1. Poisoning from quinidine and the other sodium-channel antagonist antidysrhythmics have the potential for significant cardiotoxicity.

2. Hypertonic sodium bicarbonate is considered the treatment of choice for intraventricular conduction defects and ventricular dysrhythmias that result from quinidine and other sodium-channel antagonist antidysrhythmic poisoning.

3. Hypotension that accompanies quinidine and other sodium channel antidysrhythmic poisoning usually responds to careful crystalloid challenges. If hypotension is unresponsive to fluid boluses, consider norepinephrine.

REFERENCES
1. Kolecki PF, Curry SC. Poisoning by sodium channel blocking agents. Crit Care Clin Med Toxicol 13:4:829-848, 1997.
2. Kim SY, Benowitz NL: Poisoning due to class 1A antiarrhythmic drugs. Quinidine, procainamide, and disopyramide. Drug Safety 5:393-420, 1990.

PATIENT 34

A 7-year-old with rapidly progressive paralysis

A 7-year-old girl presents with the chief complaint of weakness. This morning she was noted to have an unsteady gait and difficulty feeding herself. Over the following 8 hours she became unable to stand and was brought to the emergency department by her mother. She has not had any recent fevers or upper respiratory tract infections. She denies headache, nausea, vomiting, or visual disturbances. She has not had constipation or urinary retention. No one else in the household is sick. There are no prescription, herbal, or over-the-counter medications in the house. She lives in a suburb in the northeastern United States and has not traveled recently. The township provides the water supply. She lives alone with her mother who is employed at a doctor's office. She has no medical history and has been developing normally.

Physical Examination: Temperature 36.7° C, pulse 74/min, respirations 14/min, blood pressure 107/52 mmHg. General: well-appearing, nontoxic. HEENT: pupils 5 mm and reactive to light, mucous membranes moist. Chest: lungs clear. Cardiovascular: regular rate and rhythm. Abdomen: soft without masses, normal active bowel sounds. Extremities: warm and well perfused. Skin: normal color without diaphoresis, no rash. Neuromuscular: alert and cooperative; ptosis of left eye, limited lateral gaze of left eye, no nystagmus, left peripheral facial nerve palsy (see figure) remainder of cranial nerves intact; sensory exam normal; 3/5 strength upper extremities and 1/5 strength lower; deep tendon reflexes absent; cerebellar signs absent.

Laboratory Findings: Hemogram: WBC 5600/μL, hemoglobin 13.0 g/dL, platelets 253,000/μl. Coagulation profile: PT 14.7 sec., aPTT 32.5 sec. Serum chemistries: Na^+ 144 mEq/L, K^+ 3.7 mEq/L, Cl^- 108 mEq/L, CO_2 27 mEq/L, BUN 14 mg/dL, Cr .8 mg/dL, Glu 99 mg/dL, Ca^+ 9.3 mg/dL. Creatine kinase 198 U/L. Lumbar puncture: WBC 1/hpf, RBC 0/hpf, protein 14 mg/dL, glucose 52 mg/dL. Non-contrast head CT: normal.

Question: What is poisoning this patient?

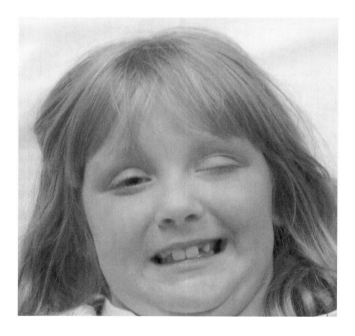

Diagnosis: Upon closer examination an engorged tick is found on the scalp, under her hair.

Discussion: Tick paralysis is generally a disease of school-age children. Theoretically this epidemiological phenomenon is simply a matter of size. The smaller weight of children is felt to give a higher dose effect to the toxin as compared to larger adults. However, there have been a few reported cases in adult patients from Australia. In addition, the disease seems to predominate in young girls with long hair, presumably due to difficulty in seeing the tick. The peak incidence occurs in the spring and summer when tick exposure is highest. There is a geographic predilection for the western United States, Canada, and Australia in particular, but the disease has been reported across the U.S. Despite the enormous number of individuals bitten by ticks each year, the disease is exceedingly rare. In Washington State there were only 33 reported cases from 1946 to 1996. It may be an unrecognized disease, however, simply from poor awareness or lack of reporting.

The cause of tick paralysis is felt to be release of a neurotoxin into the blood of the affected victim by an attached female tick after prolonged feeding. In North America the most common offending ticks are *Dermacentor variabilis* (American dog tick) and *Dermacentor andersoni* (Rocky Mountain wood tick), *Amblyomma americanum* (Lone Star tick), and *Ixodes scapularis* (deer tick). The toxin produced by Dermacentor is also called **ixobotoxin** and is thought to affect the sodium flux across axonal membranes, sparing the neuromuscular junction, ultimately preventing release of acetylcholine (Ach). In Australia the most common causative organism is the tick *Ixodes holocyclus* that produces a family of toxins termed **holocyclotoxins**. It tends to cause a more severe and rapidly progressive form of the disease by inhibiting Ach release from the neuromuscular junction itself. In both ixobotoxin and holocyclotoxin poisoning there is normal response of the post-synaptic neuromuscular junction to Ach, but failure of the pre-synaptic junction to release Ach in response to an evoked potential.

Initially the attached tick feeds very slowly to prepare itself for the rapid increase in size it will undergo. Subsequently the tick promptly consumes enormous amounts of blood, increasing its body weight some 100–200 times. This time of rapid feeding coincides with maximal toxin production, and hence symptoms begin 3–4 days after the tick has begun feeding. These include a prodome of fatigue, anorexia, vomiting, and muscle pain. Children are frequently described as "ataxic" or "clumsy" initially, when in fact the problem is neuromuscular weakness of the lower extremities. This rapidly progresses, in a matter of hours to days, to involve the trunk and upper extremities. Hence, tick paralysis generally presents with an **ascending paralysis** without causing bowel or bladder dysfunction. Deep tendon reflexes are either markedly reduced or absent, again usually in an ascending order. Bulbar signs and symptoms, including ophthalmoplegia, facial paralysis, dysarthria, and difficulty swallowing are generally very late findings. Failure to identify the disease can lead to weakness of the respiratory muscles and hypoventilation as well as loss of the gag reflex.

The workup of tick paralysis is limited to an excellent history and a meticulous physical exam. There are no commonly available laboratory tests to make the diagnosis. The offending tick is commonly found in the scalp, in particular behind the ears where they favor feeding. Many patients undergo extensive diagnostic evaluations including imaging studies and lumbar puncture. Although a rare diagnosis, in a very small minority of patients with new-onset weakness, the pain, cost, and potential morbidity of these tests can be avoided by a **careful physical exam**. If a lumbar puncture is performed, the cell count and the protein and glucose levels are normal.

Removal of North American ticks results in a rapid and often dramatic resolution of symptoms. Within a couple of hours strength begins to return, and symptoms are generally completely resolved within 24–36 hours. The tick should be removed with a pair of tweezers or forceps by applying steady linear pressure while grasping the head. Time-honored methods such as alcohol, petroleum, acetone, or a heated match or pin are less effective and potentially injurious.

Supportive therapy, including mechanical ventilation, may be necessary until symptoms resolve. Canine-derived antitoxin is generally reserved for veterinary use due to the high potential for acute reaction. There may be some role for its use in severe, life-threatening cases, but it does not have an immediate effect. In addition, it may only be effective early in the disease. There are several different formulations of the serum, making dosing recommendations difficult.

The most effective means of management in humans is primary prevention with proper outdoor attire, thorough examination after outdoor activities, and liberal use of topical insect repellents (acaricides). Removing the tick during the slow-feeding stage, before large amounts of toxin are produced, completely avoids any potential paralysis.

Complications related to the disease are generally due to a delay in diagnosis. Early reports of mortality have been as high as 10% from respiratory paralysis. These deaths probably could have been prevented by early diagnosis, making awareness of the disease imperative. It should be remembered that the vectors responsible for tick paralysis are also potential carriers of other tick-borne illnesses, including Rocky Mountain spotted fever, babesiosis, ehrlichiosis, tularemia, tick-borne relapsing fever, Colorado tick fever, and Lyme disease.

In the present patient, the tick was identified as a *Dermacentor variabilis* female that had been feeding for 6 days. It was removed with a pair of forceps, and the child's symptoms completely resolved within 18 hours.

Clinical Pearls

1. The clinician must always keep tick paralysis in the differential of any child with acute onset, rapidly progressive, ascending paralysis to reduce unnecessary testing and morbidity.

2. Ticks can be hard to find, particularly in children with thick, long hair. Search carefully behind the ears, in the axilla, pubic region, and auditory canals.

3. Removal of North American ticks results in prompt recovery, and anti-toxin has limited utility.

REFERENCES

1. Greenstein P: Tick paralysis. Med Clin North Am 86(2):441-446, 2002.
2. Felz MW, Smith CD, Swift TR: A six-year-old girl with tick paralysis. New Engl J Med 342(2):90-94, 2000.
3. Goetz CG, Meisel E: Biological neurotoxins. Neurol Clin 18(3):719-40, 2000.
4. Grattan-Smith PJ, Morris JG, Johnston HM, et al: Clinical and neurophysiological features of tick paralysis. Brain 120(Pt 11):1975-1987, 1997.

PATIENT 35

A 2-year-old boy with a swollen mouth

A 2-year-old boy began crying after playing in the living room of his home. His grandmother found that he had been playing with one of her large houseplants (see figure), located in a planter on the floor. The grandmother denies any antecedent illness and denies emesis. The child is crying softly and intermittently places one or both of his hands in his mouth. He has been developmentally normal and has no previous medical history. There are no medications, cleaning agents, or other chemicals located in the house.

Physical Examination: Temperature 37.5° C rectally, pulse 120/min, respirations 22/min, blood pressure 112/75 mmHg. General: well-developed, well-hydrated, developmentally appropriate; easily consolable by grandmother. HEENT: atraumatic; normal pupils, conjunctiva; normal nares; lips and oral mucosa erythematous, with mild edema and no notable ulcers or sloughing; anterior tongue is mildly edematous; scant drooling. Chest: normal. Cardiovascular: normal. Abdomen: normal. Neuromuscular: normal.

Questions: What is the immediate concern? What is the management for this exposure?

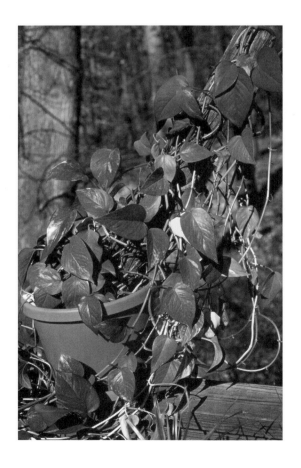

Diagnosis and Treatment: The child has had an exposure to dumbcane (*Dieffenbachia* spp.) The immediate concern is oral and, possibly, airway swelling. If there are no immediate threats to life, the treatment is symptomatic and supportive care.

Discussion: Approximately 10% of calls to U.S. poison centers involve exposures to plants, making this the fourth most common poisoning exposure encountered. Almost 85% of these exposures occur in children who are less than 6 years of age and involve oral ingestions. Children often begin using their newly developed mobility to access the wide variety of colorful household plants that offer a tempting enticement for both manual and oral exploration. Tens of thousands of plant species exist that can be sources of exposure. Unless one is a botanist or works in a herbarium, identification can be difficult. A number of resources, both print and electronic, exist to facilitate identification of the species. Fortunately, the most common species found in the home have limited toxicity. Some examples of the most common household species include dumbcane (*Dieffenbachia* spp.), holly (*Ilex* spp.), jade plants (*Crassula* spp.), philodendron (*Philodendron* spp.), and poinsettia (*Euphorbia pulcherrima*). The majority of these cause no toxicity. Of these, dumbcane, philodendron, and the peace lily (*Spathiphyllum* spp.) contain various concentrations and packaging of **calcium oxalate crystals**, which contribute to their unique toxicity.

The plant in this case is dumbcane. It is a varietal of the *Dieffenbachia* spp., and members of this genus are referred to by a number of common names, such as mother-in-law's tongue, dumbplant, tufroot, and poisonous arum. It is an extremely popular houseplant, due to its ease of cultivation, hardiness, and colorful foliage. All parts of the plant contain idioblasts, which are specialized pressure-sensitive organelles containing raphides, small needle-like crystals of calcium oxalate. When stimulated by a mechanical force, such as biting or chewing, the idioblasts discharge the raphides as projectiles. They can travel two to three times the length of the idioblast. Each of the raphides has a small groove, which is thought to contain proteolytic enzymes similar to some found in snake and scorpion venom, and also has small barbs. The highest concentration of idioblasts in *Dieffenbachia* spp. is found in the stalk of the plant.

When these raphides penetrate tissue, they induce a local irritation due to the combination of local histamine release and a minor contribution of the proteolytic enzymes. The symptoms develop rapidly and include redness, swelling, and local pain. The rapid development of pain limits and typically prevents repeat pediatric exposures. The location of the exposure often determines its severity. Though extremely rare, large oral exposures can produce a significant local reaction that can lead to serious swelling of the pharynx—potentially compromising the airway. Ocular exposure may produce a chemical conjunctivitis and corneal abrasion. The delicate tissues of the **mouth and eye** are particularly sensitive. However, exposures to other areas of the skin do not manifest any effects due to the inability of the calcium oxalate needles to penetrate.

Once any airway concerns are addressed, treatment for *Dieffenbachia* exposures is primarily symptomatic. The great majority of these cases can be managed at home. Ocular exposures should be managed like other chemical exposures with copious irrigation with normal saline. After treatment, a careful assessment for corneal abrasions should be performed. For oral exposures, topical cooling with cold drinks, ice, or frozen juice bars relieves most patient's discomfort and may improve any swelling. Oral antihistamines to swish and spit, as a topical anesthetic, are typically unnecessary. There is no role for systemic antihistamines or steroids unless significant airway edema has resulted.

The present patient was given a frozen juice bar, and after he was calm and distracted, a thorough physical examination was performed. After 4 hours of observation, his condition had not deteriorated and he was discharged home with follow-up the next day with his pediatrician. The grandmother was instructed to remove the plant from the child's reach and given literature on other ways to minimize poison exposures for her grandchild.

Clinical Pearls

1. Most common household plant species are nontoxic or only mildly toxic. Many exposures can be managed at home, preferably with consultation with the regional poison center.

2. *Dieffenbachia* spp. cause local toxicity by way of calcium oxalate crystals that penetrate the thin tissue of the lips and mouth, producing pain and swelling.

3. Treatment of *Dieffenbachia* plant exposures is primarily symptomatic, with topical cooling or irrigation.

REFERENCES

1. Tagwireyi D, Ball DE: The management of Elephant's Ear poisoning. Hum Exp Toxicol 20(4):189-192, 2001.
2. Pedaci L, Krenzelok EP, Jacobsen TD, Aronis J: *Dieffenbachia* species exposures: An evidence-based assessment of symptom presentation. Vet Hum Toxicol 41(5):335-338, 1999.
3. Krenzelok EP, Jacobsen TD: Plant exposures: A national profile of the most common plant genera. Vet Hum Toxicol 39(4):248-249, 1997.
4. Lawrence RA: Poisonous plants: When they are a threat to children. Pediatr Rev 18(5):162-168, 1997.
5. Chiou AG, Cadez R, Bohnke M: Diagnosis of *Dieffenbachia*-induced corneal injury by confocal microscopy. Br J Ophthalmol 81(2):168-169, 1997.
6. Gardner DG: Injury to the oral mucous membranes caused by the common houseplant, *Dieffenbachia*. A review. Oral Surg Oral Med Oral Pathol 78(5):631-633, 1994.

WEB-BASED PLANT IDENTIFICATION RESOURCES

1. Cornell University, Ithaca, New York.www.ansci.cornell.edu/plants/index.html
2. Munro DB: Canadian Poisonous Plants Information system. Government of Canada. sis.agr.gc.ca/pls/pp/poison?p_x=px
3. Oklahoma State University Environmental Health and Safety Department: Online Safety Library—Poisonous Plants, Animals, and Arthropods. www.pp.okstate.edu/ehs/links/poison.htm

PATIENT 36

A 16-year-old boy with painful, bullous skin lesions

A 16-year-old boy with no significant medical history is brought to the emergency department (ED) with a painful, pruritic rash of 12-hour duration. He states that earlier in the day he had been hiking in the woods near his house. He noted the rash on his arms and upper chest several hours after returning home. He was taken to his primary care physician, who diagnosed contact dermatitis from poison ivy and prescribed hydoxyzine for itching and a two-week course of prednisone. When blisters began to form and pain developed, he was brought to the ED. On further questioning, the boy admits that he had been hiking in an abandoned military installation and had found what appeared to be old, rusted artillery shells partially buried in the soil. A yellow-brown oily liquid was leaking from one, which he inadvertently got on his arms and chest.

Physical Examination: Temperature 37.9° C, pulse 96/min, respirations 16/min, blood pressure 135/80 mmHg, oxygen saturation 98% in room air. General: healthy-appearing, in intense pain. HEENT: mild, bilateral conjunctival injection; pupils symmetrical and reactive; visual acuity 20/20 bilaterally; airway patent without edema. Chest: clear. Cardiovascular: regular rate without murmurs. Abdomen: nontender; bowel sounds normal. Genitourinary: mild erythema without vesicles or bullae. Extremities: no wounds, deformities, or edema. Skin: intense erythema with multiple vesicles and bullae on upper chest and both forearms. Neuromuscular: normal.

Laboratory Findings: Hemogram: WBC 15,400/μL, hemoglobin 12.3 g/dL, platelets 254,000/μL. Coagulation profile: PT 12.3 seconds, PTT 27.0 seconds. Serum chemistries: sodium 136 mEq/L, potassium 3.7 mEq/L chloride 98 mEq/L, bicarbonate 24 mEq/L, BUN 15 mg/dL, creatinine 1.2 mg/dL, glucose 90 mg/dL. Urinalysis: normal. Chest radiograph: normal.

Questions: Given the history and time course of symptom development, what is the most likely cause of the patient's skin findings? What is the appropriate management?

Diagnosis and Treatment: Cutaneous exposure to sulfur mustard. Management includes decontamination, pain control, wound debridement, application of a topical antibiotic cream, tetanus prophylaxis, and wound management.

Discussion: Sulfur mustard is a vesicant, meaning it is capable of producing severe blisters on the skin and mucous membranes. Other vesicants include Lewisite (an arsenical) and phosgene oxime. Sulfur mustard was used extensively as a chemical weapon on the battlefield during World War I. It has also been used in subsequent armed conflicts, including the Iran-Iraq war from 1979 to 1988. It is now considered a potential weapon for use by terrorist organizations against civilian populations.

Sulfur mustard is a yellow to brown, oily liquid that can be aerosolized with a spray device or when combined with an explosive. Its name derives from its odor of garlic or mustard. It is highly viscous and can persist on surfaces for up to a week. It penetrates skin and mucous membranes in a matter of minutes, a process that is enhanced by moisture. It has multiple mechanisms of action, including alkylation of cellular molecules, formation of highly reactive cyclic ethylene sulfonium ions, inhibition of glycolysis, and glutathione depletion with resultant lipid peroxidation, enzyme inactivation, and cell death. The eyes and skin, especially the moist skin of the groin and axillae, are most sensitive. However, all tissues of the body can be affected.

Clinical effects of mustard depend on the route of exposure. There is usually a latent period of 4 to 12 hours before onset of symptoms. However, after exposure to high doses symptoms may develop more rapidly. Skin manifestations include erythema, edema, necrosis, and the formation of vesicles and bullae. Toxicity increases with ambient temperature. After inhalation, sore throat, hoarseness, cough, dyspnea, bronchospasm, and chest discomfort may develop, and in severe cases respiratory failure and death can result. Eye exposure leads to severe pain, photophobia, blurred vision, tearing, blepharospasm, conjunctival injection, periorbital edema, and corneal vesicle formation with sloughing. Despite this, permanent vision loss is rare. Systemic manifestations of sulfur mustard exposure include nausea, vomiting, diarrhea, and bone marrow suppression. An increased risk of malignancies of the skin and respiratory tract has been reported among long-term survivors. Death from sulfur mustard exposure is rare, with historical mortality rates of less than 5%.

Diagnostic studies contribute little to the initial management of sulfur mustard victims. A complete blood cell count may reveal an initial leukocytosis, which is followed by leukopenia and thrombocytopenia in the case of bone marrow suppression. A chest radiograph may demonstrate evidence of chemical pneumonitis or pneumonia.

Because there is no antidote for sulfur mustard, management is supportive. Unless patient decontamination is initiated within 1 to 2 minutes of exposure, skin absorption is unpreventable. However, health care providers are at risk of secondary contamination; therefore, patient decontamination is still appropriate. This involves removing the patient's clothes and washing the skin with copious amounts of soap and water. Secure patient clothing and belongings in double biohazard bags. Staff should wear chemical-resistant suits with eye and respiratory protection. Once decontamination is complete, assess the airway, and insert an endotracheal tube if edema or severe respiratory distress is present. Administer oxygen to patients with respiratory symptoms. Bronchodilators are indicated to treat bronchospasm.

Management of skin lesions is similar to care of burn victims and includes debridement, application of topical antibiotics, pain control, and vigilance for secondary infections. Although fluid requirements are generally less than those of thermal burn victims, hydration status and electrolytes should be monitored. Administer tetanus prophylaxis when indicated. Irrigate exposed eyes with copious amounts of water, and administer topical antibiotics and mydriatics if corneal defects are noted. In the case of large exposures, obtain serial blood counts to detect bone marrow suppression. Patients with any but the mildest exposure should be admitted, often under the care of a plastic surgeon, burn specialist, or ophthalmologist. Hematology consultation may also be required.

In the present case, because the patient was wearing the same clothing he had on at the time of exposure, he was moved to a decontamination shower outside the ED where he removed his clothing and showered with copious amounts of soap and water. His clothes were bagged to prevent cross-contamination. Intravenous access was established and morphine given for pain control. Bullae were debrided, and silver sulfadiazine cream was applied. Because of mild conjunctival injection, the eyes were irrigated with 2 L of saline. A follow-up slit lamp examination revealed very mild corneal edema and erosions bilaterally. Cycloplegic and antibiotic eye drops were administered. The patient was current with tetanus immunizations, so additional prophylaxis was not required. Plastic surgery and ophthalmology consultation was requested, and the patient was admitted for pain control and wound care. The local law enforcement agency was contacted regarding the artillery shells. The military subsequently decontaminated the site at the abandoned base.

Clinical Pearls

1. Clinical manifestations of sulfur mustard toxicity develop several hours after initial exposure. A careful history is needed to make the diagnosis.

2. While decontamination rarely prevents sulfur mustard absorption, it should still be performed to prevent secondary exposure of health care workers.

3. Because the fluid requirements of sulfur mustard victims are less than those of victims of thermal burns, aggressive fluid resuscitation is rarely needed.

4. Consider sulfur mustard exposure an act of terrorism until proven otherwise, and notify law enforcement officials early in the patient's care.

REFERENCES

1. Vilensky JA, Redman K: British anti-Lewisite (dimercaprol): An amazing history. Ann Emerg Med 41:378-383, 2003.
2. Centers for Disease Control and Prevention: Facts about sulfur mustard. 2003. www.bt.cdc.gov/agent/blister/mustardgas/basics/facts.asp.
3. Dire DJ: CBRNE—Vesicants, Mustard: Hd, Hn1-3, H. 2003. www.emedicine.com/emerg/topic901.htm.
4. Safarinejad MR: Ocular injuries caused by mustard gas: Diagnosis, treatment, and medical defense. Military Medicine 166: 67-70, 2001.
5. Cieslak TJ: A field-expedient algorithmic approach to the clinical management of chemical and biological casualties. Military Medicine 165:659-662, 2000.
6. Sidell FR, Urbanetti JS, Smith WJ, et al: Vesicants. In Sidell FR, Takafuji ET, Franz DR (eds): *Medical Aspects of Chemical and Biological Warfare*. Falls Church, VA, Office of the Surgeon General, 1997, pp. 197-228.
7. Borak J, Sidell FR: Agents of chemical warfare: Sulfur mustard. Ann Emerg Med 21:303-308, 1992.

Fred M. Henretig, MD

PATIENT 37

A 7-month-old boy with a necrotizing skin lesion

A 7-month-old boy presents with a lesion of 2-days' duration just above his left elbow. Initially it began as a painless, red macule with slight associated swelling. The next day the swelling increased, and the lesion became papular with slight serous drainage. He was taken to his pediatrician who prescribed amoxicillin/clavulanate for a presumed infected insect bite. However, on re-examination the next day, the lesion looks worse, and the child is admitted to the hospital for intravenous antibiotics and possible surgical drainage.

Physical Examination: Temperature 37.2° C. General: alert, no apparent distress. Extremities: a 2-cm open lesion with surrounding erythema and induration just above left elbow; clear yellow drainage; surrounding painless swelling.

Laboratory Findings: Hemogram: WBC 28,100/μL (47% neutrophils), Hct 42.5%, platelets 409,000/μL. Serum chemistries: sodium 128 mEq/L, potassium 4.9 mEq/L, BUN 14 mg/dL, creatinine 0.6 mg/dL.

Initial Hospital Course: The child undergoes incision and drainage, which reveals no abscess, but 10 mL of dark red fluid is expressed from the lesion. He is begun on intravenous ampicillin-sulbactam. Despite these measures, the swelling progresses and fever ensues; clindamycin is added. By hospital day 5 the lesion has evolved to a 4.5 × 5 cm erythematous plaque with a central 1-cm black eschar (see figure). The arm has diffuse, marked edema from hand to shoulder.

Questions: What caused this child's lesion? What is the differential diagnosis for progressive cutaneous lesions marked by eschar formation?

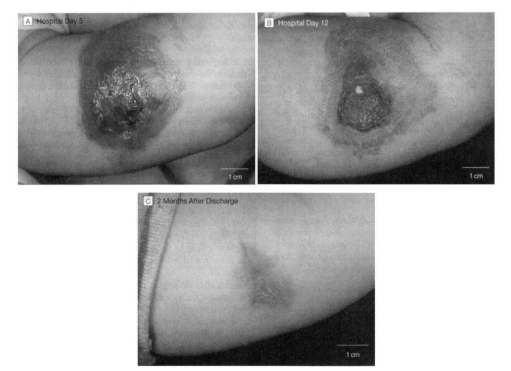

Figures from Freedman A, Olubunmi A, Chang MW, et al: Cutaneous anthrax associated with microangiopathic hemolytic anemia and coagulopathy in a 7-month-old infant. JAMA 287:869-874, 2002; with permission.

Diagnosis: Cutaneous anthrax

Discussion: Many readers who followed closely the terrorist events of 2001 in the U.S. will recognize this case. This infant, a resident of New York City, was the only pediatric victim of the mail-borne anthrax attacks, and his illness was widely reported in the media. His mother worked for a national television studio and had visited her office with him one day before his lesion began. Subsequently, of course, anthrax spores were discovered there. Of interest, the working diagnosis for much of his hospitalization was brown recluse spider bite, an envenomation that is decidedly uncommon in the northeast U.S. Additional common diagnoses to be considered in the evaluation of necrotic skin lesions include other spider bites and Lyme disease (see table).

Anthrax is caused by the gram-positive, spore forming *Bacillus anthracis*. Cutaneous anthrax occurs when organisms gain entry into skin, particularly through abrasions or cuts. Vegetative anthrax bacteria elaborate two protein toxins, edema toxin and lethal toxin, which account for much of its virulence (and justify, along with the disease's potential confusion with brown recluse spider bites, our inclusion of this case here). The skin lesion begins with the appearance of a papule at the inoculum site, which then progresses over a few days to a vesicle, then an ulcer and finally to a depressed, black eschar. The surrounding tissue becomes markedly edematous but not particularly tender, distinguishing this infection from typical cellulitis. It is usually quite amenable to therapy with a variety of antibiotics, and, with timely institution of treatment, is rarely fatal. In the 2001 attack, all 11 patients with cutaneous anthrax survived.

This child's subsequent hospital course was complicated by microangiopathic hemolytic ane-mia with thrombocytopenia, coagulopathy, renal insufficiency, and hyponatremia. These systemic manifestations are not typically reported in otherwise uncomplicated cases of cutaneous anthrax, thus raising the possibility of a particular vulnerability in infancy. Fortunately, he improved with steroid therapy, blood product transfusions, and intensive supportive care and was discharged home on hospital day 17. His diagnosis was confirmed by the Centers for Disease Control with a polymerase chain reaction from serum drawn on hospital day 2 and positive immunohistochemical testing done on skin biopsy tissue.

Major Causes of Cutaneous Eschars

Bites

Loxosceles sp.
Other spiders
  Tegenaria agrestis (hobo spider)
  Phidippus sp. (jumping spider)
  Cheiracanthium sp. (yellow sac spider)
  Argiope aurantia (orange argiope)
  Lycosa sp. (wolf spiders)
  Peucetia viridans (green lynx spider)
  Dolomedes sp. (fishing spider)

Infections

Cutaneous anthrax
Scrub typhus
Rickettial spotted fevers
Rat bite fever
Lyme disease
Tularemia
Ecthyma gangrenosum

Miscellaneous

Focal vasculitis
Warfarin-induced skin necrosis

Clinical Pearls

1. All skin lesions that progress to black eschars are not brown recluse spider bites!

2. These are strange times; clinicians need to be vigilant for unusual presentations or clustering of patients that might suggest an intentional spread of disease.

3. Agents of bioterrorism may have differing, and particularly, more fulminant clinical courses in infants and young children than have been classically described in adults.

REFERENCES

1. Freedman A, Afonja O, Chang MW, et al: Cutaneous anthrax associated with microangiopathic hemolytic anemia and coagulopathy in a 7-monthold infant. JAMA 287:869-874, 2002.
2. Henretig FM, Cieslak TJ, Eitzen EM Jr: Biological and chemical terrorism. J Pediatr 141:311-326, 2002.
3. White S, Henretig F, Dukes R: Medical management of vulnerable populations and co-morbid conditions of victims of bioterrorism. Emerg Med Clin North Am 20:365-392, 2002.

PATIENT 38

A 77-year-old woman with nausea, vomiting, and dizziness

A 77-year-old woman with a history of myocardial infarction, congestive heart failure (CHF), hypertension, and non–insulin-dependent diabetes mellitus presents complaining of several days of dizziness, nausea, and vomiting. There is no chest or abdominal pain. No fevers, chills, or cough are reported. Her medications include glyburide, coumadin, digoxin, isosorbide dinitrate, furosemide, and potassium.

Physical Examination: Pulse 42/min and regular, respirations 16/min, blood pressure 145/92 mmHg. Chest: normal. Cardiovascular: normal. Abdomen: normal. Neurological: normal cranial nerves, motor and sensory function; intact but slow rapid alternating movements and finger-nose-finger.

Laboratory Findings: Serum chemistries: sodium 139 mEq/L, potassium 5.6 mEq/L, chloride 97 mEq/L, bicarbonate 27 mEq/L, BUN 51 mg/dL, creatinine 1.7 mg/dL, glucose 147 mg/dL. EKG (see figure): sinus bradycardia with 2:1 AV block and left bundle branch block.

Question: What is the cause of this patient's symptomatic bradydysrythmia?

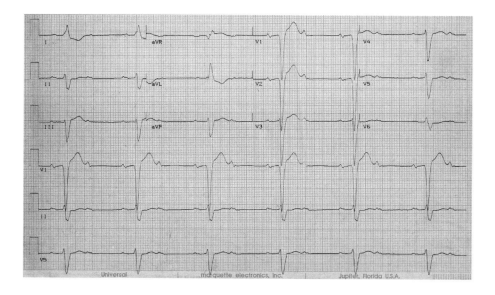

Answer: Digoxin toxicity

Discussion: Digoxin is a cardiac glycoside used to suppress supraventricular tachydysrythmias and improve the symptoms of CHF. Numerous types of cardiac glycosides can be found in nature, including in plants like foxglove (*Digitalis* spp; see figure), yellow oleander (*Nerium* spp.), red squill (*Urginea* spp.), and lily of the valley (*Convallaria* spp.) and in animals like the *Bufo alvarius* toad. Cardiac glycosides effect cells by inactivating the **sodium-potassium adenosine triphosphate (Na-K ATPase) pumps**. These Na-K ATPase pumps are found throughout the body, but inhibition of those found on the myocardial cells manifest the pharmacological effects of these compounds. The pumps maintain the electrical gradient across the membrane by pumping sodium extracellularly and potassium intracellularly. When inhibited, the intracellular sodium rises, triggering a sodium-calcium exchanger to remove the sodium and raise intracellular calcium. This increases myocardial contractility and alters the membrane potential, ultimately improving inotropy and inhibiting conduction through the AV node. Poisoning exaggerates these effects, causing bradydysrhythmias and increasing automaticity, thereby producing tachydysrhythmias. In addition, extracellular serum potassium increases.

Clinically, digoxin manifests toxicity with a combination of gastrointestinal (GI) symptoms such as nausea and vomiting; neurological symptoms such as dizziness, headache, confusion, and delirium; and potentially life-threatening cardiac dysrhythmias. Any number of dysrhythmias can be seen, including frequent PVCs (the most common dysrhythmia seen in cardiac glycoside poisoning), all grades of AV blocks, and ventricular tachycardia. Only an atrial tachycardia with a rapid ventricular response would *not* be consistent with this diagnosis. Hypotension is uncommonly seen except in the most severe poisonings. If present, hypotension should prompt the clinician to think about poisoning with other drugs commonly prescribed in patients with heart disease and CHF, such as antihypertensives. Underlying medical problems or conditions, such as age, heart disease, renal insufficiency, hypoxia, electrolyte disturbances (specifically hypokalemia, hypomagnesemia, and hypercalcemia), and concombinant medications such as calcium channel or beta blockers or various antidysrythmics, increase a patient's susceptibility to digoxin poisoning.

It is important to recognize that, just as with aspirin and theophylline, there are both acute and chronic presentations of digoxin poisoning. *Acute poisonings* are usually the result of intentional suicide ingestions. Initial symptoms include nausea and vomiting, and early dysrhythmias are typically vagally mediated with AV nodal blocks. Over time, automaticity increases, as does the risk of ventricular tachycardia. Early in the acute setting, serum digoxin levels may be dramatically elevated in an otherwise clinically well-appearing patient. As this digoxin distributes into tissue, however, signs of toxicity (e.g., GI and cardiac manifestations) occur. Hyperkalemia appears to be an effective screening marker for acute digoxin poisoning.

Chronic digoxin poisoning is much more difficult to diagnose and requires a high index of suspicion. It most often is seen in elderly patients with multiple medical problems including heart disease. The symptoms and signs develop and progress over days, not hours as seen in acute poisoning, and GI and neurological symptoms are most prominent. Anorexia, nausea, and nonspecific dizziness or generalized weakness for several days may be misinterpreted as a viral syndrome or gastroenteritis. Some patients may

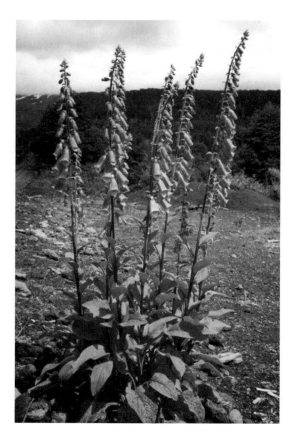

be treated for infectious etiologies, based on symptoms of confusion or altered mental status. Dysrhythmias are later in the course, and ventricular dysrhythmias appear to be more common in chronically poisoned patients. As opposed to acute poisoning, the potassium may be elevated, normal, or low depending on the patient's underlying renal function and the use of diuretics. This patient's presentation was typical of many chronically poisoned patient's and the significant EKG changes and a careful review of her medication list prompted the clinician to check the serum digoxin level. It was markedly elevated at 7.7 ng/nL. The patient's renal insufficiency, which had developed over the past few months, decreased her clearance of digoxin and was the most likely reason she became poisoned.

Treatment of digoxin poisoning begins the same as any poisoning. If asymptomatic, focus should be on obtaining an accurate history of the ingestion and its timing, GI decontamination with oral activated charcoal, and continuous cardiac monitoring. In symptomatic patients, focus should initially be on the ABCs of resuscitation and assessment and treatment of cardiac toxicity. Bradydysrhythmias may respond to atropine or pacing. In the setting of digoxin poisoning, internal cardiac pacing is associated with a higher complication rate—it can induce ventricular dysrhythmias, possibly due to direct mechanical stimulation of the pacer wire on an irritable myocardium with its enhanced automaticity—so **external pacing** is preferred. For tachydysrhythmias, phenytoin has traditionally been the drug of choice. Type 1A antidysrhythmics, such as quinidine or procainamide, are *contraindicated* because they suppress AV nodal conduction and may actually enhance digoxin's toxicity.

For most patients with cardiac glycoside poisoning, the drug of choice is **digoxin-specific Fab (dig Fab) fragments** (see table). These antibody fragments are widely distributed throughout the tissues, and they bind and remove the digoxin from the Na-K ATPase; this complex is then renally eliminated. This therapy is extremely well tolerated, but the rare adverse effects may include hypokalemia, CHF, and a rash or flushing that may represent a mild hypersensitivity reaction. There are no cases of severe hypersensitivity, such as anaphylaxis or serum sickness, reported. Digoxin-specific Fab fragments dosing is based on either calculating the amount of digoxin ingested or, more commonly, the serum digoxin level. To calculate the number of vials required to treat a patient the serum digoxin level is multiplied by the patient's weight in kilograms and this number is divided by 100 (typically, the calculation is rounded up to the next whole vial). For example, in this patient who weighed approximately 60 kg and who had a serum digoxin level of 7.7 ng/mL, it was determined to infuse 5 vials of dig Fab (# of digFab vials = serum digoxin level × patient's weight in kg/100 = 7.7 × 60/100 = 4.6 vials). In critically ill patients when the clinical presentation is suspicious for digoxin poisoning, 10 vials (400 mg) of dig Fab are recommended empirically before any serum digoxin levels are known. While these antibody fragments are manufactured specifically for digoxin, they have been clinically effective in patients who have been poisoned by other cardiac glycosides from plants and animals. In poisonings involving other cardiac glycosides, serum digoxin assays may be positive, helping to confirm the exposure, but cannot be used to calculate digoxin Fab dosing. Therefore, in these cases empiric dosing must be used.

Hyperkalemia is a marker of acute digoxin poisoning. This is because Na-K ATPase pumps are located throughout body tissues, not just in the myocardium, so when digoxin levels rise, potassium is unable to be adequately returned intracellularly, and serum levels rise. In fact, in acutely poisoned patients, a serum potassium > 5.0 mEq/L is an indication for treatment with dig Fab. If digoxin poisoning–induced hyperkalemia is life threatening, standard treatment with intravenous sodium barcarbonate and dextrose and insulin should be used in conjunction with dig Fab. Intravenous calcium salts, however, have been suggested to be specifically *contraindicated* because of the potential for further elevating already high intracellular calcium levels and inducing cardiac tetany. In the setting of digoxin poisoning, moderate hyperkalemia is effectively treated by dig Fab.

Indications for Administration of Digoxin-Specific Antibody Fragments

- Any life-threatening dysrhythmia when the clinical situation suggests a cardiac glycoside poisoning
- Chronically poisoned patients with several systemic symptoms, which may include noncritical bradydysrhythmia, gastrointestinal symptoms, mild cognitive changes, or new renal insufficiency
- Serum potassium >5.0 mEq/L in acute digoxin overdose
- Serum digoxin level >15 ng/mL
- Excellent history of digoxin ingestion involving >10 mg in adult, 4 mg in child

---

The present patient received 5 vials of digoxin-specific Fab fragments infused over 30 minutes. Two hours later, her nausea and bradycardia had improved, and her EKG had become a normal sinus rhythm with a rate of 60/min without heart block. She was admitted to the step-down cardiac intensive care unit and was discharged in the morning with normal vitals, feeling much improved.

Clinical Pearls

1. Digoxin is the most common source of cardiac glycoside poisoning, but other sources are found in nature (e.g., foxglove, lily of the valley, and oleander plant).

2. Chronic digoxin poisoning may present with nonspecific symptoms including nausea, vomiting, dizziness, and relative bradycardia.

3. Hyperkalemia is a marker for severe acute digoxin poisoning.

4. Indications for digoxin-specific FAB antibodies include life-threatening digoxin-induced dysrhythmias, significant hyperkalemia >5.5 mEq/L associated with an elevated digoxin level, and critically ill patients with a clinical presentation suggestive of digoxin poisoning.

REFERENCES

1. Hauptman PJ, Kelly RA: Digitalis. Circulation 99:1265-1270, 1999.
2. Rich SA, Libera JM, Locke RL: Treatment of foxglove extract poisoning with digoxin-specific Fab fragments. Ann Emerg Med 22:1904-1907, 1993.
3. Taboulet P, Baud FJ, Bismuth C: Acute digitalis intoxication: Is pacing still appropriate? J Toxicol Clin Toxicol 31:261-273, 1993.
4. Kelly RA, Smith TW: Recognition and management of digitalis toxicity. Am J Cardiol 69:108-109, 1992.
5. Moorman JR, Pritchett EL: The arrhythmias of digitalis intoxication. Arch Intern Med 145:1289-1293, 1985.

PATIENT 39

A 5-month-old male collie dog with coma

A 5-month-old male collie presents to the veterinary emergency service (ES) approximately 9 hours after ingesting an unknown quantity of a horse anthelmintic containing moxidectin (2%). Two hours after ingestion, the dog was lethargic. There was a rapid progression to ataxia, followed by generalized seizures. Upon presentation to a local veterinarian, the dog was comatose and cyanotic and was placed on a portable, volume-limited ventilator (100% O_2) prior to transport to the ES.

Physical Examination: Temperature 40.1° C (normal 37.5–39° C), pulse 100/min (60–80/min). General: comatose. Chest: respirations shallow and rapid, increased bronchovesicular sounds. Cardiovascular: cardiac auscultation normal, normal sinus rhythm, normal pulses. Neuromuscular: comatose; all myotactic, flexor, perineal (anal), and cranial nerve reflexes absent with exception of weak pupillary light reflex.

Laboratory Findings: WBC 21,800/μL (normal 6700–18,300/μL). Serum chemistries: normal. Urinalysis: normal. Arterial blood gas (100% FiO_2): PaO_2 603.2 mmHg (92.1 +/− 5.6); $PaCO_2$ 57.2 mmHg (36.8 +/− 3.0); base excess −4.3 mmol/L. Chest radiograph: heavy interstitial pattern in the caudodorsal lung regions.

Question: Moxidectin toxicity is primarily manifest through agonism of which neuronal chemical messenger?

Answer: The macrolide endectocide moxidectin agonizes release of gamma-aminobutyric acid (GABA).

Discussion: Moxidectin is a milbemycin **endectocide** used for the treatment and prevention of endoparasitism in horses and as a prophylactic heartworm medication given once a month to dogs. Other macrolide endectocides include ivermectin, selemectin, abamectin, doramectin, eprinomectin, and milbemycin oxime. These agents are fermentation products of *Streptomyces* spp. Ivermectin is the most widely used drug in the group. It has been investigated for use in humans to treat several human parasitic diseases including onchocerciasis, scabies, lymphatic filariasis, and loiasis. The macrolide endectocides have a wide margin of safety in mammals, although human and animal intoxications have been documented.

Antiparasitic activity and mammalian toxicity of the macrolide endectocides is due to their GABA agonism. *In vitro*, macrolide endectocides release GABA from vertebrate brain synpatosomes and increase binding of GABA postsynaptically via receptor upregulation. This potentiates the opening of GABA-gated chloride channels and increases chloride influx, which results in membrane hyperpolarization and impaired neurotransmission. The wide margin of safety in most mammals is due to poor penetration of these agents across the blood-brain barrier, where GABA neurotransmission occurs. However, collies, Shetland sheepdogs, English sheepdogs, and Australian shepherds are *uniquely sensitive* to macrolide endectocides. It has been hypothesized that their sensitivity is due to a lack of p-glycoprotein in the blood-brain barrier. **P-glycoprotein** serves to prevent the passage of structurally diverse, amphiphilic, hydrophobic drugs and toxicants across the barrier. Mild clinical signs have occurred in collies given a single oral dose of 90 µg/kg, whereas beagles have tolerated 1130 µg/kg daily for 1 year. Severe symptoms of intoxication in humans have been reported with ingestions of 15.4 mg/kg of ivermectin and 114.9 mg/kg of abamectin.

Clinical signs of macrolide endectocide intoxication in animals range from behavioral changes, anorexia, hypersalivation, and lethargy to focal or generalized muscle tremors, ataxia, emesis, seizures, extreme mental depression, stupor, and coma. Physical examination findings may include hypothermia or hyperthermia, bradycardia, slow respiratory rate, poor chest excursions, and cyanosis. Canine neurological examination may reveal altered states of mentation, as well as, mydriasis or miosis; loss of pupillary light, menace, and gag reflexes; hyporeflexia or hyperreflexia of myotatic and flexor reflexes; and lack of response to deep or superficial painful stimuli. Clinical signs in intoxicated people include coma, pulmonary aspiration with respiratory failure, and hypotension.

A diagnosis is based primarily on a history of exposure and compatible clinical signs (see table). Laboratory testing of biological samples is possible to confirm exposure, but concentrations associated with intoxication have not been determined.

After a potentially toxic ingestion, consideration should be given to the potential value of gastric decontamination. Ivermectin and moxidectin are excreted primarily via the feces; therefore, multiple doses of activated charcoal (AC) may be beneficial. Treatment of clinically affected animals and humans is primarily supportive in nature. Hypoventilation, as was present in this case, can be supported with proper ventilatory management. Diazepam may be contraindicated for the treatment of muscle tremors or seizures because the macrolide endectocides can increase the number and affinity of benzodiazepine binding sites. Physostigmine and picrotoxin have been evaluated for the treatment of ivermectin intoxication, but have not proven to be useful antidotes.

Differential Diagnosis of Paresis/Paralysis in Dogs

Spinal cord disorders
Neoplasia
Inflammation
Trauma
Disk extrusion
Infarction
Lower motor neuron disease
Congenital demylinating diseases
Inflammatory, immune-mediated diseases
Polyneuropathies
Botulism
Tick paralysis
Episodic weakness
Polymyositis
Myasthenia gravis
Cardiopulmonary disease
Episodic hemorrhage
Hypoglycemia
Hypoadrenocorticism
Other
Ionophore toxicosis
Skeletal muscle relaxant toxicosis

In the present case, serum, blood, adipose tissue, and feces were collected for toxicological testing. However, moxidectin was detected in only the adipose sample. This confirmed exposure, but not intoxication. At presentation, the dog exhibited respiratory acidosis ($PaCO_2$ of 57.2 mmHg) and had a mild metabolic acidosis (base excess of −4.3 mmol/L). Increasing the ventilation rate corrected the respiratory acidosis. A nasogastric tube was inserted, and a dose of AC (1 g/kg) combined with magnesium citrate (0.07 g/kg) was administered. Subsequent doses of AC were given every 4 hours for a 24-hour period. An IV infusion of metoclopramide (2 mg/kg over 24 hours) was initiated to facilitate gastric emptying. The pulmonary radiographic findings were attributed to mild neurogenic pulmonary edema. Continuing treatment consisted of positive-pressure ventilation, intravenous fluid administration, enteral feeding, and administration of amikacin sulfate. The dog was neurologically improved on day 3, although he was not able to ventilate himself adequately. Improvement continued on days 4 and 5, with more frequent periods of arousal. A continuous infusion of fentanyl (0.50 µg/kg/min) was used to permit continued comfortable endotracheal intubation. Spontaneously inspired tidal volume increased throughout days 4 and 5, and the dog was completely weaned from the ventilator on day 6. The dog was discharged from the hospital on day 10, although he was still slightly lethargic. A neurological examination 2 weeks after discharge was normal.

Clinical Pearls

1. Macrolide endectocides have a wide margin of safety in mammals due to their poor penetration into the brain, where mammalian GABA receptors are found.

2. A history of exposure, particularly in susceptible dog breeds, is important for the early recognition of intoxication. Laboratory detection of macrolide endectocides is possible but not widely available.

3. Appropriate ventilatory support and good nursing care are critical for successful case management. Pulmonary aspiration is the most serious complication of intoxication.

REFERENCES

1. Beal MW, Poppenga RH, Birdsall WJ, Huges D: Respiratory failure attributable to moxidectin intoxication in a dog. JAVMA 215:1813-1817, 1999.
2. Chung K, Yang CC, Wu ML, et al: Agricultural avermectins: An uncommon but potentially fatal cause of pesticide poisoning. Ann Emerg Med 34:51-57, 1999.
3. Hadrick MK, Bunch SE, Kornegay JN: Ivermectin toxicosis in two Australian Shepherds. JAVMA 206:1147-1152, 1995.
4. Tranquilli WJ, Paul AJ, Seward RL, et al: Response to physostigmine administration in collie dogs exhibiting ivermectin toxicosis. J Vet Pharmacol Ther 10:96-100, 1987.
5. Sivine F, Plume C, Ansay M: Picrotoxin, the antidote to ivermectin in dogs? Vet Rec 116:195-196, 1985.
6. Heit JE, Tranquilli WJ, Parker AJ, et al: Clinical management of ivermectin overdose in a collie dog. Comp Anim Prac 19: 3-7, 1980.

Constance M. Yuan, MD, PhD
Philip R. Spandorfer, MD
Leslie M. Shaw, PhD

PATIENT 40

A toddler with bizarre behavior and slurred speech

A 5-year-old girl is brought to the emergency department (ED) by her family, due to unusual behavior. The grandmother reports that the girl awoke from a nap crying and grabbing randomly in the air, with slurred speech and a wobbly gait. The grandmother thought she was flushed and warm as well. The child had been in her usual state of good health and was well appearing when she went down for the nap. There is no history of fever, upper respiratory illness, vomiting, diarrhea, or trauma. She is not taking any regular medications and has no drug allergies. The family denies any history of ingestions and states that the only medicines in the house are the grandmother's nitroglycerin and over-the-counter cold medications. The girl lives at home with her mother, father, grandmother, 2-year-old brother, and 3-year-old cousin.

When the family is questioned further, they acknowledge that the aunt had seen the child playing on the floor with some pills. However, the family continues to state that the only medications in the home are some cold preparations and nitroglycerin; they deny the presence of "nerve pills" (e.g., tricyclic antidepressants) or muscle relaxants (e.g., cyclobenzaprine). The family is asked to bring in all of the medications in the household, and the following are produced: carbinoxamine syrup, cyproheptadine tablets, hydroxyzine syrup, nitroglycerin tablets, and multivitamin tablets.

Physical Examination: Temperature 37.7° C, pulse 178/min, respirations 30/min, blood pressure 162/88 mmHg (repeat = 120/62 mmHg). Pulse oximetry, room air: 97%. General: agitated with apparent visual hallucinations. HEENT: pupils dilated and unreactive to light. Chest: normal. Cardiovascular: tachycardia, otherwise normal. Abdomen: normally active bowel sounds. Genitourinary: bladder not palpable. Skin: flushed.

Laboratory Findings: Hemogram: normal. Serum chemistries: normal. EKG (see figure): sinus tachycardia. CT scan of brain: normal. Qualitative urine immunoassay for drugs of abuse: negative for amphetamine, barbiturates, benzodiazepines, cocaine, opiate. Qualitative serum toxicology screen: positive for tricyclic antidepressants (TCAs); negative for acetaminophen, salicylate, ethanol.

Questions: Based solely on the laboratory findings, what is the likely cause of this child's symptoms? Does all of the evidence support this initial diagnosis?

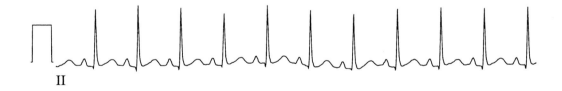

II

Diagnosis: Hallucinations, tachycardia, mydriasis, and flushing suggest an anticholinergic syndrome. The lack of QRS widening on electrocardiography and the exposure history invoke suspicion regarding the drug screen results. The toxidrome is more consistent with an antihistamine such as cyproheptadine.

Discussion: Initial management in the ED following the positive toxicological report included rapid-sequence endotracheal intubation, nasogastric administration of 1g/kg activated charcoal, and 2 mEq/kg of intravenous sodium bicarbonate for presumed TCA toxicity. Arrangements were made to transfer the child to a regional children's hospital for treatment. Shortly after arrival at the receiving hospital, the child was extubated. Her skin was still flushed, pupils were large and sluggishly reactive, and she remained tachycardic.

A toxicology consult was requested to assist with the diagnosis and appropriate management of the child. Further probing revealed that the white pills the child had been playing were cyproheptadine. A comprehensive urine drug immunoassay was negative for the presence of TCAs. A full toxicological work up, using confirmatory gas chromatography-mass spectrometry (GC-MS) methods and high-performance liquid chromatography (HPLC) assays adapted for the detection of tricyclic compounds, was performed. The total ion chromatograph of the ingested tablets revealed a prominent peak with a retention time of 11.36 minutes. The corresponding mass spectrum of this peak included a molecular ion with an m/z of 287. The full mass spectrum was highly matched (96% match quality) to a standard spectrum of cyproheptadine (see figure on next page). Subsequent GC-MS analysis of an extract of the patient's urine confirmed the presence of cyproheptadine. Similar findings were observed in HPLC analysis of the patient's serum. Results revealed a major peak with a retention time of 9.14 minutes, corresponding to cyproheptadine. TCAs were *not* detected.

This case of cyproheptadine toxicity was initially misdiagnosed as tricyclic toxicity based on the results of a preliminary rapid toxicological serum screen. Although emergency medicine physicians frequently rely on rapid toxicological screening tests to influence patient management, false-positive results are a well known phenomenon (see table), and cross-reactivity in a TCA screen has been reported in cyclobenzaprine, carbamazepine, and cyproheptadine toxicity.

Of note, TCA toxicity often induces significant abnormalities on the EKG, including sinus tachycardia, widened QRS complexes, prolonged QT intervals, and a positive terminal 40 msec right axis deviation best described as a "positive R wave in lead aVR." Additionally, TCA ingestion initially may be associated with mild anticholinergic signs as in this case, but is followed rapidly by coma and hypotension. Other than sinus tachycardia, none of these changes were observed on the patient's EKG. Furthermore, case reports of pediatric cyproheptadine overdose describe clinical symptomatology similar to that observed in this patient. Confirmatory GC-MS methods and HPLC assays adapted for the detection of tricyclic compounds can pinpoint the diagnosis.

The degree of cross-reactivity may vary in toxicological screens due to differences in the threshold of positive vs. negative test results, different methodology (depending, for example, on system/brand, the reagents used, detection method, and the affinity and specificity of the antibody used in the immunoassay). Confirmatory toxicological testing of routine rapid toxicological screens can be invaluable.

The present patient continued to improve. Flushing and tachycardia resolved overnight, and she was discharged in the morning, awake and alert.

Major Causes of False-Positive Toxicology Immunoassay Results

Presumed Drug	Potential Causes of False Positive
Tricyclic antidepressants	Carbamazepine, cyproheptadine, diphenhydramine, cyclobenzaprine, phenothiazines (several)
Amphetamines	OTC decongestants, herbal ephedrine
Marijuana	Cannabinoids derived from legal hemp food products
Phencyclidine	Dextromethorphan
Benzodiazepines	Oxaprosin

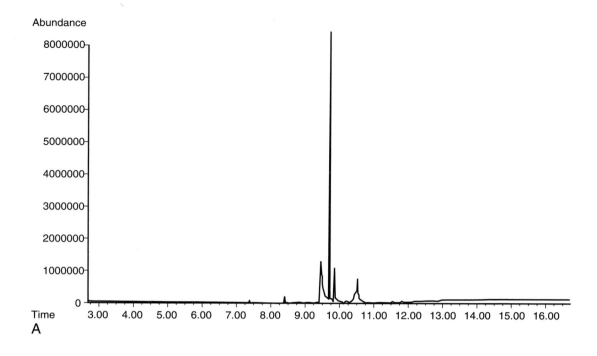

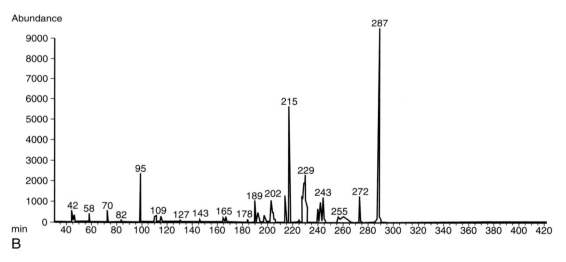

GC/MS analysis of ingested tablets. (A) Total ion chromatograph and (B) corresponding mass spectrum of the major peak showed 96% identity to cyproheptadine. (From Yuan CM, Spandorfer PR, Miller SL, et al: Evaluation of tricyclic antidepressant false positivity in a pediatric case of cyprohepatadine [periactin] overdose. Ther Drug Monit 25:299-304, 2003; with permission.)

Clinical Pearls

1. All laboratory data must be correlated with the clinical scenario.
2. Due to false-positive test results, all toxicological screens with positive results should be followed by confirmatory testing
3. Although anticholinergic signs are seen early in cyclic antidepressant poisonings, EKG findings should be present concurrently. Their absence suggests an alternative (noncyclic antidepressant) etiology of the anticholinergic findings.

REFERENCES

1. Yuan CM, Spandorfer PR, Miller SL, et al: Evaluation of tricyclic antidepressant false positivity in a pediatric case of cyproheptadine (Periactin) overdose. Ther Drug Monit 25:299-304, 2003.
2. Rainey PM: Laboratory principles and techniques for evaluation of the poisoned or overdosed patient. In Goldfrank LR, Flomenbaum NE, Lewin NA, et al (eds): Goldfrank's Toxicologic Emergencies, 7th ed. New York, McGraw-Hill, 2002, pp 69-93.
3. Matos ME, Burns M, Shannon MW: False-positive tricyclic antidepressant drug screen results leading to the diagnosis of carbamazepine intoxication. Pediatrics 105:e661-e663, 2000.
4. Blaustein BS, Gaeta TJ, Balentine JR, Gindi M: Cyproheptadine-induced central anticholinergic syndrome in a child: A case report. Pediatr Emer Care 11:235-237, 1995.
5. Wians FH Jr, Norton JT, Wirebaugh SR: False-positive serum tricyclic antidepressant screen with cyproheptadine. Clin Chem 39:1355-1356, 1993.

PATIENT 41

A 32-year-old man with crampy abdominal pain

A 32-year-old man has suffered distressing abdominal pain for 6 hours. He reports a mild headache for the last 2 days for which he took aspirin with good relief. This morning, while looking for his aspirin, he accidentally ingested his wife's new medication, pilocarpine, which she uses to treat her dry mouth secondary to her radiation therapy. Within 30 minutes, he developed excessive salivation, tearing, intermittent sweating, nausea, diarrhea, and diffuse intermittent and crampy abdominal pain.

Physical Examination: Temperature 36.8° C, pulse 42/min, respirations 22/min, blood pressure 122/70 mmHg. Oxygen saturation: 99% in room air. General: alert, awake, no distress. HEENT: profuse rhinorrhea, salivation and lacrimation; pupils 1 mm bilaterally. Chest: normal. Abdomen: soft, nontender, nondistended, with hyperactive bowel sounds. Skin: cool and diaphoretic. Neuromuscular: normal. Extremities: no fasciculations or abnormal movements.

Laboratory Findings: Hemogram: normal. Serum chemistries: normal. Chest radiograph: normal. EKG (see figure): sinus bradycardia.

Question: Can pilocarpine be responsible for these symptoms?

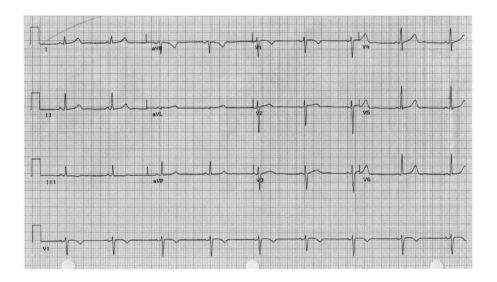

Diagnosis: Increased fluid release from exocrine glands, skin, and mucosa, with miosis and bradycardia, are the hallmarks of muscarinic toxicity and are consistent with pilocarpine poisoning.

Discussion: Pilocarpine is a direct muscarinic receptor agonist. It has been used most commonly in ophthalmology for glaucoma, but has also been used in the treatment of dry mouth associated with Sjögren syndrome and head/neck irradiation.

Understanding the physiology of pilocarpine requires a review of the cholinergic nervous system and its neurotransmitters. Acetylcholine (ACh) activates two types of cholinergic receptors—nicotinic and muscarinic. ACh's effect is dependent on the receptor types present in each end organ. Nicotinic receptors, when activated, open sodium channels to allow sodium influx and cellular depolarization. Muscarinic receptors are linked to a G-protein and have various effects depending on subtype.

ACh is stored in vesicles in presynaptic neurons. Depolarization of the neuron leads to release of the ACh into the synapse. ACh may interact with the receptors in the post-synaptic membrane and is then degraded by acetylcholinesterase to choline and acetic acid. The choline is taken up by the presynaptic membrane and then recycled into ACh to be repackaged in vesicles.

Nicotinic or muscarinic receptors are found in all four parts of the human nervous system: the parasympathetic nervous system (PNS), the sympathetic nervous system (SNS), the central nervous system, and the somatic motor system. In the PNS, nicotinic receptors exist in the ganglionic synapse, and muscarinic receptors are found in the pupils, glands, heart, and mucous membranes. Stimulation of these muscarinic receptors leads to miosis, salivation, lacrimation, urination, vomiting, diarrhea, hyperactive bowel sounds, bradycardia, bronchorrhea, and bronchospasm. The somatic motor system only contains nicotinic receptors. Stimulation of these receptors leads to muscular contraction, and, if overstimulated, fasciculations and even paralysis develops. The central nervous system contains both nicotinic and muscarinic receptors. Stimulation of these receptors produces various effects including seizures and agitation.

The SNS has preganglionic nerves, which release ACh that then binds to postsynaptic nicotinic receptors on the adrenal medulla, sweat glands, and end organs. The adrenal medulla releases norepinephrine and epinephrine into the blood stream. In the end organs, postganglionic nerves release norepinephrine. Additional postganglionic nerves release ACh in sweat glands, which binds to muscarinic receptors. Stimulation of these receptors produces sweating.

The effects of a cholinergic medication or chemical are dependent on its specificity for individual receptor types. For example, administration of succinylcholine (a depolarizing somatic muscle nicotinic receptor agonist) leads to muscular fasciculation and paralysis. Administration of pilocarpine (a direct muscarinic agonist) leads to stimulation of the PNS and stimulation of the sweat glands of the SNS. This leads to miosis, bradycardia, bronchorrhea, bronchospasm, salivation, lacrimation, urination, vomiting, diarrhea, and sweating. The organophosphate insecticides and the nerve agents inhibit the breakdown of ACh in all synapses in the body, leading to prominent muscarinic symptoms as described with pilocarpine ingestion. In addition, stimulation of ganglionic sympathetic and parasympathetic nicotinic receptors leads to either bradycardia or tachycardia, and stimulation of muscular nicotinic receptors may produce fasciculations and paralysis.

The common medications and chemicals that are active at cholinergic sites are listed in the table. Muscarinic symptoms from a direct muscarinic agonist or from an indirect agonist, such as an organophosphate, can be treated with a competitive muscarinic antagonist agent, such as atropine. Intravenous doses of 0.5–2.0 mg may be given slowly in patients with potentially dangerous toxicity (unstable or severe bradycardia, bronchorrhea, or severe bronchospasm). Caution must be taken not to administer atropine either too rapidly or in too large a dose, as anticholinergic toxicity may result.

The present patient experienced worsening bradycardia (28/minute) with mild depression in blood pressure (92/44) and was given intravenous atropine 1.0 mg over 5 minutes, with relief of the bradycardia and the muscarinic symptoms. He was admitted to the hospital, and over the next 24 hours he recovered fully, required no further atopine, and was uneventfully discharged from the hospital.

Common Cholinergically Active Agents

Nicotine receptor agonists
- Nicotine
- Methacholine
- Succinylcholine (muscular nicotine receptor subtype)

Nicotine receptor antagonists
- Vecuronium (muscular nicotine receptor subtype)
- Pancuronium (muscular nicotine receptor subtype)

Muscarinic receptor agonists
- Muscarine
- Pilocarpine
- Bethanechol
- Methacholine

Muscarinic receptor antagonists
- Atropine
- Benztropine
- Cyclobenzaprine
- Diphenhydramine
- Scopolamine
- Antihistamines
- Cyclic antidepressants
- Phenothiazines

Enhance acetylcholine release
- Yohimbine

Prevent acetylcholine release
- Clonidine
- Guanabenz
- Guanfacine
- Oxymetazoline

Acetylcholinesterase inhibitors
- Carbamate pesticides
- Donepezil
- Edrophonium
- Neostigmine
- Nerve agents (VX, soman, sarin, etc)
- Organophosphate pesticides
- Physostigmine
- Pyridostigmine
- Rivastigmine

Clinical Pearls

1. Pilocarpine and other cholinergic agents produce miosis, bradycardia, and increased fluid production from skin and mucosa. This is also known as the cholinergic toxidrome.
2. Muscarinic toxicity may be treated with the competitive muscarinic antagonist atropine.
3. There are numerous cholinergically active chemicals.

REFERENCES

1. Johnson JT, Ferretti GA, Nethery WJ, et al: Oral pilocarpine for post-irradiation xerostomia in patients with head and neck cancers. N Engl J Med 329:390-395, 1993.
2. Littmann L, Kempler P, Rohla M, Fenyvesi T: Severe symptomatic atrioventricular block induced by pilocarpine eye drops. Arch Int Med 147:586-587, 1987.
3. Epstein E, Kaufman I: Systemic pilocarpine toxicity from overdosage. Am J Ophthalmol 59:109-110, 1965.

Sandra H. Schwab, MD
Kevin C. Osterhoudt, MD

PATIENT 42

An 18-month-old boy with household cleaner ingestion

An 18-month-old boy is brought to the emergency department via fire rescue after being found unresponsive. Ninety minutes prior to hospital arrival, the child was found by family members with an open bottle of floor cleaner (see figure). According to the family, he stood in a spilled pool of cleaner and his breath and clothes smelled of the cleaner. Aside from an episode of vomiting, he initially seemed well and unaffected. A short time later he was noted to have unsteady gait, slurred speech, and drowsiness. His family called for emergency medical services when the boy was no longer arousable.

Physical Examination: Temperature 36.3° C, pulse 130/min, respirations 14/min, blood pressure 87/59 mmHg; oxygen saturation 100% in room air. General: sleeping on back with flaccid extremities. HEENT: atraumatic, pupils 5 mm to 3 mm and reactive, breath with sweet pine scent, oral mucosa without burns or ulcerations. Cardiovascular: regular rate and rhythm, strong distal pulses. Lungs: clear to auscultation. Abdomen: soft. Skin: no rash or burns. Neurological: no eye opening, withdraw to painful stimulus, and moaning with painful stimulus (Glasgow Coma Scale score = 6).

Laboratory Findings: Bedside blood dextrose: 155 mg/dL. Chest x-ray: no infiltrates. Serum chemistries: normal.

Question: What component of this common household cleaner is responsible for this child's central nervous system depression?

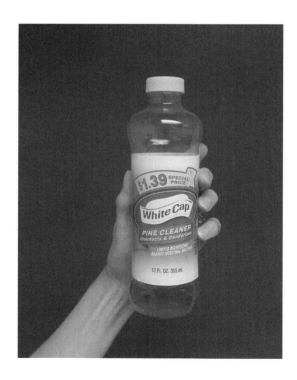

Diagnosis: Corrosive substances in some cleaners may lead to tissue injury. Many cleaners contain toxic alcohols and may cause hypoglycemia. However, the distinctive odor of his breath and clothes points the clinician to pine oil as the offending agent.

Discussion: This patient presents with the common scenario of household cleaning agent ingestion. Reports to the Toxic Exposure Surveillance System (TESS) of the American Association of Poison Control Centers demonstrate that cleaning substances account for nearly 10% of all reported human exposures to potentially toxic substances. Children historically comprise more than half of these exposures. Pine oil is used in many household products because of its disinfectant properties as well as its clean, fresh scent; it is the major toxic constituent in many household cleaner exposures.

The major component of pine oil is **terpene**, a cyclic hydrocarbon. The terpenes are naturally occurring substances found in trees, plants, and flowers. Pine oil is a wood distillate of pine trees, as is turpentine. These wood distillates are readily absorbed from the gastrointestinal tract and, unlike many other hydrocarbons, have direct central nervous system (CNS) toxicity. Most ingestions result in only mild symptoms. Pine oil ingestions greater than 1 g/kg may cause potentially lethal poisoning. From an epidemiological viewpoint, suicidal ingestions and ingestions with a product containing greater than 20% pine oil result in more severe toxicity.

Patients with pine oil ingestion frequently present with the strong odor of pine in their breath, vomitus, and urine. Early gastrointestinal irritation commonly produces vomiting and diarrhea, even with small ingestions. As with other hydrocarbon ingestions, mucous membrane irritation occurs. Although pine oil has a greater surface tension than many similar hydrocarbons, the risk of pulmonary aspiration and pneumonitis is high, especially if the patient is vomiting. The typical clinical presentation after pine oil absorption includes somnolence, lethargy, and slurred speech; coma and death are rare. Ataxia is frequently observed in children. Rare complications include bradycardia, acute renal failure, and thrombocytopenic purpura.

As with any emergency, a patent airway is the first priority. In standard trauma care paradigms a Glasgow Coma score of 6 would mandate endotracheal intubation; however, this paradigm does not necessarily apply to the intoxicated patient. CNS depression following pine oil ingestion is of finite duration. The risk of withholding intubation is the potential for further vomiting during the state of depressed mentation, which might lead to potentially fatal pulmonary aspiration. The risk of endotracheal intubation is the possibility of inducing vomiting or suffering other iatrogenic complications of the procedure. This **risk versus benefit decision-making process** must be carefully considered in the clinical setting.

After stabilization of the airway, breathing, and circulation, removal of any potentially irritating product from the skin, mucous membranes, and eyes is important. Some clinicians might consider nasogastric lavage among patients with significant pine oil ingestions presenting to medical care soon after the event. The risk of aspiration with these interventions should be given thoughtful consideration. The mainstay of treatment remains attentive supportive care. The majority of patients have only mild gastrointestinal symptoms, which resolve in several hours, and they may be released from hospital care.

There is no readily available clinical test to measure serum levels of pine oil, although gas chromatographic–mass spectrometric methods have been reported useful in special circumstances. Obtain a chest radiograph to evaluate for aspiration pneumonia and pneumonitis. Choose other laboratory tests according to the clinical situation. Osmolar gap calculations or alcohol levels might be warranted after solvent exposures. Check blood sugar in any patient with altered sensorium.

In the present case, the family reported approximately 6 ounces of the cleaner missing. The product contained 30% pine oil. The patient demonstrated continued retching while in the resuscitation room. We suspected several hours of obtundation from the exposure history. In consideration of the likelihood for continued vomiting and the possibility of subsequent aspiration, the airway was secured using rapid sequence intubation techniques. The boy was carefully monitored, and regained consciousness approximately 12 hours after his ingestion. The boy appeared well at the time of hospital discharge.

Clinical Pearls

1. Household cleaning agents account for a substantial proportion of all poison exposures.

2. Many distinctive cleaning agents contain pine oil, which belongs to the terpene class of hydrocarbons.

3. The wood-derived hydrocarbons may cause direct CNS toxicity, including somnolence, lethargy, slurred speech, ataxia, and, rarely, coma.

REFERENCES:
1. Welker JA, Zaloga GP: Pine oil ingestion: A common cause of poisoning. Chest 116:1822-1826, 1999.
2. Brook MP, McCarron MM, Mueller JA: Pine oil cleaner ingestion. Ann Emerg Med 18:391-395, 1989.

Zachary F. Meisel, MD, MPH
Jeanmarie Perrone, MD

PATIENT 43

A 57-year-old woman with depression, diarrhea, and tremors

A 57-year-old woman with a longstanding history of bipolar affective disorder and hypertension presents to the emergency department with diarrhea, vomiting, and crampy, epigastric abdominal pain of 4-day duration. She denies any fevers or chills. She has no sick contacts and no recent travel history. She lives with her son, who notes that her hands have been trembling more severely over the past week and that she has been more tired. Her medications are lithium carbonate and hydrochlorothiazide (HCTZ)–triamterene. She has been taking the same dose of lithium for many years; the HCTZ–triamterene was recently prescribed by her primary care physician for hypertension.

Physical Examination: Temperature 36.3° C, pulse 89/min, respirations 16/min, blood pressure 118/78 mmHg. General: ill-appearing, sluggish. HEENT: mucous membranes dry, pupils 3 mm reactive and equal, extra-ocular eye movements intact without nystagmus; neck moderately enlarged, nontender palpable thyroid. Chest: normal. Cardiovascular: regular rate and rhythm. Abdomen: soft, nontender, no hepatosplenomegaly. Extremities: no clubbing, cyanosis, or edema; capillary refill approx 3 seconds. Skin: warm, dry, mild tenting of skin on hands. Neuromuscular: generalized weakness with poor effort, cranial nerves II–XII intact, visual acuity grossly intact, sensation normal, deep tendon reflexes 0-1+ throughout, fine tremor in bilateral upper-extremities, no clonus, normal Babinski.

Laboratory Findings: Hemogram: WBC 13,300/μL with 71% neutrophils, no bands; hemoglobin 13 g/dL; platelets 255,000/μL. Serum chemistries: Na^+ 135 mEq/L, K^+ 3.4 mEq/L, Cl^- 102 mEq/L, bicarbonate 23 mEq/L, BUN 24 mg/dL, creatinine 1.4 mg/dL, amylase 85 U/L, lipase 200 mm/L.. Urinalysis: leukocyte esterase negative, nitrite negative, pH. 6.5, glucose negative, ketones 15 mg/dL, protein negative. Serum lithium 3.01 mmol/L. Thyroid-stimulating hormone 4.19 μIU/mL. T3 uptake 0.95. Free thyroxine index 8.0. Thyroxine 8.4 μg/dL. Creatinine kinase 119 U/L. Electrocardiogram (EKG): normal sinus rhythm at 72, normal axis and intervals, nonspecific t-wave changes in V1–V3, QRS 90 ms.

Question: How does volume status and dehydration affect lithium toxicity?

Answer: Dehydration is likely to be a cause *and* an effect of this patient's chronic lithium toxicity.

Discussion: Lithium is a light metal. It has been used to treat patients with psychiatric mood disorders since 1949 and it is still commonly used as a first-line treatment for manic-depressive illness. It is also used to treat patients with refractory headache syndromes and unipolar depression. Lithium carbonate is most commonly prescribed in a sustained-release preparation; the narrow therapeutic window sometimes leads to toxicity.

Lithium exerts its effects on the central nervous system (CNS) in multiple ways; its mechanism as a mood stabilizer remains unclear. It is eliminated entirely by the kidney. However, lithium clearance can be significantly affected by hydration status, renal function, and co-ingestions. The organ systems involved in lithium toxicity include the renal, CNS, gastrointestinal (GI), hematological, and endocrine. Thus, lithium toxicity can present with multiple clinical manifestations. The clinical presentation, pathophysiology, and outcome of lithium toxicity are often determined by the circumstance of the poisoning: *acute, chronic*, or *acute-on-chronic* (see table).

Acute lithium toxicity usually occurs in the setting of an intentional overdose in a patient who has little or no lithium in the body prior to the ingestion. Gastrointestinal symptoms including diarrhea, nausea, and vomiting are common early signs of acute lithium toxicity. CNS effects of lithium toxicity are less common in the acutely poisoned patient and are a marker of severe toxicity. CNS symptoms are varied; they may progress from early tremor, tinnitus, and dysarthria to late changes in mental status, seizures, and coma. Cardiovascular effects of severe acute lithium intoxication include hypotension and various nonspecific EKG abnormalities.

Chronic lithium toxicity often occurs in patients who have been taking therapeutic doses of lithium carbonate who then increase their dose (as prescribed or accidentally) or who have decreased clearance of the drug due to renal insufficiency, dehydration, or drug interactions. Drugs that can induce dehyration and/or decreased renal function, such as diuretics, angiotensin-converting enzyme inhibitors, nonsteroidal anti-inflammatory agents, antidepressants, and antipsychotic medications, have all been implicated in causing chronic lithium toxicity. Similarly, lithium carbonate itself causes renal impairment (even at therapeutic levels causing nephrogenic diabetes insipidus in up to 20% of all patients maintained on the drug) and thus may induce a self-promoting cascade of lithium toxicity.

Chronic lithium toxicity is often more clinically severe than acute toxicity. Mildly elevated serum levels of lithium can result in significant morbidity in the patient who is on daily lithium because the total body burden of lithium is

Presentation and Treatment of Lithium Toxicity

	Acute Toxicity	Chronic Toxicity	Treatment
Serum level	>4.0 mmol/L	>1.5 mmol/L	
GI symptoms	Diarrhea, vomiting	Nausea, mild diarrhea	IV fluids, whole bowel irrigation (for acute ingestions)
Neurologic symptoms	Tremors, weakness, tinnitus, ataxia, altered mental status, coma, seizure, choreoathetosis	Same as acute	Hemodialysis
Renal symptoms	Prerenal azotenmia	Nephrogenic DI, interstitial nephritis	
Cardiovascular symptoms	Hypotension, prolonged QTc, myocarditis	Same	IV hydration
Endocrine symptoms	—	Hypothyroidism, goiter (may occur at therapeutic levels)	Thyroxine replacement

DI=diabetes insipidus.

136

already high. Often, these patients will have few or mild GI effects. In contrast, neurological manifestations of lithium toxicity may be the presenting and predominant symptoms in this patient group. Similar to severe acute intoxication, the CNS symptoms of chronic lithium poisoning are (early) tremor, tinnitus, and dysarthria; and (late) changes in mental status, seizures, hyperthermia and coma. Any patient that presents with CNS symptoms of lithium toxicity is at risk for permanent and severe neurological injury.

In addition to neurological abnormalities in the poisoned patient, long-term lithium therapy can cause leukocytosis, hypothyroidism with goiter (50% prevalence), and polyuria with nephrogenic diabetes (as previously discussed).

Acute-on-chronic lithium toxicity often presents with clinical elements of both acute and chronic toxicity. This scenario commonly occurs when someone on chronic lithium therapy ingests extra lithium tablets or becomes unable to clear the drug due to acute renal insufficiency. Such patients may present with both GI and CNS effects. Lithium toxicity may be particularly severe.

The evaluation and treatment of patients who have lithium toxicity include basic emergency principles of airway, breathing, and circulatory support as necessary. Laboratory studies including serum lithium levels, electrolytes, renal function tests, and a complete blood count are commonly obtained. Thyroid function tests may be helpful in the chronically toxic patient in whom hypothyroidism is suspected. As in nearly all cases of suspected drug toxicity, an EKG should be considered as well. Patients with serum lithium levels of >4.0 mmol/L in the acute setting and >1.5 mmol/L in the chronic setting are likely to be manifesting clinical lithium toxicity and will need medical intervention.

Normal saline hydration is an essential part of the treatment for patients with lithium toxicity. Relative hyponatremia will worsen lithium toxicity, since sodium and lithium will be passively reabsorbed in the tubules together, causing a net decrease in renal lithium excretion. Because most patients with lithium intoxication are hypovolemic (due to diarrhea, vomiting, or diabetes insipidus), volume expansion is an essential way to correct any pre-renal insufficiency and improve urinary clearance of excess lithium. In euvolemic patients without renal impairment, maintenance fluids to maintain urinary output is recommended. Evaluation and correction of any electrolyte abnormalities are indicated as well.

Gastrointestinal decontamination is indicated only for patients with acute lithium toxicity due to ingestion. Lithium does not bind to activated charcoal and thus its use is not recommended unless a co-ingestion is suspected. Whole bowel irrigation with a polyethylene glycol-electrolyte solution (e.g., Go-Lytely) may contribute to gastrointestinal clearance, especially in patients who have ingested sustained-release preparations of lithium, and is the mainstay of GI decontamination in these patients. The solution can be administered orally or via nasogastic tube at a rate of 2 L/h in the adult or at 500 mL/h in the child until the patient's stool is clear. The use of GI lavage with a large-bore orogastric (OG) tube is controversial. There are no published data comparing the clinical outcome of patients who received OG lavage to those who did not in lithium overdoses. Nevertheless, because lithium does not adsorb activated charcoal, there may be a limited indication for OG lavage in patients who have ingested large quantities of lithium within 1 to 2 hours of presentation. Cation exchange–binding resins such as sodium polystyrene sulfonate (Kayexelate) have been shown in animal studies to decrease lithium levels; however, the dose needed to accomplish this safely among lithium poisoned patients has not yet been clarified.

Hemodialysis (HD) will eliminate lithium rapidly and is indicated for patients with severe acute or severe chronic toxicity. Chronic toxicity, more often than acute toxicity, will indicate the use of HD to clear lithium from the body. Patients with acute intoxication and levels greater than 4.0 mmol/L are likely to have severe symptoms and should be treated with HD. However, there are no absolute levels that mandate this intervention. Rather, clinical manifestations including altered mental status, seizures, coma, or ataxia are indications for HD. Patients with mild tremors indicating early neurological impairment must be monitored closely if HD is not performed initially. Patients with renal failure who cannot excrete lithium and those with congestive heart failure may benefit from emergent HD.

Patient monitoring and treatment are indicated for nearly all cases of lithium toxicity regardless of whether the patient receives HD. Close evaluation of electrolytes and neurological status as well as IV fluid maintenance are the mainstays of treatment and should be performed in a hospitalized setting. Early consultation with a nephrologist and serial levels and reassessments are helpful in uncertain cases. All cases of lithium toxicity should be reported to a local or regional poison center.

The present patient was determined to have chronic lithium toxicity with an acute component as manifested by her GI symptoms. The recent addition of a diuretic to her medications may have been the inciting factor that elevated the patient's lithium level and decreased her ability to clear the drug. Diarrhea and vomiting (from the lithium) may have worsened her symptoms and caused clinical dehydration, likely pre-renal insufficiency and worsening lithium toxicity. She was given a bolus of 2 liters IV normal saline and placed on maintenance crystalloid fluids. She was also given IV antiemetics, and a Foley catheter was placed to monitor urine output.

The present patient had a significantly elevated lithium level in the presence of chronic toxicity (3.01 mmol/L) and was manifesting signs of early neurological toxicity; therefore, the use of HD was considered. After consultation with a toxicologist, it was decided to admit the patient to a monitored inpatient unit where intravenous hydration could be continued, a nephrology consult arranged, and her neurological status, lithium levels, and serum electrolyte status could be closely monitored. Her diuretics and lithium carbonate medications were held. Following hydration, her lithium level was 2.5 mmol/L, and her symptoms were improving 4 hours later. The patient was discharged from the hospital 3 days later without HD. She had a normal neurological examination and a lithium level of 0.76 mmol/L. Her antihypertensive agent was changed to a non-diuretic formulation.

Clinical Pearls

1. Chronic lithium toxicity is likely to be more severe and occurs at lower serum levels than acute toxicity.

2. IV fluids are the mainstay for treating lithium toxicity.

3. Activated charcoal will not bind lithium.

4. Whole bowel irrigation may be indicated for acute lithium ingestions. Gastric lavage is controversial and is only considered for very recent, large-quantity ingestions.

5. Neurological symptoms of lithium toxicity indicate severity and often warrant hemodialysis.

REFERENCES

1. Henry GC: Lithium. *In* Goldfrank Flomenbaum NE, Lewin NA, et al (eds): Goldfrank's Toxicologic Emergencies, 7th ed., New York, McGraw Hill, 2002, pp 894-899.
2. Osborn HH, Malkevich D: Lithium. *In* Ford MD, Delaney KA (eds): Clinical Toxicology. Philadelphia, W.B. Saunders Co., 2001, pp 532-538.
3. Timmer RT, Sands JM: Lithium intoxication. J Am Soc Nephrol 10:666-674, 1999.
4. Finley PR, Warner MD, et al: Clinical relevance of drug interactions with lithium. Clin Pharmacokin 29:172-191, 1995.
5. Okusa MD, Crystal LJ: Clinical manifestations and management of acute lithium intoxication. Am J Med 97:383-389, 1994.
6. Groleau G: Lithium toxicity. Emerg Med Clin North Am 12:511-531, 1994.
7. Bosse GM, Arnold TC: Overdoses with sustained realeased lithium preparations. J Emerg Med 10:719-721, 1992.
8. Amdisen A: Clinical features and management of lithium poisoning. Med Toxicol 3:18-32, 1988.

Jennifer Brandeis, MD
Francis DeRoos, MD

PATIENT 44

A 67-year-old man with abdominal cramping and diarrhea

A 67-year-old man with a history of hypertension, coronary artery disease, and gout presents complaining of 1 day of abdominal cramping and diarrhea. The patient states that over the past 4 days he has had an unusually painful gouty flare in his left great toe, and he has taken ibuprofen and 10 to 12 0.6-mg colchicine tablets daily to alleviate his pain. He denies fevers, chills, vomiting, weakness, and bruising.

Physical Examination: Temperature 37.6° C, pulse 120/min, respirations 20/min, blood pressure 132/94 mmHg. General: uncomfortable and ill-appearing. HEENT: oropharynx without lesions, moist mucous membranes, conjunctiva pink, sclera anicteric. Chest: clear bilaterally. Cardiovascular: tachycardic without murmurs, rubs, or gallops. Abdomen: soft, nondistended, mildly tender diffusely without rebound or guarding. Genitourinary: nontender rectal exam with guaiac-positive, brown stool. Extremities: non-tender muscles. Neuromuscular: motor ⅗ in all extremities, sensation intact to light touch and pin prick.

Laboratory Findings: Hemogram: WBC 3400 /μL, hemoglobin 45.6 g/dL. Serum chemistries: sodium 146 mEq/L, potassium 4.2 mEq/L, chloride 94 mEq/L, bicarbonate 21 mEq/L, BUN 28 mg/dL, creatinine 1.3 mg/dL. Electrocardiogram: sinus tachycardia; otherwise unchanged from previous.

Question: What could explain both this patient's gastrointestinal (GI) complaints and his relative neutropenia?

Diagnosis and Treatment: A thorough history and high clinical suspicion are imperative to diagnosing colchicine toxicity in its early stages. Excessive colchicine use, or a failure to adjust dosing in patients with comorbidities, may cause significant poisoning, with initial signs being only generalized GI complaints that may progress to multi-system organ failure.

Discussion: Colchicine is an alkaloid extracted from the bulb of *Colchicum autunmale* and from the tubers of *Gloriosa superba*, both members of the lily family. It is approved for treatment of gout and for prophylaxis in the management of familial mediterranean fever. Other experimental uses include treatment of chronic hepatitis B, hepatic cirrhosis, and Sweet's syndrome, and as a mild antimitotic agent.

The **dosing** of colchicine is fairly confusing because it is based upon both symptoms and a maximum daily limit. The recommended dose of oral colchicine for the treatment of an acute gouty flare is 1.2 mg initially, followed by 0.6 mg every 2 hours until relief of pain or until GI symptoms occur or until a maximum dose of 6.0 mg is reached. Intensive regimens of colchicine treatment should not be repeated for at least 3 days after a course of oral treatment. Among elderly patients or patients with coexisting hepatic disease or renal insufficiency defined as a glomerular filtration rate <50 mL/min or serum creatinine >1.6 mg/dL, a maximum dose of no more than 3.0 mg daily is recommended to minimize potential toxicity. The recommended intravenous dose of colchicine is 1.0 mg IV followed by 0.5 mg IV every 6 hours until relief of pain or until a maximum dose of 4.0 mg is reached. Onset of the effects of intravenous colchicine is about 8 hours. Intravenous colchicine should *never* be administered to patients with renal or liver disease. A 7-day "holiday" from colchicine must occur before resuming its use either orally or IV.

As much as 20% of this drug is excreted unchanged via the kidneys while the remainder is metabolized via deacetylation by the liver, with significant amounts of both drug and metabolite excreted in the bile. Alternative gout treatments, such as nonsteroidal anti-inflammatory agents (NSAIDs) or brief bursts of oral steroid treatment, should be considered for these high-risk patients, but co-administration of NSAIDs and colchicine may not be ideal because NSAIDs reduce renal blood flow and compete with colchicine at the site of renal excretion. The present patient was taking too large of a dose for his age and other medical conditions, resulting in his poisoning.

Colchicine functions intracellularly by blocking the polymerization of tubulin into microtubules. Therapeutically this inhibits leukocyte migration and the resulting inflammation and ultimately pain associated with gouty arthritis. In overdose, this disruption of cell division manifests across multiple organ systems, particularly those with high turnover rates such as the intestinal epithelium, bone marrow, and hair follicles. In addition, colchicine has direct toxic effects on muscle cells, particularly those of the myocardium.

Early signs of colchicine toxicity include nausea, vomiting, diarrhea, and stomach pain. These symptoms may occur within 1 to 6 hours of ingestion and may result in volume depletion and hypotension. Diagnosis rests purely with a known or suspected **history of ingestion** and **high clinical suspicion**, as drug levels have not proved clinically useful. Aggressive supportive care and gastric decontamination must be instituted in this early phase. Multiple doses of oral activated charcoal may be useful even 24 hours after ingestion because of the significant enterohepatic circulation of colchicine. Unfortunately, intestinal ileus may develop as a side effect of the poisoning and limit the ability to administer multiple doses of activated charcoal. Colchicine-induced diarrhea should *not* be treated, since the drug is eliminated in the stool.

Admission to an **intensive care unit** is indicated in all cases of colchicine toxicity. This is because after the significant GI distress and diarrhea, there is a real risk of myocardial dysfunction including hypokinesis and sudden asystolic cardiac arrest that is poorly understood but can be lethal. In addition, severely poisoned patients may develop multiple organ system failure including noncardiogenic pulmonary edema, oliguric renal failure, and rhabdomyolysis. This typically occurs during the first 3 days after an acute poisoning and is the time when most fatalities occur. Chronically overdosed patients may present with a more prolonged and less acute course. Nervous system disturbances such as polyneuropathy, delirium, cerebral edema, and seizures have been seen during this period as well. The present patient was initially treated with volume resuscitation, cardiac monitoring, and opioid analgesics for his pain. Over the next 24 hours he remained hemodynamically stable but his diarrhea continued, and fever developed.

Hematological manifestations may include an initial peripheral leukocytosis followed by severe pancytopenia, which is secondary to bone marrow suppression similar to that occurring under high dose chemotherapy. This is most pronounced 4 to 7 days after ingestion. Disseminated intravascular coagulation as well as overwhelming sepsis has resulted from these effects on the hematopoietic system. Case reports regarding the use of granulocyte colony–stimulating factor (G-CSF) to treat the colchicine-induced pancytopenia have been encouraging. In the present patient, after his WBC dropped to 800/µL on day two, bacterial cultures were obtained, and he was treated with empiric antibiotics and G-CSF. Three days later his WBC had rebounded to 5300/µL.

For patients who receive prompt intensive care and recover from significant colchine overdoses, signs of improvement are most often evident by the 10th day. A prolonged convalescent period generally follows over the next 1 to 2 weeks. Alopecia may present on about the 12th day after ingestion, and a rebound leukocytosis may also be noted even without the use of G-CSF. The present patient was discharged from the hospital on day 10 with alopecia. His colchicine prescription was not renewed, but he was offered opioid analgesics and an NSAID to treat any subsequent gouty attacks.

The devastating effects of colchicine toxicity and the significant devotion of resources to the monitoring and treatment of these cases have spurred research for more definitive treatment of these cases. Immunotherapy advances have enabled the development of colchicine-specific Fab antibodies that are very similar to digoxin-specific antibody fragments. While not yet approved for use within the United States, research indicates that this treatment may restore the function of tubulin in cells impaired by the effects of colchicine and limit these life-threatening effects in those unfortunate patients who intentionally, mistakenly, or inadvertently overdose on colchicine.

Clinical Pearls

1. Colchicine toxicity follows a typical pattern of early GI symptoms, cardiac instability, leukopenia, and alopecia. Most fatalities occur early in the course of poisoning due to hemodynamic collapse.

2. Thorough history taking and clinical suspicion are needed to diagnose cases of colchicine toxicity.

3. Profound colchicine-induced neutropenia may respond to G-CSF administration.

4. Careful attention to dosing and explicit instructions can minimize the risk of inadvertent colchicine poisoning among gouty patients.

REFERENCES

1. Baud F, Sabouraud A, Vicaut E, et al: Treatment of severe colchicine overdose with colchicine-specific Fab fragments. N Engl J Med. 332:642-645, 1995.
2. Hood R: Colchicine poisoning. J Emerg Med 12:171-177, 1994.
3. Katz R, Chuang L, Sutton J: Use of granulocyte colony stimulating factor in the treatement of pancytopenia secondary to colchicine overdose. Ann Pharmocother 26:1087-1088, 1992.
4. Stapczynski J, Rothstein R, Gaye W: Colchicine overdose: Report of two cases and review of literature. Ann Emerg Med 10:364-368, 1981.

M. Bradley Falk, MD
Francis DeRoos MD

PATIENT 45

A 32-year-old car wash employee with finger pain

A previously healthy, 32-year-old man presents complaining "my fingers really hurt." For the past 10 hours, while at work, he has developed increasingly intense burning of his right index, middle, and ring fingers. He cannot recall any specific trauma or exposure. He is employed at a car wash, and recently he began "detailing" cars; today he was working on bumpers and hubs.

Physical Examination: Temperature 37.2° C, pulse 79/min, respiratory rate 18/min, blood pressure 150/84 mmHg. Oxygen saturation: 99% in room air. General: holding fingers in obvious discomfort. Neuromuscular: normal. Extremities: right hand with mild edema and erythema involving distal index, middle, and ring fingers (see figure); affected digits tender to palpation; marked pallor of associated nailbeds; good capillary refill and radial pulse; radial, median and ulnar sensory and motor function intact.

Laboratory Findings: Hemogram: normal. Serum chemistries: Ca 9.2 mg/dL, Mg 2.1 mg/dL. EKG: Normal sinus rhythm, axis and intervals without acute injury pattern. Radiograph of right hand: no fractures or other bony abnormalities.

Question: What caused this patient's pain?

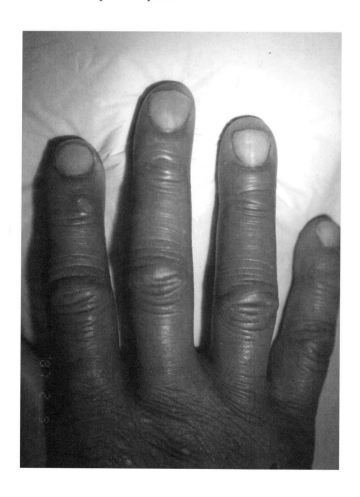

Diagnosis: The combination of the patient's occupational exposure risks and significant pain despite limited clinical findings strongly suggests a hydrofluoric acid exposure.

Discussion: Hydrofluoric acid (HF) is an inorganic acid with many industrial uses including glass etching, brick cleaning, electroplating, and rust removal. Dermal exposures, particularly involving the hand, are by far the most common type of exposure; however, ocular, inhalational, and oral routes have all been reported. The injury HF causes is distinctly different from the direct coagulation necrosis caused by "typical" acids. HF is a weak acid, so it remains relatively undissociated and nonpolar, which allows it to better penetrate the skin. Once in the tissue, its equilibrium shifts as the strongly reactive flouride ion begins binding to free calcium and phosphorus and precipitating in the tissues as fluorapatitie $[3(Ca_3(PO_4)_2Ca(F_2)]$. This causes the pain and tissue injury, and in patients who have been exposed to high concentrations or who have large surface area exposures, severe hypocalemia and hypophosphatemia can result, precipitating fatal dysrhythmias.

Onset of symptoms is related to the concentration of the HF to which the patient is exposed. For relatively low concentrations of 3-12%, like those found in rust removers, pain may develop several hours after exposure. Higher concentrations (>20%) causes more immediate pain. Higher concentrations of the acid and larger surface areas of exposure are associated with a greater risk of systemic hypocalemia, hypophosphatemia, hyperkalemia, and potentially fatal dysrhythmias. For patients who have been exposed to low concentrations for long periods of time, as was the case with this patient, bony destruction may occur, supporting the use of radiological imaging.

The classic presentation of an HF exposure is one of an extremely distressed patient with a paucity of physical examination findings. As the injury progresses, erythema, nailbed discoloration, or small white vesicles may develop. In chronic exposures, diffuse erythema, tissue bogginess, and tenderness may be present.

The initial management of any significant HF exposure includes decontamination (careful removal of clothing and copious irrigation of the involved area), attention to the ABCs (airway, breathing, and circulation), establishment of a peripheral intravenous catheter, supplemental oxygen administration, and cardiac monitoring. An EKG should be obtained and electrolytes assessed, including calcium and magnesium. Radiographs are indicated in patients with chronic exposures or those with inhalational exposures.

The mainstay of treatment for all HF exposures is to present exogenous cations so that the electronegative fluoride anion can bind to those rather then tissue stores of cations. Calcium is used, either topically or parenterally to essentially "mop up" these destructive fluoride ions, produce symptomatic improvement, and halt further injury. For patients with minor exposures or symptoms, a topically applied gel of 2.5% calcium gluconate is often effective. The gel is made by mixing a standard "amp" of calcium gluconate from the adult resuscitation cart (25 mL of a 10% solution) with 75 mL of a water-soluble lubricant. For fingertip, finger, and hand exposures, a latex glove filled with this gel is an efficient and effective method of applying the gel. For more severe pain, or if the topical treatment is ineffective in relieving pain, subcutaneous or intradermal infiltration with 10% calcium gluconate may help. A dose of 0.5 mL/cm^2 of involved skin is recommended and is ideal for upper arm or thigh exposures. Intradermal infiltration is not recommended for fingertip exposures because the injection increases tissue pressure and therefore causes increased pain and possible vascular compromise. Another approach is to place an arterial catheter (radial or brachial artery) and administer 10% calcium gluconate (10 mL of 10% calcium gluconate diluted in 40 mL D5 and infused over 4 hours). While this technique is relatively invasive and can be complicated by vascular compromise, arterial thrombosis, and infection, it can provide significant pain relief and minimize tissue injury and should be attempted in severely affected patients. Remember to provide adequate doses of parenteral opioid analgesics, and consider nerve blocks if intra-arterial infusion is required.

The present patient was treated with topical calcium gluconate gel in a glove and opioid analgesics, with good improvement in his pain. Upon outpatient follow-up 24 hours later, he had some persistent dysesthesias but was overall much improved. In addition, there was now some darkening of the fingertips on his affected digits.

Clinical Pearls

1. Suspect hydrofluoric (HF) acid exposure in the setting of car washes, glass etching, brick cleaning, and electronics.

2. Do not be mislead by a normal physical appearance of an exposed region in a patient complaining of severe, localized pain who was exposed to acid.

3. Remember that small exposures of highly concentrated HF can rapidly produce profound hypocalcemia, hypophosphatemia, and hyperkalemia and induce life-threatening dysrhythmias.

REFERENCES

1. Graudins A, Burns MJ, Aaron CK: Regional intravenous infusion of calcium gluconate for hydrofluoric acid burns of the upper extremity. Ann Emerg Med 30:604-607, 1997.
2. Bertolini JC: Hydrofluoric acid: A review of toxicity. J Emerg Med 163-168, 1992.
3. Henry JA, Hla KK: Intravenous regional calcium gluconate perfusion for hydrofluoric acid burns. J Toxicol Clin Toxicol 30:203-207, 1992.
4. Cummings CC, McIvor ME: Fluoride-induced hyperkalemia: The role of Ca^{2+} dependent K^+ channels. Am J Emerg Med 6: 1-3, 1988.
5. Greco RJ, Hartford CE, Haith LR Jr, *et al*: Hydrofluoric acid-induced hypocalcemia. J Trauma 28:1593-1596, 1988.

PATIENT 46

A 15-year-old boy with altered mental status

A 15-year-old previously healthy boy is brought to the emergency department after being found unresponsive by his father. The father states that he last saw his son the night before, at which time an argument had ensued. He found his son unresponsive in bed with vomitus around his mouth and holding his upper extremities in a tonic flexed position. Emergency medical services were mobilized, and the patient was endotracheally intubated in the field by paramedics using rapid-sequence techniques. Medications in the home include desipramine, quinapril (Accupril), simvastatin (Zocor), pioglitazone (Actos), and ibuprofen. Mom is currently hospitalized for "chemical abuse."

Physical Examination: Temperature 36.5° C, pulse 149/min, blood pressure 90/40 mmHg; oxygen saturation 100% on 100% inspired oxygen; weight 70 kg. General: well-developed, unresponsive and artificially ventilated. HEENT: atraumatic, pupils mid-position and reactive, oropharynx with endotracheal tube in place. Chest: clear to auscultation. Cardiovascular: tachycardic, regular rhythm, no murmurs, gallops, or rubs. Abdomen: normoactive bowel sounds, soft, nondistended. Extremities: good pulses and brisk capillary refill; light green vomitus found on right arm. Neuromuscular: paralyzed and sedated, symmetrical deep tendon reflexes, intact cranial nerves.

Laboratory Findings: Hemogram: WBC 6500/µl, hemoglobin 3.5 g/dL, platelets 203,000/µL. Coagulation profile: PT 12.7 seconds, aPTT 29.2 seconds, fibrinogen 118, fibrin split products negative. Serum chemistries: sodium 140 mEq/L, potassium 3.7 mEq/L, chloride 102 mEq/L, bicarbonate 19 mEq/L, BUN 13 mg/dL, creatinine 1.3 mg/dL, glucose 240 mg/dL, calcium 8.6 mEq/L, magnesium 1.9 mEq/L, phosphorus 5.8 mEq/L. Arterial blood gas (100% FiO_2): pH 7.19, $PaCO_2$ 51 mmHg, PaO_2 498 mmHg, base excess −9.3, osmolality 310 mEq/L. Toxicology testing: serum negative for salicylate, acetaminophen, and ethanol; urine immunoassay negative for common drugs of abuse. Electrocardiogram: sinus tachycardia, QRS 0.98 ms, QT_c 0.457 ms, ST depressions II, III, avF, V3-6. Chest radiograph: perihilar pulmonary edema bilaterally, endotracheal tube in good position (see figure).

Question: Which of the available drugs was most likely responsible for this boy's toxic syndrome?

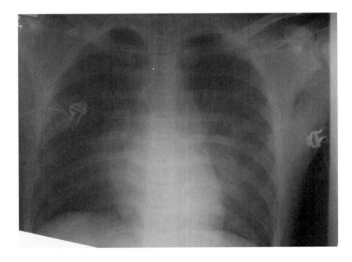

Diagnosis: Ibuprofen overdose

Discussion: Ibuprofen is commonly taken in overdose, but rarely causes serious toxicity. However, patients with massive ingestions can develop life-threatening processes including coma, seizures, metabolic acidosis, acute renal failure, gastrointestinal (GI) bleeding, liver dysfunction, and hemodynamic instability.

Ibuprofen is a nonsteroidal anti-inflammatory (NSAID) medication available over the counter that has anti-inflammatory, antipyretic and analgesic properties. It primarily inhibits prostaglandin synthesis. It is rapidly absorbed by the GI tract and with a single therapeutic dose has a peak concentration within 1 to 2 hours of ingestion. The serum half-life is 1 to 2.5 hours and does not appear to be prolonged after overdosage. It is highly protein bound (99%) and has a small volume of distribution (0.18 L/kg). Elimination is via hepatic metabolism, with excretion of inactive metabolites via the kidney.

In therapeutic doses, the most common side effects of taking ibuprofen include GI discomfort and rashes. In overdose, GI symptoms such as nausea, vomiting, and epigastric pain usually predominate. In large overdoses, ibuprofen can become a central nervous system (CNS) depressant and cause signs and symptoms ranging from mild sedation to coma. It is postulated that ibuprofen may have a central "opioid" effect. Interestingly, some animal studies have suggested that naloxone can reverse the analgesic effects of NSAID. Anecdotal reports exist describing reversal of ibuprofen-induced CNS depression with naloxone.

Renal failure is a potential but uncommon complication of overdosage. It may develop as a result of decreased renal blood flow secondary to inhibition of prostaglandin production and typically resolves with standard support measures. Dialysis is rarely required. Metabolic acidosis has also been reported after ibuprofen overdose and is likely to be multifactorial in etiology. Respiratory complications may include development of an eosinophilic pneumonia and noncardiogenic pulmonary edema. It is speculated that prostaglandin inhibition plays a role in the development of acute respiratory distress syndrome associated with ibuprofen. Serum ibuprofen levels have not been found to have prognostic value, and are not routinely available.

The present patient was given activated charcoal for gastric decontamination, and his metabolic acidosis was corrected with sodium bicarbonate. Intravenous fluids restored intravascular volume. Over the next 12 hours the boy regained alertness, and his artificial airway was discontinued. He subsequently admitted to eating thirty 600-mg tablets of ibuprofen about 5 hours prior to presentation. Gas chromatography with mass spectroscopy of the vomitus found on the patient detected nearly pure ibuprofen. An initial serum ibuprofen level was 1707.5 mg/L. Upon recovery, the boy was diagnosed with major depression and was discharged to a psychiatric hospital.

Clinical Pearls

1. Massive ingestion of ibuprofen can lead to life-threatening complications including coma, seizures, metabolic acidosis, acute renal failure, gastrointestinal bleeding, liver dysfunction, and hemodynamic instability.

2. Routine ibuprofen levels are not of prognostic value.

3. Patients who ingest less that 100 mg/kg of ibuprofen are unlikely to become symptomatic.

4. Patients who are not symptomatic within 4 hours of ibuprofen ingestion are unlikely to subsequently become symptomatic.

REFERENCES

1. Easley RB, Altemeier III WA: Central nervous system manifestations of an ibuprofen overdose reversed by naloxone. Pediatr Emerg Care 16:39-41, 2000.
2. Seifert SA, Bronstein AC, McGuire T: Massive ibuprofen ingestion with survival. J Toxicol Clin Toxicol 38:55-57, 2000.
3. Nonsteroidal anti-inflammatory drugs In Ellenhorn MJ (ed): Ellenhorn's Medial Toxicology, 2nd ed. Baltimore, MD, Williams and Wilkins, 1997, pp 196-206.
4. Zuckerman GB, Uy CC: Shock, metabolic acidosis, and coma following ibuprofen overdose in a child. Annals Pharmacother 29:869-871, 1995.
5. Le HT, Bosse GM, Tsai Y: Ibuprofen overdose complicated by renal failure, adult respiratory distress syndrome and metabolic acidosis. J Toxicol Clin Toxicol 32:315-320, 1994.
6. McElwee NE, Veltri JC, Bradford DC, et al: A prospective, population-based study of acute ibuprofen overdose: Complications are rare and routine serum levels not warranted. Ann Emerg Med 19:657-662, 1990.

Robert Marsan, Jr. BS
Francis DeRoos MD

PATIENT 47

A 26-year-old woman with nausea and vomiting after eating mushrooms

A 26-year-old woman presents with nausea and vomiting. Three hours prior to presentation she ate a meal consisting primarily of sautéed mushrooms that her uncle recently collected (see figure). Her uncle immigrated from Hungary, where he was an accomplished woodsman and mushroom forager, about 18 months ago. Last week she had eaten a few of these same mushrooms and had developed some mild nausea and 1 day of loose stools, but no fevers, vomiting, or abdominal pain.

Physical Examination: Temperature 36.8° C, pulse 94/min, respirations 16/min, blood pressure 110/68 mmHg. General: uncomfortable and actively vomiting. HEENT: anicteric, mucosa dry. Abdomen: nondistended, nontender, normally active bowel sounds. Neuromuscular: alert, awake, cooperative, motor/sensory intact, reflexes normal and symmetrical.

Laboratory Findings: Serum chemistries: HCO_3^- 23 mmol/L, anion gap 9 mmol/L, normal hepatic aminotransferases. Coagulation profile: normal.

Question: Which component of the history is most important for predicting this patient's prognosis?

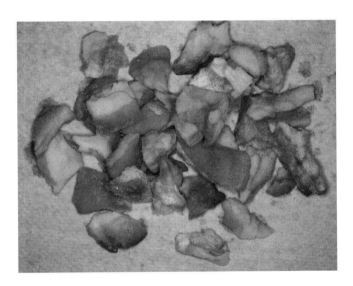

Answer: Time frame. Typically the first symptoms in mushroom poisoning are gastrointestinal (GI) in nature. Symptoms that begin within the first 4 hours are almost always self-limited and consist most commonly of nausea, vomiting, and loose stools. Those that develop after 6 hours ominously suggest ingestion of highly toxic mushrooms (e.g., hepatotoxic).

Discussion: Approximately 10,000 cases of mushroom ingestion exposures are reported to United States poison control centers each year. Common exposure scenarios include curiosity-driven toddler ingestions, foragers collecting mushrooms for food (particularly among several immigrant populations), and use of mushrooms for their hallucinogenic properties. Of these, roughly 5% result in moderate poisoning and 0.3% result in severe toxicity including hepatic failure and death. Cyclopeptide-containing mushrooms account for over 90% of the annual deaths from mushroom ingestions worldwide. In the U.S. they are commonly found in the cool coastal areas of the western states, and less commonly within mid-Atlantic and northeastern forests.

Mushrooms are fungi that consist of a branching network of mycelium, a fruiting body, and spores. The fruiting body, the component usually ingested, is highly variable among species, and only a trained mycologist can accurately differentiate them. Of the 10,000 or so varieties of mushrooms that have been identified, only 52 cause serious symptoms, and only 32 have been associated with fatalities. Therefore, accurate **identification** of mushrooms may help with treatment; your regional poison center may be helpful in this regard. However, often this is not feasible, and treatment is based on signs, symptoms, and regional knowledge of local mushroom flora. Occasionally, poisonous mushrooms can appear almost identical to edible mushrooms from other parts of the world, as may have been the case with this patient. Because mushroom gathering is a common part of many cultures throughout the world, recent immigrants to the U.S. are at greatest risk of serious injury from mushrooms.

Poisonous mushrooms can be separated into two main categories based on the time of onset of initial GI symptoms: those that produce nausea and vomiting early, typically within 4 hours after ingestion, and those that do not produce GI symptoms until at least 6 hours after ingestion. These **"late presenting" mushrooms** are responsible for hepatic and renal failure and the few mushroom deaths annually in the U.S.

Mushroom species that cause **early-onset gastroenteritis** are the most common type encountered. Several different toxins have been isolated from this type including hemolysin and bolesatine. Ingestion of these mushrooms typically produces symptoms such as crampy abdominal pain, vomiting, and diarrhea within 1 to 4 hours after ingestion. This gastroenteritis is generally self-limited, but may be severe enough to cause significant dehydration and mild GI distress and persist for up to 48 hours. Treatment is supportive, with intravenous fluids and antiemetic pharmacotherapy as needed. Persistent, worsening, or recurrent symptoms should alert the physician that the ingestion may involve multiple varieties of mushrooms.

Some mushrooms cause rapid **neurological symptoms** as well. Symptoms occur within hours and are seen in foragers or in patients who ingest mushrooms for their hallucinogenic effects. The main neurological toxins encountered in these various mushrooms are psilocybin, ibotenic acid, and muscarine. Psilocybin is found in *Psilocybe* or "magic" mushrooms, resembles LSD mechanistically, and is both an agonist and antagonist at multiple serotonergic receptors in the brain. It produces altered perception, changes in mood, hallucinations, and distortion of time. Ibotenic acid, which is found in *Amanita muscaria* and *A. pantherina*, can be converted to muscimol, which inhibits GABA and alters serotonin and catecholamine levels, producing visual hallucinations, myoclonus, and even seizures. Muscarine is found in many *Clitocybe* and *Inocybe* mushrooms. Muscarine stimulates postganglioninc cholinergic receptors and induces the cholinergic toxidrome remembered by the mnemonic SLUDGE (salivation, lacrimation, urination, diarrhea, gastrointestinal upset, emesis). In addition, bradycardia, bronchospasm, and miosis are part of this cholinergic toxidrome.

These neurological effects typically present within 30 minutes and last 2 to 6 hours. Treatment is supportive. Benzodiazepines can be titrated carefully to treat anxiety, agitation, and seizures. Atropine can be used to reverse muscarinic symptoms but should generally only be used when severe bradycardia or respiratory distress from severe bronchorrea and excessive salivation is present.

Mushrooms of the Coprinum family, known as "inky caps," contain coprine which, after being hydrolated during cooking, can inhibit hepatic acetaldehyde dehydrogenase. This produces the **"disulfiram reaction"** after ingesting ethanol, which manifests as flushing, diaphoresis, headache, tachycardia, nausea, and vomiting. This enzyme inhibition may be present for up to 2 days following ingestion of a significant amount of Coprinum mushrooms. It is treated like any disulfiram reaction with IV hydration, antiemetics, and monitoring of serum electrolytes.

The vast majority of morbidity and mortality from mushroom poisoning come from mushrooms that cause late-onset of symptoms—specifically, the **cyclopeptide-containing mushrooms**. These include a number of species such as *Amanita phalloides* ("death cap"), *A. verosa* ("destroying angel"), *A. verna, Galerina autumnalis* ("autumn skullcap"), *G. venenata, Lepiota helveola,* and *L. chlorophyllum*. There are two well-characterized cyclopeptides found in *A. phalloides*. Alpha-amanitin, an amatoxin, is a heat-stabile octapeptide, which is absorbed by the intestinal mucosa and taken to the liver. There it binds to RNA-polymerase II and inhibits protein synthesis, causing rapid destruction of hepatocytes, acute hepatitis, and liver failure. Because alpha-amatoxin undergoes repeated cycles of enterohepatic circulation, there is some support for the use of multiple doses of activated charcoal when treating these patients. Phallatoxins are also found in *Amanita* species. They cause disruption of cell membranes along with inhibition of protein synthesis and are likely responsible for the initial GI upset seen with these mushrooms. Cyclopeptide-containing mushroom poisoning is often described in stages, with GI distress as the first stage. The second stage of poisoning occurs after the GI symptoms have improved somewhat, but prior to manifestation of significant signs and symptoms of hepatic injury and dysfunction. The third stage of hepatic and sometimes renal dysfunction typically begins 48 to 72 hours after ingestion. Signs and symptoms include right upper quadrant abdominal tenderness, jaundice, asterixis, coagulopathy, electrolyte abnormalities, and encephalopathy. Death can occur in up to 25% of patients from worsening hepatic and renal failure, typically within 4 to 9 days after ingestion.

Patients may present during the initial gastroenteritis or during the period of hepatic failure. In the first case, it is critical to determine an accurate ingestion history—specifically, the timing relative to ingestion and onset of symptoms. While treatment is generally supportive and symptom oriented regardless of the mushroom ingested, for those at high risk for cyclopeptide ingestions, because of the significant risk of death, aggressive yet poorly studied treatments may be considered. These include multiple doses of activated charcoal, high-dose penicillin G, thioctic acid, cimetidine, and early hemoperfusion. All patients are likely to benefit from fluid replacement and frequent monitoring for hypoglycemia at a minimum of every 2 hours, along with baseline and daily liver function tests (LFTs), electrolytes, and coagulation studies for 3–5 days. Once LFT abnormalities are present, they should be monitored 2–4 times per day. Prompt referral or transfer to a transplant center is advisable if encephalopathy or progressive coagulopathy develop. Orthotopic or auxillary liver transplants have been successful in preserving or maintaining life during the recovery phase of amanita poisoning. Patients can be discharged after LFTs begin to normalize or after negative observation for signs and symptoms of toxicity for 24 hours.

The present patient likely ate poisonous mushrooms that appeared similar to edible mushrooms her Hungarian uncle knew about in Europe. Her gastroenteritis symptoms began within 3 hours, suggesting that this was not a hepatotoxic mushroom ingestion. She was treated with 3 L of normal saline and intravenous antiemetic drugs, and in 4 hours was feeling much improved and able to tolerate fluids without producing nausea or vomiting.

Clinical Pearls

1. In general, U.S. patients who present with gastrointestinal symptoms within a few hours of a mushroom ingestion are at little risk of hepatic injury.

2. Treatment of most mushroom poisonings is supportive, with hydration and symptomatic relief.

3. If ingestion of cyclopeptide-containing mushrooms, such as an *Amanita phalloides* or *Galerina autumnalis,* is suspected, monitoring of hepatic and renal function is warranted. If abnormalities such as hypoglycemia, coagulopathy, or encephalopathy develop, strongly consider referral to a liver transplant center.

REFERENCES

1. Shih RD: Plants, mushrooms, and herbal medications. In Marx JA (ed): Rosen's Emergency Medicine: Concepts and Clinical Practice, 5th ed. St. Louis, Mosby, 2002, pp 2198-2207.
2. Schneider SM: Mushrooms. In Ford MD (ed): Clinical Toxicology. Philadelphia, W.B. Saunders, 2001, pp 899-907.
3. Rosenthal P: Auxiliary liver transplantation for toxic mushroom poisoning. J Pediatr 138:449-450, 2001.
4. Pomerance HH, Barness EG, Kohli-Kumar M, et al: A 15-year-old boy with fulminant hepatic failure. J Pediatr. 137(1): 114-118, 2000.
5. Anonymous: From the Centers for Disease Control and Prevention. *Amanita phalloides* mushroom poisoning—northern California, January 1997. JAMA 278:16-17, 1997.

PATIENT 48

A 2-year-old boy who ingested his grandmother's blood sugar pills

A 2-year-old boy is discovered with an open bottle of sustained-release glyburide (5-mg) tablets. He was not witnessed eating any of the tablets, but five are unaccounted for after counting the pills. The Poison Control Center recommended hospital evaluation since even one ingested glyburide tablet might produce symptomatic hypoglycemia. Five hours after presumed ingestion the boy becomes lethargic, sweaty, and tachycardic. His blood sugar is noted to be 42 mg/dL. He is fed juice, and intravenous fluids containing 10% dextrose are administered. Despite such supportive therapy, the symptomatic hypoglycemia is persistent.

Physical Examination: Temperature 36.8° C, pulse 134/min, respirations 20/min, blood pressure 98/58 mmHg. General: somnolent. HEENT: slight mydriasis of pupils. Chest: normal. Cardiovascular: tachycardia. Abdomen: soft. Skin: diaphoretic.

Laboratory Findings: Serum chemistries: HCO_3^- 19 mEq/L, glucose 35 mg/dL. Urinalysis: small ketones.

Question: What antidotal therapy might be a reasonable next step in the effort to maintain euglycemia in this patient?

Treatment: Octreotide is a synthetic somatostatin analogue useful for the treatment of refractory hypoglycemia resulting from sulfonylurea overdose.

Discussion: Exploratory drug ingestion during childhood represents a large proportion of the poison exposures reported to Poison Control Centers each year. Fortunately, it is uncommon for young children, without intent of self-harm, to become seriously ill following such an exposure to pharmaceutical agents. Some drugs are of theoretical risk to toddler-aged children after ingestion of only a single dose (see table), and oral hypoglycemic agents of the sulfonylurea class are on that list.

Sulfonylurea drugs, such as glyburide, glipizide, tolbutamide, and chlorpropamide, lower blood glucose by stimulating pancreatic insulin secretion, enhancing insulin receptor sensitivity, and inhibiting glycogenolysis. Most children who will become hypoglycemic after glyburide ingestion will do so within 8 hours, but the overnight fast may be a particularly vulnerable period.

The routine use of prophylactic intravenous dextrose solutions is not recommended, as this practice may mask the onset of toxic hypoglycemia. Symptomatic hypoglycemia is, perhaps, best treated through enteral administration of carbohydrates. Feed the patient! Patients unable to drink or in need of extra sugar administration, may be treated with intravenous dextrose. As bolus dosing of dextrose may lead to a compensatory insulin release, a continuous infusion of dextrose may be theoretically preferable.

Diazoxide was once considered first-line therapy for sulfonylurea-induced refractory hypoglycemia, but poor efficacy and significant side effects were frequently encountered. Recently, the drug octreotide has been used with success in this setting and has become the favored treatment for refractory hypoglycemia from glyburide overdose. No formal dosing trials have been performed. Administration of 2 mcg/kg (maximum 50 mcg) of octreotide intravenously or subcutaneously is a reasonable starting dose, and may be repeated every 12 hours as needed.

The present patient was fed, administered 10% dextrose intravenously, and given 2 mcg/kg of octreotide with subsequent stabilization of his blood glucose. No further doses of octreotide were deemed necessary, and intravenous fluids were weaned over the next 18 hours. The patient was well upon hospital discharge.

Drugs That Can Be Dangerous to a Young Child in Only One or Two Doses

Benzocaine	Lindane
Beta-adrenergic antagonists (especially propranolol)	Methadone
	Phenothiazines
Calcium channel antagonists	Quinidine
Camphor	Quinine
Chloroquine	Sulfonylureas
Clonidine	Theophylline
Cyclic antidepressants	
Diphenoxylate	

Adapted from Osterhoudt KC: The toxic toddler: Drugs that can kill in small doses. Contemp Pediatr 17:73-88, 2000.

Clinical Pearls

1. Even a single sulfonylurea dose can cause symptomatic hypoglycemia in a toddler-aged child.

2. Prophylactic intravenous dextrose after an exploratory sulfonylurea ingestion may mask the onset of hypoglycemia.

3. Octreotide is a useful pharmacological adjunct for the treatment of refractory hypoglycemia often seen after sulfonylurea poisoning.

REFERENCES

1. Osterhoudt KC: This treat is not so sweet–exploratory sulfonylurea ingestion by a toddler. Pediatr Case Rev 3:215-217, 2003.
2. Howland MA: Antidotes in depth: octreotide. In Goldfrank LR, Flomenbaum NE, Lewin NA, et al (eds): Goldfrank's Toxicologic Emergencies, 7th ed. New York, McGraw-Hill, 2002, pp. 611-613.
3. Spiller HA: Management of sulfonylurea ingestions. Pediatr Emerg Care 15:227-230, 1999.

Angela Mills, MD
Jeanmarie Perrone, MD

PATIENT 49

A 22-year-old woman found somnolent in a public restroom

A 22-year-old woman was found somnolent with shallow respirations lying in a public restroom with a syringe in her arm. Paramedics were summoned and assisted her respirations with bag-valve-mask while intravenous access was obtained. Naloxone, 0.4 mg, was administered intravenously. The patient became more alert en route to the hospital.

Physical Examination: Temperature 37.3° C, pulse 58/min, respirations 8/min, blood pressure 110/70 mmHg. General: young, thin, awake. HEENT: pupils pinpoint bilaterally. Chest: shallow breaths, clear to auscultation. Cardiovascular: regular without gallops or murmurs. Abdomen: normal. Extremities: normal. Skin: "track marks" to bilateral upper extremities (see figure). Neuromuscular: normal.

Laboratory Findings: Hemogram: WBC 7000/μL, hemoglobin 15 g/dL, platelets 380,000/μL. Serum chemistries: sodium 142 mEq/L, potassium 4.3mEq/L, chloride 106 mEq/L, bicarbonate 24mEq/L, BUN 21 mg/dL, creatinine 0.9 mg/dL, glucose 75 mg/dL. Arterial blood gas (room air): pH 7.32, $PaCO_2$ 50, PaO_2 55. Urine toxicology screen: positive for opioids. Electrocardiogram: sinus bradycardia, normal intervals. Chest radiograph: normal.

Question: What findings suggest that the patient will respond to naloxone?

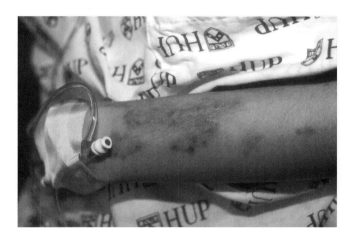

Diagnosis: Somnolence, respiratory depression, and small pupils suggest heroin overdose.

Discussion: Naloxone is an opioid antagonist that will reverse the respiratory depression and lethargy associated with opioid poisoning. The triad of central nervous system depression, hypoventilation, and miosis comprises the **opioid toxidrome**. The initial management of opioid intoxication is assessment of airway patency, ventilation, and perfusion. If there is adequate ventilation, then observation is sufficient until lethargy resolves. Patients with respiratory depression merit bag-valve-mask ventilation followed by administration of naloxone, an opioid antagonist. The recommended initial dose of naloxone is 0.2–0.4 mg intravenously followed by a higher dose (1–2 mg up to 10 mg) if there is no response within 1–3 minutes. Low doses are used initially to prevent the precipitation of acute opioid withdrawal among opioid-dependent individuals. Naloxone may also be given by intramuscular, subcutaneous, and endotracheal routes, if necessary.

History and physical examination are sufficient to make the diagnosis of opioid poisoning. Ancillary studies are usually unnecessary; however, they may be indicated to evaluate for complications of opioid toxicity. Laboratory testing is typically unremarkable, with the possible exception of respiratory acidosis with hypoxemia on arterial blood gas analysis. Intravenous heroin use may lead to noncardiogenic pulmonary edema, which may be visualized on chest radiography. Most qualitative urine toxicology screens detect opioids. Certain specific screens can differentiate heroin from morphine or methadone, thereby distinguishing opioids prescribed in hospital from those taken illicitly prior to hospital arrival. A differential diagnosis of opioid toxicity may include hypoglycemia, hypoxemia, hypothermia, intracranial hemorrhage or infarct, and intoxication with other drugs including sedative-hypnotic agents, clonidine, phenothiazines, and tramadol.

Patients who respond to naloxone and maintain adequate respirations should be observed in the emergency department for 3–4 hours. Naloxone loses efficacy in 20–40 minutes, and if inadequate ventilation recurs, repeat doses or continuous infusion may be needed. Endotracheal intubation may be beneficial if there is poor oxygenation, an inability to ventilate, or continued hypoventilation despite naloxone. Naloxone may precipitate an acute withdrawal syndrome characterized by agitation, hypertension, tachycardia, piloerection, lacrimation, emesis, diarrhea, and abdominal cramping. Other complications of intravenous drug use include endocarditis, rhabdomyolysis, cellulitis and skin abcesses, and infection with HIV and hepatitis.

Heroin and other opioid abuse (Oxycontin, Percocet) account for much morbidity and many preventable deaths in the United States. Heroin is more lipid-soluble than other opioids, allowing rapid absorption across the blood-brain barrier and leading to the drug's euphoric and toxic effects. Heroin often contains adulterants or contaminants that may lead to further toxicity. Deaths from heroin intoxication are associated with concomitant use of other drugs, especially alcohol, and the use of heroin after abstinence. The majority of heroin-related fatalities occur in long-term heroin users with significant opioid dependence.

The present patient received a second dose of naloxone in the emergency department due to increasing lethargy and inadequate respirations. The patient was subsequently observed for 4 hours and then discharged with referral to a substance abuse program.

Clinical Pearls

1. The opioid toxidrome is characterized by lethargy, respiratory depression, and miosis.

2. Opioid-like drugs, such as clonidine and tramadol, may mimic the opioid toxidrome, but manifest an inadequate or partial response to naloxone.

3. Small initial doses of naloxone (0.2–0.4 mg) should be used in adults, to avoid precipitating withdrawal in opioid-dependent individuals.

4. As the duration of naloxone is shorter than that of many opioids, it is prudent to observe patients who respond to naloxone for the recurrence of opioid toxicity.

REFERENCES

1. Nelson LS: Opioids. In Goldfrank LR, Flomenbaum NE, Lewin NA, et al (eds): Goldfrank's Toxicologic Emergencies. New York, McGraw-Hill, 2002, pp 901-923.
2. Hantsch CE, Gummin DD: Opioids. In Marx JA, Hockberger RS, Walls RM, et al (eds): Rosen's Emergency Medicine. St. Louis, Mosby, Inc., 2002, pp 2180-2186.
3. Sporer KA: Acute heroin overdose. Ann Intern Med 130:584-590, 1999.
4. Kanof PD, Handelsman L, Aronson MJ, et al: Clinical characteristics of naloxone-precipitated withdrawal in human opioid-dependent subjects. J Phamacol Exper Ther 260:355-363, 1992.
5. Hoffman JR, Schriger DL, Luos JS: The empiric use of naloxone in patients with altered mental satus: A reappraisal. Ann Emerg Med 20:246-252, 1991.

PATIENT 50

A 2-year-old girl with vomiting and metabolic acidosis

A 2-year-old girl has been vomiting for a few hours and recently has developed diarrhea. Her parents are concerned because she is becoming progressively lethargic. She has had no symptoms of a viral upper respiratory infection and has not had fever.

Physical Examination: Temperature 37.8° C, pulse 157/min, respirations 30/min, blood pressure 88/48 mmHg. General: ill-appearing, pale, somnolent. HEENT: normal. Chest: normal. Cardiovascular: tachycardia. Abdomen: diffusely tender without guarding or rebound tenderness. Extremities: capillary refill mildly delayed. Skin: diaphoretic. Neuromuscular: intact cranial nerves.

Laboratory Findings: Hemogram: WBC 16,200/μL, hemoglobin 11.2/dL, platelets 468,000/μL. Serum chemistries: sodium 138 mEq/L, potassium 4.0 mEq/L, chloride 100 mEq/l, bicarbonate 15 mEq/L, glucose 152 mg/dL. Urinalysis: trace ketones, trace glucose. Stool for occult blood: positive. Abdominal radiograph: see figure.

Questions: What drug ingestion is responsible for this girl's illness? What antidotal therapy is warranted?

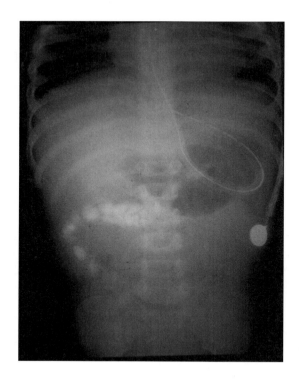

Diagnosis and Treatment: The radiographic opacities corroborate a suspicion of iron poisoning. In addition to intravenous fluids and good supportive care, therapy with deferoxamine is warranted.

Discussion: A child with recalcitrant vomiting, central nervous system (CNS) depression, tachycardia, and metabolic acidosis presents a broad differential diagnosis including medical, surgical, and toxicological maladies. Important considerations might include gastroenteritis, diabetic ketoacidosis, Reye's syndrome, bacterial infection, and intussusception. Exploratory drug ingestions that can present in this fashion include salicylate, theophylline, digoxin, and iron intoxication. Several drugs may be opaque when visualized radiographically (see table), and the appearance of the radiograph in this case suggests iron poisoning.

Highly concentrated iron is often prescribed in large quantities to anemic patients in the form of ferrous sulfate and to pregnant patients in the form of prenatal vitamins. These preparations may not be thought of as "serious" medications by parents, as they often are formulated in a manner that resembles candy. Acute iron poisoning has long been a leading cause of pediatric overdose mortality, but this situation appears to be improving since the 1997 United States Food and Drug Administration mandate that products containing more than 30 mg of elemental iron per dose need to be distributed in unit dose packaging.

Toxins That May Be Opaque with Plain Radiography

"Body packer" drug ingestions
Calcium carbonate
Chloral hydrate and halogenated hydrocarbons
Fluorinated psychotropic medications (e.g., trifluoperazine)
Metals iron, lead, mercury
Some sustained-release and enteric-coated preparations

Toxicity from iron can be expected if more than 20 mg/kg of elemental iron is ingested, and severe toxicity is expected at doses above 60 mg/kg. Severe acute iron poisoning is a multi-system illness including gastrointestinal irritation, shock, metabolic acidosis, CNS depression, and sometimes hepatotoxicity, coagulation dysfunction, and pulmonary toxicity. Hyperglycemia and leukocytosis commonly accompany iron poisoning; however, these findings are not sensitive or specific enough to be used diagnostically. A serum iron level, obtained 4–6 hours after ingestion, may help in prognostication and therapeutic decision making. A serum iron concentration of >500 µg/dL usually correlates with clinical toxicity. In the absence of a serum iron level, the presence of a wide anion gap metabolic acidosis may be the best laboratory marker for toxicity.

Iron binds poorly to activated charcoal, but whole bowel irrigation (WBI) can be considered. The effectiveness of WBI can often be monitored radiographically. Shock, dehydration, and acidosis should be managed with aggressive intravenous fluid and electrolyte therapy. Chelation therapy with intravenous deferoxamine will hasten excretion of iron in the urine. Candidates for deferoxamine administration include ill iron-poisoned patients, patients with 4- to 6-hour serum iron concentrations >500 µg/dl, and patients with large ingestions and positive radiography. Typical recommended deferoxamine dosing is 15–30 mg/kg/hr until clinical improvement is noted, serum iron drops to less than 150 µg/dL, and metabolic acidosis resolves.

The present patient was treated with intravenous fluids, antiemetic drugs, and nasogastric WBI with Golytely at 500 ml/hr. Her serum iron level at presentation was 612 µg/dL. Deferoxamine was administered for 18 hours. The child seemed to have some persistent anorexia and abdominal discomfort, but otherwise recovered uneventfully.

Clinical Pearls

1. Iron poisoning in children may mimic many other illnesses with gastrointestinal symptoms and should be considered in young children with recalcitrant vomiting and acidosis.

2. Pregnancy is a high-risk period for exploratory iron ingestion by toddler-aged children.

3. The presence of a wide anion gap metabolic acidosis may be the best laboratory predictor of iron toxicity.

4. Special laboratory methods are needed to accurately measure serum iron levels in the presence of deferoxamine therapy.

REFERENCES

1. Perrone J: Iron. In Goldfrank LR, Flomenbaum NE, Lewin NA, et al (eds): Goldfrank's Toxicologic Emergencies, 7th ed. New York, McGraw-Hill, 2002, pp 548-562.
2. Henretig FM, Drott HR, Osterhoudt KC: Acute iron poisoning. In Shaw LM (ed): The Clinical Toxicology Laboratory: Contemporary Practice of Poisoning Evaluation. Washington, AACC Press, 2001, pp 401-409.

PATIENT 51

A 16-year-old boy with bizarre behavior

After a night out with friends, a 16-year-old boy returned home confused and "not himself." During transport to the hospital he became agitated and combative. The patient does not provide any explanation for his behavior. He has a history of depression and illicit drug use and is prescribed venlafaxine, 150 mg daily.

Physical Examination: Temperature 37.1° C, pulse 138/min; respirations 20/min; blood pressure 145/81 mmHg. General: anxious and fearful; repeatedly says "look at it" or "look at them" and then becomes tearful. HEENT: pupils are 5 mm, equal, and reactive; neck is supple. Chest: normal. Cardiovascular: tachycardia with normal rhythm and no ectopy. Neuromuscular: awake, alert, and answers simple questions appropriately; motor function is grossly intact.

Laboratory Findings: Hemogram: normal. Serum chemistries: normal. Blood ethanol level: undetectable. Urine immunoassay for drugs of abuse: positive for cannabinoids.

Questions: What drug might be the cause of this patient's agitation? How should he be managed?

Diagnosis and Treatment: The patient's behavior is likely due to intoxication with a hallucinogen, such as lysergic acid diethylamide (LSD). He should be placed in a quiet room and spoken to in a calm manner. The benzodiazepine class of drugs may be useful for managing severe agitation.

Discussion: LSD is the most potent of a class of drugs known as hallucinogens or psychedelics. Specifically, LSD is a synthetic **lysergamide**; morning glory plants are a source of naturally occurring compounds of this class. The **indolealkylamines** include N,N-dimethyltryptamine, the ultra–short-acting agent referred to as the "businessman's high," and psilocybin, which is derived from several species of hallucinogenic mushrooms. Mescaline, from the peyote cactus, and MDMA, a synthetic drug better known as ecstasy, are **phenylethylamines**. Drugs acting by different mechanisms but still classified as hallucinogens include marijuana and anticholinergic agents. The lysergamides, indolealkylamines, and phenylethylamines are believed to act by a common mechanism. Each has a structural similarity to serotonin (5-HT) and acts as an agonist at serotonin receptors or causes serotonin release. Hallucinogenic potency has been specifically linked to affinity for $5-HT_2$ receptors.

LSD has had an illustrious history following its accidental synthesis in 1938. The drug was used as an "entactogen" to aid in psychotherapy prior to its widespread use and subsequent banning in the 1960s. It is extremely potent, with usual doses of 20 to 80 μg impregnated on tiny sheets of blotter paper for oral consumption (see figure). It is long acting, with duration of effect around 12 hours. The drug is also sold in liquid, pill, or powder forms and is typically ingested orally.

LSD, like other hallucinogens, can cause profound alterations in perception and awareness. The user may experience distortions in time perception, intensified sensory input, and thought disorder. Colors may appear brighter, halos appear around objects, body parts such as faces appear distorted, and vivid geometric images called **pareidolias** may be visible. Synesthesia, which involves blending of sensory input so that colors seem to be heard and sounds visualized, may occur. Hallucinations are most commonly visual, but may involve any of the senses.

The LSD-intoxicated patient may demonstrate mild sympathomimetic stimulation including tachycardia, tachypnea, hypertension, diaphoresis, and mydriasis. Patients are usually awake and alert and able to give a history of their drug use, though they may appear distracted, internally stimulated, or agitated and need to be refocused. Diagnosis is usually based solely on the history and clinical presentation. Hallucinogen intoxication may be differentiated from other causes of drug-induced agitation by the *absence of delirium*.

LSD use may result in a number of toxic effects, the most common being dysphoria and a severe anxiety reaction or "**bad trip**." The anxiety may be precipitated by the hallucinations, depersonalization, and disordered thought. There is some debate surrounding the extent of longer-lasting psychiatric effects from the drug. Long-term

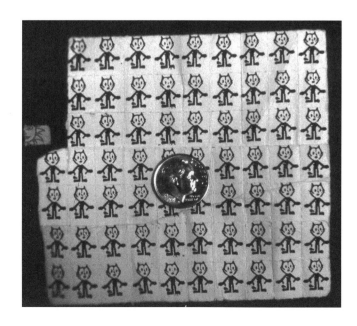

psychotic episodes after use are likely related to preexisting psychiatric disease. In **"flashbacks,"** formally termed hallucinogen persisting perception disorder, patients relive perceptual disturbances such as hallucinations that were experienced with the drug's initial use. These episodes can be quite distressing for some patients; they may occur for several years, and there is no effective therapy. Laboratory testing for the drug is rarely available, and detection is difficult due to the minute quantities ingested. Drug screening may be useful to rule out any coingestants and to narrow the differential diagnosis.

Treatment of LSD intoxication primarily involves decreasing the patient's sensory input and anxiety. Many clinicians favor the "talkdown" method: the patient is placed in a quiet area and calmly spoken to, reoriented, and reassured. This requires the continued presence of a person to help interpret sensory misperceptions. Severely agitated or anxious patients may require physical and chemical restraint. Benzodiazepines, such as lorazepam, may be given intravenously or intramuscularly and titrated to effect. Some recommend the concurrent use of an antipsychotic agent, such as haloperidol, to achieve more effective and rapid sedation. There may be a theoretical role for the use of atypical antipsychotic agents for acute LSD intoxication. These agents are generally potent antagonists at 5-HT$_2$ receptors, where LSD is thought to exert its most important effect. The only currently available parenteral atypical antipsychotic agent is ziprasidone, and there are no published data concerning its use in this type of patient.

The current patient was placed in a quiet room and treated with two doses of lorazepam intramuscularly for a total dose of 4 mg. He was subsequently calm, with resolution of his tachycardia and hypertension. He admitted to using LSD earlier in the evening. After 6 hours of observation in the emergency department, the patient appeared essentially normal and was discharged to home.

Clinical Pearls

1. LSD is an extremely potent and long-acting hallucinogen.

2. The LSD-intoxicated patient may be alert and oriented on exam, but also anxious and exhibiting signs of sympathetic excess such as mydriasis and tachycardia. True delirium is absent.

3. Most patients with LSD "toxicity" seek care when the altered sensory input has become overwhelming and precipitates fear and anxiety. They may be safely and effectively treated by decreasing the sensory input: place them in a quiet area with someone who can speak calmly and reassuringly to them.

REFERENCES

1. Tucker JR, Ferm RP: Lysergic acid diethylamide and other hallucinogens. In Goldfrank LR, Flomenbaum NE, Lewin NA, et al (eds): Goldfrank's Toxicologic Emergencies, 7th ed. New York, McGraw-Hill, 2002, pp 1046-1053.
2. Blaho K, Merigian K, Windberry S, et al: Clinical pharmacology of lysergic acid diethylamide: Case reports and review of the treatment of intoxication. Am J Ther 4:211-221, 1997.
3. Abraham HD, Aldridge AM, Gogia P: The psychopharmacolgy of hallucinogens. Neuropsychopharmacol 14:285-298, 1996.
4. Schwartz RH: LSD: Its rise, fall, and renewed popularity among high school students. Ped Clin North Am 42:403-413, 1995.
5. Aghajanian GK: Serotonin and the action of LSD in the brain. Psych Ann 24:137-141, 1994.
6. Miller PL, Gay GR, Ferris KC, Anderson S: Treatment of acute, adverse psychedelic reactions: "I've tripped and I can't get down." J Psych Drugs 24:277-279, 1992.

Anthony W. Rekito, MD
Francis DeRoos, MD

PATIENT 52

A 37-year-old man with a severe coagulopathy

A 37-year-old man was found unconscious in his bed. A cup of green powder was nearby on his nightstand. When paramedics arrived, the patient was noted to be in ventricular fibrillation and respiratory arrest. He was immediately treated with cardiopulmonary resuscitation (CPR), endotracheal intubation, epinephrine, dextrose, naloxone, and thiamine. The patient rapidly regained a sinus rhythm, and he was promptly transported to the emergency department.

Physical Examination: Pulse 120/min; blood pressure 80/50 mmHg. General: unconscious, being ventilated, Glasgow Coma Scale score of 6 (withdraws to pain). HEENT: pupils 4-5 mm and sluggishly reactive to light. Chest: clear to auscultation. Cardiovascular: regular tachycardia without murmur or gallop. Abdomen: normal. Genitourinary: gross hematuria. Rectal: guiac + brown stool. Skin: multiple bruises.

Laboratory Findings: Hemogram: WBC 21,000/μL, hemoglobin 10 g/dL, Hct 28%, platelets 243/μL. Coagulation profile: PT > 30 seconds, PTT > 120 seconds. Serum chemistries: normal. Urinalysis: gross hematuria. Arterial blood gas (100% Fio_2): pH 7.18, $Paco_2$ 38, Pao_2 320. Repeat arterial blood gas after IV fluids (40% Fio_2): pH 7.38, $Paco_2$ 38, Pao_2 139. Head CT (see figure): multiple intracerebral hemorrhages with edema and mass effect.

Questions: What is the most likely identity of the poisonous green powder that led to the coagulopathy and fatal hemorrhage? What is the appropriate therapy for this type of poisoning?

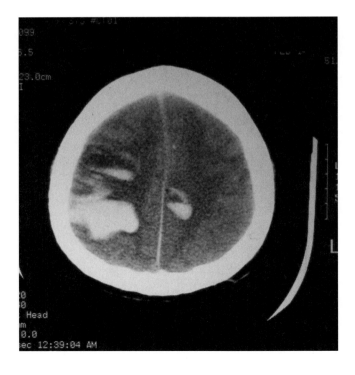

Diagnosis and Treatment: In addition to the green powder at the patient's bedside, the family also found several empty boxes of rat/mouse poison in the garbage. Appropriate care includes resuscitation with crystalloid and packed RBCs (as needed) and reversal of the anticoagulation effects with fresh frozen plasma and high doses of vitamin K_1.

Discussion: **Superwarfarin rodenticides** are responsible for over 90% of rodenticide exposures reported to poison centers in the United States annually. Prior to the widespread use of these relatively safe rodenticides, many extremely toxic compounds had been used as rodenticides (see table) and some can still be found in barns and garages across the U.S. today. All of these rodenticides have significant toxic potential to both rodents and humans alike, and each has unique clinical manifestations that are beyond the scope of this case discussion. We will focus on superwarfarin exposures and poisoning.

Warfarin was the first anticoagulant used as a rodenticide, but because of its relatively short half-life (< 24 hrs), its effective use required rodents to repeatedly ingest the bait or poison over days. In addition, rodents in large cities such as Chicago and New York developed resistance to warfarin, rendering them essentially immune to these baits. Over the past 30 years, more effective anticoagulant rodenticides have been developed, including superwarfarins and indandione derivatives. The superwarfarins include the 4-hydroxycoumarins: brodifacoum, diphenacoum, and bromadiolone. Of these, **brodifacoum** is the compound found in most products sold over the counter in the United States.

The superwarfarins' mechanism of action is identical to that of warfarin, but their half-life is significantly longer. Activation of clotting factors II, VII, IX, X, protein C, and protein S requires vitamin K_1 as a cofactor. The warfarins act by inhibiting vitamin K quinone reductase and vitamin K 2,3-epoxide reductase, preventing the reactivation of inactive vitamin K into the active vitamin K_1. A coagulopathy does not become evident until a clotting factor level falls below 30% of baseline, and because factor VII has the shortest half-life (5 hours), a measurable effect is not evident until at least 15 hours after exposure. Clinical bleeding may develop **2 to 3 days after ingestion**.

The superwarfarins are more lipophilic and occupy the hepatic warfarin-binding sites with greater affinity than their predecessors. The half-life of brodifacoum is approximately 120 days, compared to 24 hours for warfarin. Therefore, *the anticoagulant effect of superwarfarins persists for months*, and this increased potency and prolonged activity make superwarfarins highly toxic.

By far the most dramatic, and potentially fatal, superwarfarin rodenticide exposures involve intentional adult ingestions such as in this case. Fortunately, these cases are extremely unusual. In fact, of the almost 20,000 cases of rodenticide exposures reported to poison centers annually, no more than 5 or 6 are fatal. If a patient presents within a few hours after ingesting a large amount of anticoagulant rodenticide, oral activated charcoal might be considered as a decontamination strategy, and his or her coagulation/bleeding status should be assessed (liver function tests, complete blood count, and coagulation profile [PT/PTT]). Unfortunately, many of these suicidal patients do not present to medical attention until days after their ingestions when severe anticoagulation and bleeding have developed. Clinical

---

"BRATS PANIC" Mnemonic for Rodenticide Chemicals[*]

Chemical	Mechanism of Action
Bromethalin barium carbonate	Uncouples oxidative phosphorylation in the brain/depolarizing neuromuscular blockade
Red squill	Digitalis-like glycoside
Arsenic	Arsenic poisoning
Thallium	Thallium poisoning
Sodium monofluoroacetate/ Strychnine	Inhibits Krebs cycle/glycine antagonist in nervous system
Phosphorus/PNU (Vacor)/ phosphides of zinc	Cellular poison/destroys pancreatic islet cells/phosphine gas
ANTU	Pulmonary edema in adult Norway rats
Norbromide	Intense vasoconstriction in rats
Indandiones	Long-acting coumarin-like compounds
Coumarins/Cholecalciferol	Anticoagulants/hypercalcemia

[*]Modified from initial RATS PANIC mnemonic created by Dr. Jack Snyder, for a teaching session at the Poison Control Center at Philadelphia.

manifestations may include ecchymoses, hematomas, epistaxis, gingival bleeding, gross hematuria, vaginal bleeding, gastrointestinal (GI) bleeding or hemoptysis. In these patients, massive pulmonary, GI, or intracranial hemorrhage typically results in death.

Treatment modalities for anticoagulant ingestion are highly variable and are based upon presentation. The hemorrhaging anticoagulated patient should be resuscitated with oxygen, intravenous fluids, and blood transfusions for volume and fresh frozen plasma or factor concentrates to stop the bleeding. In addition, large doses of vitamin K_1 (phytonadione) should be administered to replace the depleted active vitamin K_1 stores. Remember that vitamin K_1 is active, and after it "activates" the clotting factors, it needs to be recycled by two enzymes to be effective again. This reactivation is what warfarin and the long-acting anticoagulants block. An initial dose of 150 to 200 mg vitamin K_1 orally or via NG tube is reasonable in these patients. This is much larger than the 1 or 2 mg IV that is typically recommended to partially reverse a mildly supratherapeutic but asymptomatic patient on therapeutic warfarin. The intravenous route of vitamin K is controversial because of the reported risk of anaphylactoid reactions and should only be given by slow push at a rate of 1 mg/min. Therefore, some physicians prefer subcutaneous injection (10 mg) when oral administration is not feasible.

The present patient was the recipient of maximal resuscitative efforts focused on decreasing intracerebral pressure with hyperventilation, mannitol, and steroids. The bleeding process was stopped with vitamin K_1 and fresh-frozen plasma. Nevertheless, the patient died within 24 hours.

The management of the *asymptomatic* but measurably anticoagulated adult is somewhat more complex. In these situations, the patient can be treated with oral vitamin K_1 at 50 to 100 mg three times a day for at a minimum of 4 to 6 weeks. This dose may need to be increased if the PT/PTT is not effectively corrected within the first few days of therapy. Hospital admission is typically considered initially to provide a safe environment and intensive psychiatric evaluation and treatment, and, most importantly, to ensure continued compliance with the oral vitamin K_1 regimen and routine coagulation studies. After 4 to 6 weeks, a trial without vitamin K_1 therapy can be performed with close monitoring of coagulation. If there is evidence of recurrent anticoagulation, the vitamin K_1 therapy should be reinstituted for 1 to 2 weeks before repeating the withdrawal trial.

By far the most common rodenticide exposure is an exploratory pediatric ingestion of an unknown but presumably small quantity of an anticoagulant rodenticide. These patients are asymptomatic and rarely develop clinical bleeding or even laboratory evidence of measurable anticoagulation. They do not require any initial laboratory studies, but one dose of activated charcoal may be reasonable depending on the exposure history. Some recommend follow-up in 48 to 72 hours to assess for any evidence of clinical bleeding such as bruising, hematuria, or blood in the stool. These patients should *not* be given any vitamin K_1 initially because this will alter any ability to assess for anticoagulation in 2 to 3 days, and will commit the patient to either multiple repeat physician visits or several weeks of vitamin K_1 therapy. Remember that a patient who presents with any symptoms shortly after a rodenticide ingestion may have ingested other, much less common or discontinued rodenticides—many of which are highly toxic. Consultation with a poison center or clinical toxicologist is recommended, particularly for those patients with marked clinical symptoms initially because this is not consistent with superwarfarin toxicity.

With proper management and avoidance of bleeding complications, full recovery is common. Anticoagulant rodenticide poisonings can range from minor accidental ingestion, to chronic bleeding, to life-threatening hemorrhage and may require long-term therapy.

Clinical Pearls

1. Exploratory pediatric exposures require no laboratory testing emergently, but rather repeat clinical assessment in 48 to 72 hours after exposure.

2. Suicidal or depressed patients with spontaneous bleeding should raise suspicion concerning a possible rodenticide ingestion.

3. Among patients with significant clinical symptoms *immediately following* an unknown rodenticide exposure, anticipate toxins other than superwarfarins that initially present *without* symptoms.

REFERENCES

1. Burkhart KK: Anticoagulant rodenticides. In Ford, Delaney, Ling, Erickson (eds): Clinical Toxicology. Philadelphia, WB Saunders, 2001, pp 848-853.
2. Bruno CR, Howland MA, McKeeking A, Hoffman RS: Long-acting anticoagulant overdose: Brodifacoum kinetics and optimal vitamin K dosing. Ann Emerg Med 36:262-267, 2000.
3. Hui CH, Lie A, Lam CK, et al: Superwarfarin poisoning leading to prolonged coagulopathy. Forensic Science Intern 78: 13-18, 1996.
4. Lipton RA, Klass EM: Human ingestion of "superwarfarin" rodenticide resulting in prolonged anticoagulant effect. JAMA 252:3004-3006, 1988.

PATIENT 53

A 46-year-old firefighter with profound weakness

A firefighter presents on his day off complaining of severe weakness and profound fatigue of 2-month duration. Both problems have been increasing in severity, and his wife has finally forced him to seek medical attention. His medical history is unremarkable. He takes no medications, does not smoke, and does not use illicit drugs. He drinks a case of beer over several weekends each month but does not become "intoxicated."

Physical Examination: Temperature 37.7° C, pulse 115/min, respirations 19/min, blood pressure 100/70 mmHg. Pulse oximetry: 96% in room air. General: awake and oriented to person, place, and time. HEENT: pale conjunctiva. Chest: clear. Cardiovascular: tachycardia, otherwise normal. Abdomen: normal. Neuromuscular: normal. Skin: warm and dry, no rashes.

Laboratory Findings: Hemogram: WBC 27,000/μL, hemoglobin 9.8 g/dL, blood smear consistent with acute myelogenous leukemia (AML).

Questions: Could occupational factors be associated with this patient's AML?

Answer: Yes. Studies of workers in a number of industries with documented **benzene** exposure have revealed a substantially increased risk for the development of acute myelogenous leukemia.

Discussion: Benzene is one of the most important and ubiquitous industrial chemicals in the world today. It is used primarily in the production of other chemicals including styrene and cyclohexane, as well as synthetic rubber, lubricants, pharmaceuticals, and various agricultural chemicals. Benzene is also found as a natural constituent of petroleum. Currently, gasoline in the United States contains less than 2% benzene by volume; however, substantially more benzene is contained in gasoline used in other countries where the benzene concentration may exceed 3–5%.

Firefighters may become exposed to benzene while fighting fires wherein any of the above chemicals or materials are being combusted. While most firefighters employ effective **respiratory protection** during the fire suppression phase of firefighting, strict respiratory protection may not be used at all times by these workers. Since benzene is very efficiently absorbed by both inhalation and ingestion routes, airborne benzene from fires could indeed pose a threat to firefighters. Absorption through the skin may also occur, but skin is not usually considered to be a primary route for exposure. Studies show that roughly half of the amount of benzene that has been inhaled is absorbed after a 4-hour exposure to approximately 50 ppm benzene in air.

Following absorption, benzene is distributed throughout the body, but it is concentrated in the **bone marrow**. It is also found in tissues with high perfusion rates or high lipid content. Benzene is initially metabolized in the liver and later in the bone marrow. Although the total quantity of benzene metabolites is greater in blood than in marrow, the concentrations of those metabolites in the marrow can be substantially higher than in blood. When metabolized in the liver, benzene is oxidized to form phenol, which is its major metabolite. Additional metabolic products include catechol, hydroquinone, and 1,2,4-trihydroxybenzene.

The primary target organ for chronic benzene toxicity is the bone marrow. The metabolites of benzene are thought to be responsible for the marrow toxicity, although the identity of the ultimate bone marrow toxicant is not yet identified. Theoretically, once in the bone marrow, benzene metabolites may bind covalently to cellular macromolecules and thus cause interruption of cell growth and cell replication. The primary histological type of leukemia associated with benzene exposure is AML; however, erythroleukemia and acute myelomonocytic leukemia have also been reported to be associated with benzene exposure. In addition, benzene exposure has been associated with the development of aplastic anemia. A latency period of 5–15 years for benzene-induced leukemia has been identified.

Benzene-induced depression of blood elements tends to slowly reverse once exposure is terminated. However, the situation can be grave once marrow aplasia or leukemic transformation has occurred. Chemotherapy and bone marrow transplants are therapeutic options for leukemia and aplastic anemia, respectively. In the case described here, the firefighter underwent antologous bone marrow transplantation followed by matched donor transplant. Unfortunately, he eventually succumbed to recurrent AML.

Clinical Pearls

1. At adequate doses and situations of exposure, benzene can act as a leukemogen and is associated with the development of acute myelogenous leukemia.

2. Various workers may have medically important exposures to benzene, including those in the petroleum industry, chemical manufacturing, firefighting, and rubber manufacturing.

3. Workers may be monitored with regard to benzene exposure by the use of urine phenol levels.

REFERENCES

1. Caux C, O'Brien C, Viau C: Determination of firefighter exposure to polycyclic aromatic hydrocarbons and benzene during firefighting using measurement of biological indicators. Appl Occup Environ Hygiene 17:379-386, 2002.
2. Kacew S, Lemaire I: Recent developments in benzene risk. J Toxicol Environ Health Part A 61:485-498, 2000.
3. Krewski D, Snyder R, Beatty P, et al: Assessing the health risks of benzene: A report on the benzene state-of-the-science workshop. J Toxicol Environ Health Part A 61:307-338, 2000.
4. Finkelstein MM: Leukemia after exposure to benzene: Temporal trends and implications for standards. Am J Ind Med 38:1-7, 2000.

PATIENT 54

A victim of a subway "explosion"

During a Monday morning rush hour, a 21-year-old woman became aware of an unusual odor as she exited from her subway train, and she experienced nausea, dyspnea, and dizziness. She observed other persons collapsed in the vicinity and attempted to help one victim with CPR until paramedics arrived. She soon lost consciousness herself and was transported to the emergency department (ED) by a rescue squad.

Physical Examination: General: unconscious. Vital signs: pulseless, apneic. Neurological: pin-point pupils.

Initial Hospital Course: Cardiopulmonary resuscitation was promptly initiated, and the patient was intubated. After 5 minutes, spontaneous respiration and pulse reappeared. She was transferred to the intensive care unit.

Shortly before this patient arrived, the ED had been alerted (at 8:16 AM) of an "explosion" and likely toxic gas release at the subway. By 8:28 AM the first subway victim arrived and, like many to follow, complained only of eye pain and dim vision. More severely affected patients soon appeared, and over the next 1½ hours, 500 additional subway victims poured in, with three in full cardiopulmonary arrest, including the patient above. Of 111 moderately or severely ill patients, the symptoms that predominated were ocular (miosis, dim vision, eye pain); respiratory (dyspnea, cough, wheeze, tachypnea); gastrointestinal (nausea, vomiting, diarrhea); neurological (headache, weakness, muscle fasciculations, altered consciousness, seizures); nasal (rhinorrhea, sneezing); and psychological (agitation).

Questions: What is the cause of the subway victims' symptoms? Are there any strategies available to mitigate such a catastrophe as best as possible?

Diagnosis: Mass exposure to sarin, a potent military organophosphate nerve agent

Discussion: Many readers will recognize this grim scenario and know it is not from a sci-fi horror movie. Rather, this was just one hospital ED's experience on March 20, 1995, when a Japanese doomsday religious cult, Aum Shinrikyo, released sarin in the Tokyo subway system. This constellation of symptoms is characteristic of organophosphate poisoning, and its pattern recognition, particularly in an epidemic number of patients presenting contemporaneously, is crucial for emergency physicians in this day and age.

On that one day in Tokyo, more than 5000 persons sought medical treatment, hundreds were hospitalized, and 12 deaths ensued. Many authorities think the death toll could have been much higher. The agent was released by evaporation only, without any effort at mechanically aerosolizing it. Further, the Tokyo subways are believed to have especially excellent ventilation systems. In the wake of the September 11, 2001, attacks on the U.S. World Trade Center and Pentagon, and the subsequent intentional spread of anthrax spores through the U.S. mail, there is no doubt that physicians and hospitals require some education and preparedness for a similar chemical weapons attack in our nation.

The medical consequences and epidemiology of a chemical attack would mimic more conventional disasters, but with some important differences (see table). It would combine elements of a traditional mass disaster, such as an earthquake, and those of more everyday hazardous materials incidents. Casualties would occur immediately, and the attack would likely be recognized rapidly. Initial first responders would be police, fire, and emergency medical services personnel, who would be at considerable personal risk in extracting and decontaminating these victims before providing initial care and transportation to hospitals. It is quite likely that many less ill patients would self-transport to hospital, often without initial decontamination, as was observed in Tokyo.

The general management of contaminated victims begins with triage, emergent resuscitation, if needed, and decontamination performed by healthcare providers garbed in appropriate personal protective equipment (PPE). Decontamination is particularly important in the treatment of victims of liquid nerve agent and vesicant exposures. Appropriate PPE for hospital-based providers consists of nonencapsulated, chemically resistant body suit, boots and gloves with a full-face air purifier mask/hood. This process would typically occur in a special decontamination-treatment area outside the hospital ED. In brief, airway and cardiopulmonary support, including endotracheal intubation, and emergent antidotal therapy should be provided as necessary and contaminated clothing removed as soon as possible. Simple disrobement removes up to 90% of contamination hazard. This is accompanied or immediately followed by more meticulous decontamination. For vapor-exposed patients, this is effected principally by clothing removal and hair-washing. In contrast, patients with liquid dermal exposure require more thorough decontamination. Their skin and clothing pose a significant risk to ED staff. The clothing should be carefully removed and double-bagged. Patients with ocular exposure should have copious eye irrigation with water or saline. The skin and hair should be washed copiously, but gently, with soap and tepid water. Previously, some authorities have recommended 0.5% sodium hypochlorite (dilute bleach) for skin decontamination of nerve agents and vesicants based on military doctrine. However, this may be a skin irritant, thus increasing permeability to agents, and its use is time-consuming and not proven superior to thorough soap and water washing. Further, there is little experience with this approach in infants and young children who, unlike battlefield casualties, may be involved in a civilian terrorism scenario.

The toxicity and management of nerve agent exposures overlap considerably with that of the organophosphate pesticides (see Patient 28). Other important classes of chemical compounds that are of concern as chemical weapons include cyanogens (see Patient 9) and vesicant agents (see Patient 36). In addition, some anti-terrorism experts consider the pulmonary agents, such as chlorine and phosgene, and the riot-control agents ("tear gases") as potential threats as well. The major toxic effects and principal management considerations for all of these agents are summarized in the table on next page.

Characteristics of Chemical Attacks: Potential Differences in Comparison to "Routine" Hazardous Materials Incidents

Intent to cause mass casualties
More toxic substances
Initial substance identification delayed
Greater risk to EMS first responders
Overwhelming numbers of patients
Many "worried well"
Mass hysteria, panic
Discovery of dispersal device

EMS = emergency medical services.

Major Chemical Agents of Terrorism—Summary of Management Considerations

Agent	Toxicity	Clinical Findings	Onset	Decontamination[1]	Management
Nerve agents: tabun, sarin, soman, VX	Anticholinesterase: muscarinic, nicotinic and CNS effects	Vapor: miosis, rhinorrhea, dyspnea; Liquid: diaphoresis, vomiting; Both: coma, paralysis, seizures, apnea	Seconds: vapor; Minutes–hours: liquid	Vapor: fresh air, remove clothes, wash hair; Liquid: remove clothes, copious washing skin, hair with soap and water, ocular irrigation	ABCs; Atropine: 0.05 mg/kg IV[2], IM[3] (min 0.1 mg, max 5 mg), repeat q2-5 min prn for marked secretions, bronchospasm; Pralidoxime:25 mg/kg IV, IM (max 1 g IV; 2 g IM), may repeat within 30-60 min prn, then again Q1 hr for 1 or 2 doses prn for persistent weakness, high atropine requirement; Diazepam: 0.3 mg/kg (max 10 mg) IV; Lorazepam: 0.1 mg/kg IV, IM (max 4 mg); or Midazolam: 0.2 mg/kg (max 10 mg) IM prn seizures, or severe exposure
Vesicants: Mustard	Alkylation	Skin: erythema, vesicles; Eye: inflammation; Respiratory tract: inflammation (both mustard and lewsite)	Hours	Skin: soap and water; Eyes: water (Both: major impact only if done within minutes of exposure)	Symptomatic care
Lewisite	Arsenical		Immediate pain with Lewisite		(Possibly BAL 3 mg/kg IM Q4-6 hrs for systemic effects of Lewisite in severe cases)
Pulmonary agents: Chlorine Phosgene	Liberate HCl, alkylation	Eyes, nose, throat irritation (especially chlorine); Respiratory: bronchospasm, pulmonary edema (especially phosgene)	Minutes: eyes, nose, throat irritation, bronchospasm; Hours: pulmonary edema	Fresh air; Skin: water	Symptomatic care

Agent	Mechanism	Onset	Signs and symptoms	Decontamination	Treatment
Cyanide	Cytochrome oxidase inhibition: cellular anoxia, lactic acidosis	Seconds	Tachypnea, coma, seizures, apnea	Fresh air Skin: soap and water	ABCs, 100% oxygen Na^+ bicarbonate prn metabolic acidosis Na^+ nitrite (3%): **Dose (ml/kg) for estimated Hgb (g/dL)** 0.33 12 (est. for average child) 0.39 14 (max 10 mL) Na^+ thiosulfate (25%): 1.65 mL/kg (max 50 mL)
Riot control agents: CS, CN (Mace), capsaicin (pepper spray)	Neuropeptide substance P release; alkylation	Seconds	Eye: tearing, pain, blepharospasm Nose and throat irritation Pulmonary failure (rare)	Fresh air Eyes: lavage	Ophthalmics topically, symptomatic care

[1]Decontamination, especially for patients with significant nerve agent or vesicant exposure, should be performed by health care providers garbed in adequate personal protective equipment. For ED staff, this consists of non-encapsulated, chemically resistant body suit, boots, and gloves with a full-face air purifier mask/hood.

[2]Intraosseous route is likely equivalent to intravenous.

[3]Atropine might have some benefit via endotracheal tube or inhalation, as might aerosolized ipratropium.

Key: ABCs = airway, breathing and circulatory support; BAL = British Anti-Lewisite; Hgb = hemoglobin concentration; est.= estimated hemoglobin concentration; max = maximum; min = minimum; prn = as needed.

Adapted from Henretig FM, Cieslak TJ, Eitzen EM Jr: Biological and clinical terrorism. J Pediatr 141:311-326, 2002.

Once the etiology of the present patient's illness was recognized, she was treated aggressively with atropine and pralidoxime. She regained consciousness, was extubated by the second hospital day, and was discharged by day 6, apparently neurologically intact and without overt sequelae. Overall, of the 640 patients who were admitted to this one hospital from the sarin attack, all but two are believed to have recovered fully. Unfortunately, the other two victims who had presented in cardiopulmonary arrest were less fortunate. One failed to respond to CPR after 30 minutes, and was pronounced dead. The other had return of spontaneous circulation after 15 minutes, but was extremely acidotic (pH 6.589), sustained severe hypoxic brain damage, and died on hospital day 28.

Clinical Pearls

1. The rapid appearance of multiple casualties should sound the alarm of a potential terrorist act.

2. EDs and staff need to: be prepared with the appropriate knowledge base to recognize the clinical "toxidromes" of the important chemical weapons; stock adequate supplies for supportive care and antiodotal therapy; and have in place a hospital and community–wide disaster plan that can rapidly provide the surge capacity to mitigate outcome if such a catastrophe were to occur.

REFERENCES

1. Henretig FM, Cieslak TJ, Eitzen EM Jr: Biological and chemical terrorism. J Pediatr 141:311-326, 2002.
2. Henretig F: Biological and chemical terrorism defense: A view from the "front lines" of public health. Am J Public Health 91:718-720, 2001.
3. Macintyre AG, Christopher GW, Eitzen E Jr, et al: Weapons of mass destruction events with contaminated casualties: Effective planning for health care facilities. JAMA 283:242-249, 2000.
4. Henretig FM, Cieslak TJ, Madsen JM, et al: The emergency department response to incidents of biological and chemical terrorism. In Fleisher GF, Ludwig S (eds): Textbook of Pediatric Emergency Medicine, 4th ed. Philadelphia, Lippincott Williams & Wilkins, 2000, pp 1763-1784.
5. American Academy of Pediatrics: Chemical and biological terrorism and its impact on children; A subject review. Pediatrics 105:662-670, 2000.
6. US Army Medical Research Institute of Chemical Defense: Medical Management of Chemical Casualties, 3rd ed. Aberdeen Proving Ground, MD, 1999.
7. Brennan RJ, Waeckerle JF, Sharp T, Lillibridge SR: Chemical warfare agents: Emergency medical and emergency public health issues. Ann Emerg Med 34:191-204, 1999.
8. Okumura T, Takasu N, Ishimatasu S, et al: Report on 640 victims of the Tokyo subway sarin attack. Ann Emerg Med 28: 129-135, 1996.

Jason C. Stillwagon, MD
Richard Hamilton, MD

PATIENT 55

A 19-year-old woman with bipolar disorder and newly altered mentation

A 19-year-old woman develops a change in mental status. She has a history of bipolar disorder and is currently taking 250 mg of divalproex sodium three times daily. Her mother discovered her in the bedroom with vodka and an empty pill bottle next to her bed. She is lethargic and speaking incoherently about hurting herself. She progresses to obtundation and is endotracheally intubated to protect her airway from aspiration.

Physical Examination: Temperature 36.8° C, pulse 118/min; respirations 12/min; blood pressure 105/62 mmHg. General: obtunded. HEENT: pupils 3 mm and reactive, pharynx clear, mucosa dry, neck supple. Chest: clear. Heart: tachycardia, no murmurs. Abdomen: soft, non-tender, normal bowel sounds. Extremities: normal. Skin: normal. Neuromuscular: localizes to pain.

Laboratory Findings: Hemogram: normal. Coagulation profile: INR 1.4. Serum chemistries: AST 123 U/L, ALT 72 U/L, ammonia 174 µM/L, otherwise normal. Urine pregnancy test: negative. Toxicology: serum acetaminophen level <10 mg/L; serum salicylate 0.9 mg/dL; serum valproic acid level 133 mg/L; serum ethanol level 48 mg/dL; serum qualitatively negative for tricyclic antidepressants. EKG: sinus tachycardia, otherwise normal. CT brain scan: normal.

Question: What is the cause of this patient's neurological deterioration?

Diagnosis and Treatment: Valproate-induced encephalopathy is caused by a number of mechanisms. It is primarily treated with gastrointestinal (GI) decontamination and supportive care, but evidence suggests that carnitine supplementation may also be beneficial.

Discussion: Valproic acid (VPA) is a carboxylic acid primarily used to treat seizure disorders and bipolar affective disorder. VPA is extensively metabolized (>95%) by the liver, where it is converted to propionate and other active metabolites. It is available as valproic acid, sodium valproate, and divalproex sodium. Available forms are oral, intravenous, and extended release.

VPA metabolism must be examined to comprehend the mechanism of toxicity (see figure). VPA is metabolized via two pathways: beta (β-oxidation in the mitochondria and omega (ω-oxidation in the endoplasmic reticulum. β-oxidation starts with the carnitine-dependent transport of valproyl-CoA. The β-oxidation of valproyl-CoA produces the metabolites 2-en-VPA-CoA and 3-keto-VPA-CoA. When levels of VPA are excessive, these metabolites can rob the mitochondria of the CoA needed for the β-oxidation of fatty acids, which subsequently accumulate and produce hepatic steatosis. In addition, if carnitine stores are deficient (for example, from VPA-induced impairment of carnitine absorption from the renal tubules) metabolism shifts toward ω-oxidation and the production of the toxic metabolite 4-en-VPA. This metabolite inhibits the enzyme necessary for the breakdown of ammonia into urea and, as a result, ammonia levels rise. In addition, 4-en-VPA is directly hepatotoxic. This complex metabolism accounts for some of the varied manifestations of VPA toxicity—from mild reversible elevation of liver transaminases, isolated hyperammonemia, or toxic hepatitis to hepatic steatosis with a Reye's-like syndrome.

Acute ingestions may present with central nervous system affliction ranging from lethargy to coma. Serum levels may rise in a delayed fashion, and should be checked serially. Ammonia level and liver function should also be measured, especially if the patient is on chronic VPA therapy. Hyperammonemia may be seen with or without evidence of hepatotoxicity.

GI decontamination with activated charcoal may be especially important when VPA levels are noted to be rising, and multiple doses should be considered in such cases. Whole bowel irrigation may be warranted if an extended-release preparation has been ingested. An important, although poorly defined, treatment in patients with hyperammonemia or hepatic failure is L-carnitine

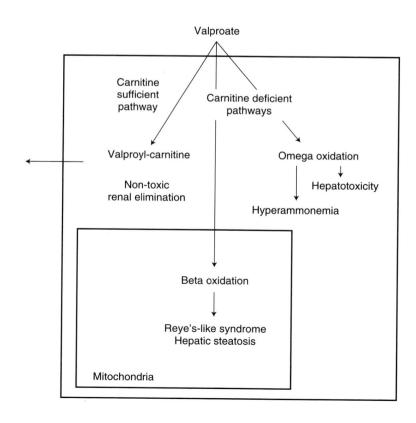

174

supplementation. Carnitine is an essential amino acid that serves as a cofactor for the β-oxidation of VPA (as well as long-chain fatty acids), thus preventing omega oxidation to toxic metabolites. There is no currently agreed-upon dosing or indication, but protective effects have been demonstrated in children on chronic VPA therapy at doses of 100 mg/kg of carnitine (up to 2 g total) divided three times daily. Case reports suggest a similar regimen may be used intravenously or orally in VPA-toxic patients with hyperammonemia, toxic hepatitis, and/or encephalopathy.

The present patient was supported with meticulous attention to her airway, breathing, and circulation. Rising serial VPA levels led to administration of multiple doses of activated charcoal, and the peak level was noted 14 hours after the ingestion. Hyperammonemia improved in a time course coinciding with carnitine therapy. The patient recovered fully.

Clinical Pearls

1. Valproic acid ingestion is a recognized cause of hepatotoxicity.
2. Valproate-induced encephalopathy can involve hyperammonemia with or without evidence of hepatotoxicity.
3. Carnitine stores are depleted in chronic valproic acid therapy.
4. Carnitine may be a useful cofactor in preventing or reversing hyperammonemia and hepatic toxicity due to VPA overdose.

REFERENCES

1. Sztajnkrycer MD: Valproic acid toxicity: Overview and management. J Toxicol Clin Toxicol 40:789-801, 2002.
2. Doyon S: Anticonvulsants. In Goldfrank LR, Flomenbaum NE, Lewin NA, et al (eds): Goldfrank's Toxicologic Emergencies, 7th ed. New York, McGraw Hill, 2002, pp 614-630.
3. Fermin B, Hack JB: Hyperammonemia and coma without hepatic dysfunction induced by valproate therapy. Acad Emerg Med 8:999-1001, 2001.
4. Ishikura H, et al: Valproic acid overdose and L-carnitine therapy. J Analyt Toxicol 20:55-58, 1996.
5. Coulter DL, Allen RJ: Secondary hyperammonemia: A possible mechanism for valproate encephalopathy. Lancet 1: 1310-1311, 1980.

PATIENT 56

A 15-year-old boy with fever, obtundation, and trembling

A 15-year-old boy with a history of mental retardation is brought to the emergency department after 2 days of progressive obtundation, fevers to 39.4° C, and intermittent trembling. Several days prior to the onset of these symptoms he was placed in a psychiatric facility for management of disruptive and aggressive behavior. His caretakers report that the patient has recently been administered haloperidol on several occasions for agitation.

Physical Examination: Temperature 38.9° C, pulse 133/min, respirations 18/min, blood pressure 161/102 mmHg. General: lethargic, responsive only to painful stimuli. HEENT: dry lips and mucous membranes, no lymphadenopathy. Chest: clear to auscultation. Cardiovascular: tachycardia, normal rhythm, no murmur or gallop. Abdomen: soft, nondistended. Extremities: warm, no edema. Skin: normal. Neurological: pupils 4 mm to 2 mm bilaterally, symmetrical increase in tone in lower extremities.

Laboratory Findings: WBC 11,200/µL with 72% neutrophils, 16% lymphocytes. Sodium 140 mEq/L, potassium 4.9 mEq/L, chloride 101 mEq/L, bicarbonate 18 mEq/L, BUN 15 mg/dL, creatinine 0.8 mg/dL, calcium 8.6 mg/dL, magnesium 3.2 mg/dL, phosphorus 6.0 mg/dL, creatine kinase 13,322 IU/L (normal 60–335 IU/L). Urine specific gravity 1.025, moderate blood, 10–25 RBC/hpf. Venous blood gas (room air): pH 7.45, $Pvco_2$ 39 mmHg, base excess +2.4 mEq/L. EKG: sinus tachycardia. Head CT: normal.

Question: What clinical syndrome describes these findings?

Diagnosis: Neuroleptic malignant syndrome (NMS)

Discussion: NMS is an uncommon but potentially life-threatening idiosyncratic reaction to antipsychotic medications (see table). Among hospitalized adults administered antipsychotic medications, its incidence ranges from 0.02% to 3.23%. Patients classically present with autonomic instability, skeletal muscle rigidity, and mental status changes after exposure to a neuroleptic drug.

The manifestations of NMS develop secondary to a dysregulation of central dopaminergic neurotransmission. A predisposition to this illness occurs among patients with organic brain disease, affective disorders, dehydration, and alcoholism. In addition, an increased risk has been associated with drug administration in depot formulations, concomitant use of lithium, and a rapid increase in neuroleptic medication dose.

Manifestations of autonomic instability may include hyperthermia, diaphoresis, tachycardia, blood pressure lability, urinary incontinence, and sialorrhea. Mental status alterations may be as subtle as agitation and confusion or as profound as obtundation and unresponsiveness. Skeletal muscle changes include rigidity, tremors, chorea, opisthotonos, trismus, nystagmus, aphonia, dysarthria, and dysphagia. Associated laboratory abnormalities include elevated creatine kinase with resultant myoglobinuria, leukocytosis, thrombocytopenia, hyperkalemia, hyponatremia, or hypernatremia.

The onset of this syndrome is typically within 2 weeks of exposure to neuroleptic therapy or after dose escalation. Symptoms typically resolve in uncomplicated cases within 2 to 14 days of diagnosis. Unfortunately, however, mortality rates as high as 12% to 20% have been reported. Life-threatening complications most commonly include renal failure or adult respiratory distress syndrome secondary to rhabdomyolysis, dysrhythmias from electrolyte abnormalities, aspiration causing respiratory failure in patients with dysphagia or altered mental status, and pulmonary embolism from rigidity and immobilization.

The diagnosis of NMS is based on a constellation of physical exam and laboratory findings in patients who have received a neuroleptic medication and in whom no general medical or mental disorder accounts for the same signs and symptoms. An initial workup in patients suspected of having NMS includes serum electrolytes, BUN, creatinine, creatine kinase, levels of urine myoglobin, and in some instances, computed tomographic imaging of the brain and lumbar puncture.

The management of patients with NMS involves withdrawal of all neuroleptic medications, vigorous hydration to avoid complications of rhabdomyolysis, and supportive care as needed. Specific pharmacotherapy may include dantrolene sodium to reduce muscle rigidity and bromocriptine to promote dopaminergic transmission.

The present patient was admitted to a pediatric intensive care unit where he was placed on aspiration precautions and given alkalinized intravenous fluids, bromocriptine, and dantrolene. He received occasional doses of a benzodiazepine for severe agitation. His creatine kinase level peaked at 19,320 on hospital day 2. He was discharged to home on hospital day 4 with normal vital signs, his baseline mental status, and a creatine kinase of 9000 IU/L.

Partial Listing of Neuroleptic Medications

Bromperidol	Loxapine	Thiothixene
Chlorpromazine	Mesoridazine	Trifluoperazine
Chlorprothixene	Molindone	
Cis-Clopenthixol	Olanzipine	
Trimethobenzamide	Perphenazine	
Clozapine	Prochlorperazine	
Ethopropazine	Promazine	
Fluphenazine	Promethazine	
Haloperidol	Risperidone	
Levopromethazine	Thioridazine	

Clinical Pearls

1. There is a broad spectrum of disease presentation among patients with neuroleptic malignant syndrome (NMS).

2. Maintain a high level of suspicion for NMS in at-risk patients who present with high fever, mental status changes, and rigidity.

3. Intensive care monitoring is essential for patients with NMS, as symptoms may be progressive and have the potential to be life-threatening.

REFERENCES

1. Ty E, Rothner A: Neuroleptic malignant syndrome in children and adolescents. J Child Neurol 16:157-163, 2001.
2. Carbone J: The neuroleptic malignant and serotonin syndromes. Emerg Med Clin North Am 18:317-325, 2000.
3. Silva R, Munoz D, Alpert M, et al: Neuroleptic malignant syndrome in children and adolescents. J Am Acad Child Adolesc Psychiatry 38:187-194, 1999.
4. Pelonero A, Levenson J, Pandurangi A: Neuroleptic malignant syndrome: A review. Psychiatr Serv 49:1163-1172, 1998.
5. Bertorini T: Myoglobinuria, malignant hyperthermia, neuroleptic malignant syndrome, and serotonin syndrome. Neurol Clin 15: 649-671, 1997.

Kevin C. Osterhoudt, MD

PATIENT 57

A 3½-month-old boy with fussiness, poor feeding, and poor tone

A 3½-month-old baby boy is evaluated in the emergency department for "being fussy" and "acting sick." He was born via a full-term, uncomplicated, vaginal delivery and had been well until 5 days prior. This breast-fed baby has had a reduction in stooling from 4 per day to only 1 per day, but his stool seems normal in consistency today. Over the past few days he has seemed "congested," and a mild "gaggy" cough has developed. For the past 24 hours he has been cranky with a "whining" cry, has not slept much, and has seemed to lose interest in nursing. Wet diapers are fewer. Fever is absent, and the baby consoles when carried by his mother.

Physical Examination: Temperature 37.1° C, pulse 152/min, respirations 38/min. General: alert, low-volume cry, expressionless face with occasional weak social smile. HEENT: anterior fontanelle flat, tympanic membranes normal, decreased tears, increased salivary pool. Chest: normal. Cardiovascular: normal. Abdomen: distended, hyperactive bowel sounds, flatulence, no masses, no organomegaly. Genitourinary: normal. Extremities: well-perfused. Skin: normal. Neuromuscular: cranial nerve function intact, poor suck, intact gag, mild hypotonia, deep-tendon reflexes present.

Laboratory Findings: Hemogram: WBC 10,700/μL, hemoglobin 12.6/g/dL, platelets 377,000/μL. Serum chemistries: Na^+ 141 mEq/L, K^+ 4.8 mEq/L, CO_2 20 mEq/L, creatinine 0.5 mg/dL. Urinalysis: specific gravity 1.020, no leukocytes or blood. Radiographic (abdominal obstruction) studies: dilated gas-filled intestine with air present from stomach to rectum. Electromyography: brief, small-amplitude, abundant motor unit potentials with incremental response to repetitive stimulation (see figure).

Question: What class of antibiotics should be avoided in the treatment of this patient?

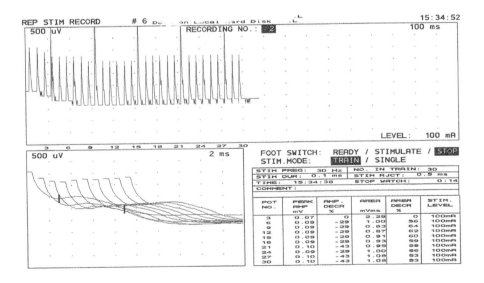

Diagnosis and Treatment: Aminoglycoside antibiotics, such as gentamicin, may potentiate the neuromuscular junction toxicity of infant botulism.

Discussion: Young infancy is an unusual time for poisoning, as newborns cannot walk or crawl to access potential poisons. Instead, consideration of a whining baby with poor feeding behaviors, cough, and congestion might suggest a simple viral syndrome as the etiology for this baby's illness. However, careful notation of this baby's affect, poor suck, distended abdomen, and hypotonia portend a more significant malady. Sepsis is to be considered; however, the baby is afebrile and consoles with the mother. Urinary tract infection is unlikely based upon a normal urinalysis result. Crankiness and abdominal distension merit thought of intussusception, and the history of diminished stooling might suggest Hirschprung's disease. However, poor suck, pooling of saliva, an expressionless face, a weak cry, and hypotonia suggest that this baby's symptomatology is derived from **weakness**. The differential diagnosis (see table) can be narrowed significantly with a good medical history and physical exam and, perhaps, with directed laboratory investigation.

Serial physical examinations note the loss of previously attained motor control of the head, a diminished gag reflex, and bilateral ptosis of the eyelids. The history of constipation and the findings of generalized weakness and cranial neuropathies in a previously healthy infant strongly suggest the diagnosis of infant botulism (see table). Aminoglycoside antibiotics are commonly prescribed empirically to septic-appearing infants but should be used with caution in infants with weakness for whom infant botulism remains a consideration.

Food-borne botulism results from the ingestion of pre-formed toxin, typically after improper canning of foodstuffs. In contrast, infant botulism typically occurs in children younger than 6 months, and involves intestinal colonization by ingested *Clostridium botulinum* spores. With spore germination, *botulinum* neurotoxin is absorbed into the bloodstream where it inhibits acetylcholine relaease at the presynaptic membranes of the neuromuscular junctions and at ganglionic and postganglionic synapses. Movements that require frequent neuromuscular transmission, such as sucking, peristalsis, and eye opening, are frequently more overtly affected.

The "gold standard" for the diagnosis of infant botulism is identification of *C. botulinum* organisms or toxin in the feces. However, most infants can be appropriately managed based upon clinical diagnosis. Electromyography (EMG) can provide diagnostic support. Clinical management should focus on support of hydration and nutrition, maintenance of ventilation and oxygenation, and prevention of secondary infections (especially aspiration pneumonia). Currently, the California Department of Health Infant Botulism Treatment and Prevention Program (www.infantbot.org)

Differential Diagnosis of Acute Floppiness During Infancy

Cortical Dysfunction
  Hypoxic / ischemic encephalopathy
  Intracranial hemorrhage
  Leukodystrophies
Anterior Horn Cell Dysfunction
  Spinal muscular atrophy
  Type II glycogen storage disease
  Poliomyelitis
Peripheral Nerve Dysfunction
  Guillain-Barré syndrome
  Metal poisoning
Neuromuscular Junction Dysfunction
  Infant botulism
  Myasthenia gravis
  Tick paralysis
Muscle Dysfunction
  Myotonic dystrophy
  Inflammatory myopathy
Systemic Illness
  Sepsis
  Meningitis / encephalitis
  Urinary tract infection
  Hypoglycemia
  Acidemia
  Electrolyte abnormality
  Cardiac failure
  Hypothyroidism
  Intussusception
  Poisoning

Symptoms and Signs of Infant Botulism

Symptoms	Signs
Constipation	Hypotonia
Poor feeding	Facial weakness
Weak cry	Diminished gag reflex
Drooling	Ptosis
Irritability	Hyporeflexia
Loss of developmental motor milestones	
Sluggishly reactive pupils	

produces a human-derived botulism immune globulin (BIG), which may be administered to infants through a Treatment Investigational New Drug protocol with the U.S. Food and Drug Administration. The average hospitalization of untreated infants may exceed 5 weeks. Preliminary use of BIG suggests that it can drastically reduce inpatient hospitalization by more than 50% and lower treatment costs.

In the present case, the infant's weakness was recognized in the emergency department, and he was admitted to an intensive care unit. An EMG demonstrated brief, small-amplitude, abundant motor unit potentials and the "staircase phenomenon" and supported the admission diagnosis of infant botulism. A nasoduodenal tube was used for nutritional support, respiratory function was monitored through measurement of negative inspiratory pressures, and BIG was administered. Bulbar weakness resolved within a week, and oral feeding was resumed within 2 weeks of diagnosis. The baby recovered uneventfully.

Clinical Pearls

1. Muscular weakness can be subtle in infants and may be manifest by weak cry, loss of head control, or failure to bring hands to the midline.

2. Constipation and the new onset of generalized weakness and cranial neuropathies strongly suggest the diagnosis of botulism among infants below the age of 6 months.

3. Aminoglycoside antibiotics can potentiate neuromuscular weakness and should be avoided in suspected cases of infant botulism.

4. Although expensive, botulism immune globulin is a beneficial and cost-effective active treatment for infant botulism.

REFERENCES

1. Davis DH, Priestley MA: A BIG treatment for a small infant with constipation and weakness. Pediatr Case Rev 2:133-140, 2002.
2. Arnon SS: Infant botulism. In Feigen RD, Cherry JD (eds): Textbook of Pediatric Infectious Diseases. Philadelphia, WB Saunders, 1998, pp 1570-1577.

Judith M. Eisenberg, MD
James R. Roberts, MD

PATIENT 58

A 32-year-old man who cannot move his neck

A 32-year-old man has had waxing and waning but progressively increasing stiffness in the left side of his neck for about 3 hours. He reports not being able to turn his head to midline, and he is becoming anxious and alarmed. He states that his tongue feels as if it is becoming swollen. The patient has had intermittent episodes of diaphoresis but denies headache, fever, vision change, shortness of breath, viral respiratory infection symptoms, chest or abdominal pain, trauma, or prior neck problems. He has no trouble walking. A mild gastroenteritis that began 2 days ago is resolving. He admits taking a single unidentified pill for nausea that he obtained from a friend who had similar gastrointestinal symptoms. He takes no prescription medications, has no significant medical history or drug allergies, and denies substance abuse.

Physical Examination: Temperature: 37.4° C, pulse 88/min, respirations 18/min, blood pressure 136/70 mmHg. General: alert and oriented, anxious, with mild discomfort in the neck. HEENT: poor muscular control of tongue, no edema; no cervical adenopathy, voice change, drooling, or stridor; head and neck intermittently turned to left, with slight extension of neck (see figure); eyes intermittently rolling upward; slight diaphoresis of forehead. Chest: normal. Cardiovascular: normal. Abdomen: normal. Extremities: no rash, edema, fasciculations, or tremor. Neuromuscular: normal.

Laboratory Findings: Urine immunoassay for drugs of abuse: negative.

Questions: What is this condition? How is it treated?

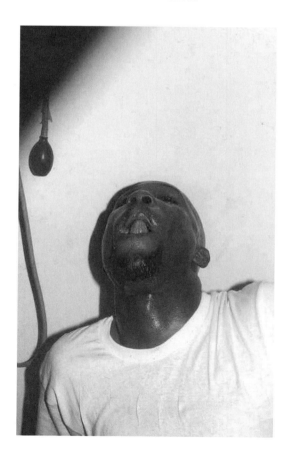

Diagnosis and Treatment: The clinical scenario is consistent with acute dystonia, in this case due to a single dose of prochlorperazine (Compazine) taken 36 hours ago. This can be treated with diphenhydramine or benztropine.

Discussion: Acute dystonia is thought to be caused by central nervous system (CNS) dopamine receptor blockade in the basal ganglia, resulting in cholinergic excess producing sustained spasms of various muscle groups. Muscles of the neck, eyes, tongue, and back are most affected, and the lower extremities are spared. Acute dystonia often occurs secondary to antipsychotic medications, such as haloperidol, as well as to structurally similar antiemetic compounds, such as prochlorperazine and metaclopramide. Serotonin agonists, including buspirone and sumatriptan, also have been implicated. Additionally, there are reports of opisthotonos with the use of antimalarial quinolones, tricyclic antidepressants, phenytoin, hemlock, phencyclidine, cocaine, lithium, and strychnine, as well as with the insect repellant delphene.

Dystonia may be confused with other drug-induced movement disorders, such as chorea, dyskinesia, akathisia, and generalized muscle rigidity (see table). Often a partial or complex seizure is suspected, especially in children. Since the symptoms often develop in psychiatric patients, dystonia can be confused with worsening of the underlying disorder, hysteria, or malingering. A single therapeutic dose of the offending drug can precipitate dystonia. The condition also can develop after the initiation of maintenance medications, usually very early in the course, with 90% occurring within 5 days. After sumatriptan therapy, the onset of stiffness may be noted within 6 hours of the first dose. Haloperidol, often sold on the street as "valium," is a common cause of acute dystonia in some areas of the U.S. Infants receiving metoclopramide (Reglan) for reflux also may experience dystonia.

Clinical presentations can vary widely, including torticollis as in this patient, retrocollis (neck hyperextension), blepharospasm, dysphagia, involuntary tongue protrusion, dysarthria, opisthotonos (retrocollis with spine hyperextension), and, rarely, stridor from laryngospasm. Oculogyric crisis is also a common presentation in which the extraocular muscles are involved, with eyes being forced into an upward or upward/lateral gaze. Opisthotonos is a severe form of this condition in which the entire body is involved, with hyperextension of the spine and the neck in retrocollis. Although the movements are involuntary, they may wax and wane, appearing to be under voluntary control. Diaphoresis is a common finding. Dystonia is frightening and uncomfortable for the patient, but it is usually not serious. Many patients think they are having a stroke. Stridor may occur but the airway remains patent, and respirations and cardiovascular function are unaffected. Whether or not dystonia of the vocal cords can produce asphyxia has been debated, but remains unproven.

Acute dystonia typically resolves with administration of diphenhydramine at a dose of 1 mg/kg IV/IM (max = 50 mg). Most clinicians prefer to use the IV route initially. If there is no improvement with the first intravenous dose, a second dose is given, and usually that is sufficient to cause resolution of the dystonia. Complete reversal of the symptoms in a few minutes is expected. Anticholinergic drugs are very effective—if symptoms do not abate, consider an alternate diagnosis. After the initial reversal, diphenhydramine should be continued orally every 6 hours for 48 hours to prevent recurrence. Alternatively, benztropine 1–2 mg IM/IV, followed by a smilar oral regimen, is quite effective and preferred by

Drug-Induced Acute Dystonia

Major Causes
Neuroleptic agents
   Phenothiazines (e.g., chlorpromazine)
   Butyrophenones (e.g., haloperiodol)
Anti-emetic agents
   Phenothiazines (e.g., prochlorperazine)
   Metoclopramide
Minor Causes (rare case reports)
Psychotropics
   Tricyclic antidepressants
   Serotonin selective reuptake inhibitor
      antidepressants
   Monoamine oxidase inhibitor antidepressants
   Risperidone
   Bupropion
   Buspirone
   Fluvoxamine
   Olanzapine
Miscellaneous
   Dextromethorphan
   Cimetidine
   Cisapride
   Ranitidine
   Sumatriptan
   Many others!!

Adapted from McCormick MA, Manoguerra AS: Dystonic reactions. In Harwood-Nuss A, Wofson AB, Linden CH, et al (eds): The Clinical Practice of Emergency Medicine, 3rd ed. Philadelphia, Lippincott Williams & Wilkins, 2001, pp 1496-1498.

some clinicians. There is some evidence that amantadine may be better than anticholinergic drugs in preventing recurrence, but no evidence exists for its use in the acute symptoms of dystonia.

The present patient provided a history of taking a single dose of a common antiemetic drug 36 hours previously, but only after a thorough drug history was elicited. Because of a delay in symptoms and the absence of an overdose scenario, even reliable patients may not remember taking 1 dose of an offending drug 2–3 days previously.

Once the antiemetic use was elicited, the diagnosis of acute dystonia secondary to prochlorperazine use was made and was confirmed when the patient's symptoms resolved with diphenhydramine administration.

In cases with classic presentation, a trial of diphenhydramine or benztropine is warranted, despite the lack of a specific history. Individuals taking street drugs are often reluctant to give the correct drug information despite the symptoms. Standard radioimmune urine drug screens will not detect the offending medications.

Clinical Pearls

1. Acute dystonia is associated with medications that cause dopamine and serotonin blockade, usually neuroleptics and antiemetics.

2. A number of movement disorders may mimic acute dystonia.

3. Onset of symptoms of acute dystonia typically occurs within 1–5 days of starting an offending medication.

4. Acute dystonia is an idiosyncratic reaction, not an allergy or overdose. The condition can be caused by a single therapeutic dose.

5. Anticholinergic antidotes should be continued for 48 hours to prevent recurrence of dystonia.

6. A therapeutic trial of diphenhydramine or benztropine is warranted in suspected cases, even without a corroborating history of medication exposure.

7. Symptoms may wax and wane, appear to be controllable, and be accompanied by diaphoresis.

REFERENCES

1. McCormick MA, Manoguerra AS: Dystonic reactions. In Harwood-Nuss A, Wofson AB, Linden CH et al (eds): The Clinical Practice of Emergency Medicine, 3rd ed. Philadelphia, Lippincott Williams & Wilkins, 2001, pp 1496-1498.
2. Venna N: Dystonia. In Noble J, Greene HL, et al (eds): Textbook of Primary Care Medicine, 3rd ed. St. Louis, Mosby, 2001, pp 1532-1534.
3. Olson KR: Emergency evaluation and treatment. In Olson KR, Anderson IB, Benowitz NL , et al (eds): Poisoning and Drug Overdose, 3rd ed. Stamford, Conn, Appleton and Lange, 1999, pp 24–25.
4. Gallagher JE, Lewin NA: Neurological principles. In Goldfrank LR, Flomenbaum NE, et al (eds): Goldfrank's Toxicological Emergencies, 6th ed. Stamford, Conn, Appleton and Lange, 1998, pp 317-319.

PATIENT 59

A 32-year-old woman who chronically sniffs glue

A 32-year-old woman is concerned about weakness. She confesses to the chronic abuse of sniffing shoe glue. She inhales the fumes by squeezing some glue onto a rag and holding the rag up to her nose. She has no other medical problems and denies the use of any other recreational drugs.

Physical Examination: Temperature 37° C, pulse 88/min, respirations 18/min, blood pressure 128/88 mmHg. HEENT: normal. Chest: normal. Cardiovascular: normal. Neurological: 2/5 muscle weakness of the arms and legs bilaterally; biceps and patella reflexes diminished bilaterally.

Laboratory Findings: Hemogram: normal. Serum chemistries: potassium 1.9 mEq/L, bicarbonate 10 mEq/L, phosphorus 1.8 mg/dL, otherwise normal. Urine immunoassay for drugs of abuse: negative. Serum ethanol: negative.

Questions: What caused this patient's weakness? What is the treatment?

Diagnosis and Treatment: This patient is suffering significant electrolyte abnormalities associated with chronic toluene abuse. These electrolyte abnormalities subsequently have caused severe muscle weakness. Treatment consists of electrolyte replacement and discontinuation of toluene abuse.

Discussion: Many different hydrocarbon solvents can be abused by inhalation. In contrast to acute hydrocarbon inhalation and potential cardiotoxicity, older patients with a history of chronic solvent abuse may suffer neurological and renal toxicity as a result of their constant exposure to these solvents. Many hydrocarbon solvents are commonly available (see table). In this case, inhaled toluene is well absorbed from the lungs and rapidly distributed to the central nervous system. The effects of toluene inhalation may last for several hours and the clinical manifestations are similar to ethanol intoxication. (See also Patient 27.)

Metabolic abnormalities have been classically described in patients who abuse toluene. Toluene is a hydrocarbon found in a variety of household products, including adhesives, spray paints, paint thinners, and varnishes. Chronic toluene abuse may cause metabolic acidosis with and without an anion gap. The elevated anion gap results from an accumulation of acidic metabolites, mainly hippuric and benzoic acids. The electrolyte abnormalities seen include hypokalemia, hypochloremia, and hypophosphatemia; these occur due to the induction of a distal renal tubular acidosis by toluene. The hypokalemia may be so great that patients suffer muscle weakness severe enough to cause rhabdomyolysis, paralysis, and respiratory failure. These metabolic abnormalities typically occur after *chronic* abuse of toluene. Complete recovery has been reported in patients during periods of avoidance. Severe hypokalemia and death associated with chronic toluene abuse have been reported. Patients suffering the medical consequences of toluene abuse often are found in a severely weakened state with paint still on their face and fingers. *Acute* ingestion of toluene has been reported to cause central nervous system depression and diarrhea severe enough to cause a non-anion gap metabolic acidosis.

The treatment for electrolyte abnormalities due to chronic toluene inhalation is discontinuation of exposure, airway management if necessary, and fluid and electrolyte replacement. Specific attention to hypokalemia is necessary, and significant deficits should be corrected, as metabolic acidosis, rhabdomyolysis, lethal arrhythmias, and death have all been reported secondary to prolonged toluene abuse. Hemodialysis along with aggressive potassium replacement has been reported as a successful treatment option for severe chronic toluene poisoning.

The present patient was admitted to the hospital, and her potassium and phosphorus were replaced both intravenously and orally. The hospital social worker referred her for outpatient drug detoxification therapy. She was discharged 2 days later with normal muscle strength and normal electrolytes.

Common Inhalants of Abuse and Their Main Chemical Constituents

Inhalants of Abuse	Chemical Constituents
Acrylic paint	Toluene
Aerosol propellant	Fluorocarbons
Anesthetics	Chloroform, nitrous oxide
Fire extinguishing agent	Bromochlorodifluoromethane
Fuel, lighter fluid, torches	Propane, butane
Gasoline	Hydrocarbons, tetraethyl lead
Glues, plastic cement, rubber cement	Benzene, carbon tetrachloride, methylethyl ketone, *n*-hexane, toluene, trichloroethylene, trichloroethane, xylene
Inks	Toluene, xylene
Paint stripper	Methylene chloride
Paints, varnishes, lacquer	Trichloroethylene, toluene
Refrigerants	Fluorocarbons
Shoe polish	Chlorinated hydrocarbons, toluene
Spot remover	Trichloroethane, trichloroethylene, carbon tetrachloride
Typewriter correction fluid (e.g., Wite-out)	Tetrachloroethylene, trichloroethane, trichloroethylene

Clinical Pearls

1. Chronic inhalation of toluene-containing products can cause severe electrolyte abnormalities including hypokalemia, hypochloremia, and hypophosphatemia and a non-anion gap metabolic acidosis.

2. Hypokalemia associated with chronic toluene abuse may be so great that patients suffer muscle weakness severe enough to cause rhabdomyolysis, paralysis, and respiratory failure.

3. The treatment for electrolyte abnormalities due to chronic toluene inhalation is discontinuation of exposure, airway management if necessary, and fluid and electrolyte replacement. Specific attention to hypokalemia is necessary, and significant deficits should be corrected, as metabolic acidosis, rhabdomyolysis, lethal arrhythmias, and death may occur.

REFERENCES
1. Kolecki P, Shih R. Inhalant abuse. In Brick J (ed): Hand book of the Medical Consequences of Alcohol and Drug Abuse. New York, The Haworth Press, 2004, pp. 303-318.

PATIENT 60

A 74-year-old man with difficulty breathing

An elderly gentleman is brought to the emergency department by ambulance with an exacerbation of his usual resting shortness of breath. He is slightly cyanotic and in mild respiratory distress. He takes no cardiac medications, has never smoked, and has no history of heart disease. His wife tells you that he worked "in the shipyards" during World War II and that his doctor told them he "may have lung problems" as a result of that work.

Physical Examination: Temperature 37.2° C, pulse 98/min, respirations 27/min, blood pressure 140/100 mmHg. General: awake and oriented, but uncomfortable due to difficulty breathing. HEENT: no neck vein distention; trachea midline. Chest: few very dry crackles heard at both bases, no rales, breath sounds equal. Heart: normal. Abdomen: nontender. Extremities: no edema. Skin: warm and dry with slight peri-oral cyanosis.

Laboratory Findings: Pulse oximetry: 92% on 2 L of oxygen. Chest radiograph: Several pleural plaques as well as a diffuse interstitial pattern of lung disease. There are no pleural effusions and no signs of congestive heart failure. CT scan: honeycombing of lung (see figure).

Question: What is the cause of this man's shortness of breath?

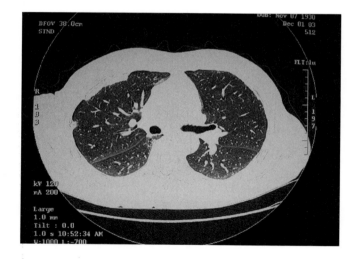

Diagnosis: Based on the patient's work history in conjunction with his presenting findings, it is most likely that he has asbestosis with an acute exacerbation.

Discussion: Asbestosis is a diffuse interstitial fibrosis involving the parenchyma of the lung and may be seen in individuals who have had heavy and unprotected exposures to asbestos, usually in occupational settings. Studies have shown a strong dose-response relationship between the degree of exposure and the prevalence and severity of asbestosis. In addition, a latency period of 20–40 years has been identified before patients manifest clinical evidence of this disease. Initially following exposure, there are no immediate symptoms due to inhalation of asbestos fibers, as the latency period must pass before clinically detectable disease develops. While this discussion focuses on asbestosis, two important neoplasms, bronchogenic carcinoma and pleural or peritoneal mesothelioma, are also considered asbestos-related diseases.

The primary complaint of patients in whom asbestosis has developed is shortness of breath; cough usually does not manifest early in the course of the disease. Patients often have late inspiratory rales at the lung bases, and pulmonary function tests demonstrate a restrictive pattern with decreased diffusion capacity. The chest x-ray shows small, irregular opacities in the lower lobes (if these are seen in the upper lobes, the diagnosis is less likely). So-called **honeycombing** of the lung may be seen on chest CT and is the only reliable chest CT finding for asbestosis. Pleural plaques also may be seen on plain chest x-rays, but these are only markers of past exposure to asbestos. They do not provide information regarding the extent or prognosis of the disease. The definitive diagnosis of asbestosis requires histological examination of lung tissue demonstrating characteristic findings, which include **peribronchial fibrosis** and the presence of so-called **asbestos bodies**.

In the present patient, his work history is critical to making the presumptive diagnosis. During the World War II era, amphibole asbestos was used as an insulation material in many areas aboard naval vessels. Workers toiling in certain areas in the shipyards of the day sometimes had extensive and unprotected exposures to high concentrations of amphibole asbestos. Amphibole asbestos is one of two broad categorizes of asbestos and encompasses several varieties of asbestos. The table below lists the various types of asbestos that are generally recognized. Anyone with a work history consistent with heavy, unprotected, inhalational amphibole asbestos exposure more than 20 years ago may be at risk for the development of asbestosis, and these patients may present to the emergency department for evaluation of respiratory difficulties.

Treatment involves definition of the degree of respiratory compromise, supplemental oxygen as needed and supportive care. Counsel these patients not to smoke and of course to avoid asbestos exposure in the future. Admission may be required if they do not respond to supportive care in the emergency department.

Asbestos Taxonomy

Serpentine group
Chrysotile
Amphibole group
Amosite
Anthophyllite
Tremolite
Croccidolite
Actinolite

Clinical Pearls

1. The development of asbestosis usually requires a latency period of at least 20 years following heavy, unprotected exposure.

2. Pleural plaques provide a clue that the patient may have been exposed to asbestos in the past.

3. Asbestosis usually presents with shortness of breath *not* associated with cough.

REFERENCES
1. Mossman BT, Gee JB: Asbestos-related diseases N Eng J Med 320:1721, 1989.
2. American Thoracic Society: The diagnosis of nonmalignant diseases related to asbestos. Am Rev Resp Dis 134:363, 1986.

Allison A. Muller, PharmD
Fred M. Henretig, MD

PATIENT 61

A 14-month-old girl with "Halloween candy poisoning"

A 14-month-old girl became irritable and lethargic, and then was unable to recognize her parents. Three hours prior to onset of symptoms, she was awake and alert, eating Halloween candy. Medical history includes varicella infection 3 weeks ago and a fall from a table 3 days ago without loss of consciousness. She is on no medications; however, the medications available within the house include acetaminophen, acyclovir, alprazolam, brompheniramine-pseudoephedrine, clonidine, diphenhydramine, naproxen, paroxetine, and sertraline. She presents to the emergency department with altered mentation and pinpoint pupils. Among the parents' initial concerns is the possibility of malevolent Halloween candy tampering.

Physical Examination: Temperature 36.9° C, pulse 99/min, respirations 16/min, blood pressure 66/34 mmHg. Pulse oximetry (room air): 98%. General: obtunded. HEENT: small pupils. Chest: normal. Cardiovascular: normal. Abdomen: normally active bowel sounds. Genitourinary: Foley catheter draining very clear, dilute urine. Neuromuscular: opens eyes and withdraws extremities to deep painful stimuli.

Laboratory Findings: EKG: see figure. Urine immunoassay for drugs of abuse: negative.

Question: From the list of drugs available within the home, which is most likely responsible for the patient's change in mental status?

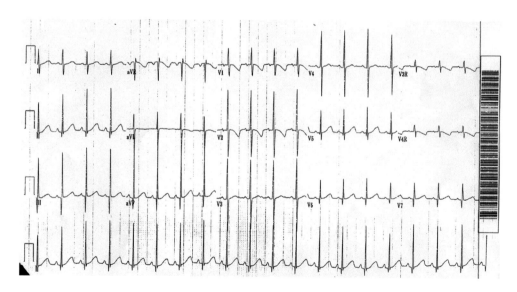

Diagnosis: Clonidine

Discussion: Clonidine is a centrally acting alpha-2 agonist widely used in the treatment of hypertension. Clonidine is also now used in the treatment of behavioral disorders, migraine headaches, and narcotic withdrawal. It is available in parenteral and oral dosage forms as well as a transdermal system. The transdermal system contains excess clonidine to provide an adequate concentration gradient for drug delivery. Three different strengths are available: 0.1 mg/24 hr, 0.2 mg/24 hr, and 0.3 mg/24 hr. They contain 2.5, 5.0, and 7.5 mg of clonidine, respectively. Even after 7 days of wear, these patches contain up to 50% of the initial drug concentration.

Clonidine's mechanism in exerting antihypertensive and central nervous system (CNS) effects appears complex. It is an alpha-2 agonist in the CNS, inhibiting neurons in the vasoregulatory center of the medulla, with resulting decrease of central sympathetic outflow. Some animal data suggest that the release of an endogenous opioid may accompany clonidine's inhibition of sympathetic outflow. There also appear to be imidazoline-specific receptors in the medulla that may interact with clonidine, leading to hypotensive effects independent of adrenergic mechanisms. Finally, clonidine seems to affect nitric oxide and gamma-aminobutyric acid activity.

In clonidine overdose, the resulting symptoms of toxicity manifest as CNS depression, miosis, bradycardia, hypotension, hypothermia, and respiratory depression. Thus, the presentation of the clonidine-poisoned patient may mimic that of an opiate overdose. However, in large overdose, clonidine may also stimulate peripheral alpha-1 receptors, resulting in early, transient, seemingly paradoxic hypertension. Severe symptoms can occur in children with as little as 0.2 mg of clonidine. Respiratory effects (e.g., hypoventilation, apnea) are often responsive to tactile stimulation. Typically, the CNS, respiratory, and cardiovascular depression resolves over 12–36 hours.

The management of clonidine toxicity primarily involves gastric decontamination and supportive care. Decontamination with activated charcoal (1 g/kg) is appropriate for patients presenting within 1–2 hours of ingestion. In cases of patch ingestion, subsequent treatment with whole bowel irrigation (200–500 ml/hr) may be beneficial. Supportive care consists of attention to the "ABCs" and the potential use of naloxone. As noted, the respiratory depression of clonidine toxicity is relatively stimulus-responsive and may be treated adequately with close monitoring and frequent auditory or tactile stimulation as needed. However, tracheal intubation may be required in severe cases. Bradycardia and hypotension may necessitate additional therapy in such patients, with intravenous fluids, atropine, or dopamine as needed. In the past, some authors have recommended the alpha-antagonist tolazoline as a specific antidote for the cardiovascular toxicity of clonidine. However, its efficacy has been inconsistent, and few physicians are familiar with it today, so it is not a first-line agent. Transient hypertension seen early after large clonidine overdoses is rarely severe enough to require specific therapy.

The role of naloxone is controversial. The success of such therapy varies from reversal of none to all opioid-associated signs and symptoms. Some authors believe that this variability in success is a factor of insufficient dosing and suggest that larger doses of naloxone (0.1 mg/kg, or 5–10 mg in adults) may be required to reverse symptoms of severe clonidine toxicity. Naloxone treatment can lead to the predominance of clonidine's peripheral alpha-adrenergic stimulation and may result in exaggerated hypertension. This has been reported following naloxone administration in clonidine-poisoned children. In our view, an initial trial dose of naloxone of 0.1 mg/kg is warranted. If a salutary response occurs, repeat doses or infusion can be instituted.

In the present patient, the EKG revealed normal sinus rhythm. Opiate toxicity was excluded on the basis of the negative urine immunoassay. Clonidine poisoning was suspected clinically from toxidrome evaluation (lethargy, miosis, and hypotension), and the diagnosis was supported by the discovery of her clonidine exposure. Whole bowel irrigation enhanced elimination of the patch and provided final confirmation of the ingestion ("the proof was in the poop!"). In this case, 1 mg of naloxone was administered and did result in a marked improvement in mental status. She subsequently went on to complete recovery.

Clinical Pearls

1. A clonidine transdermal patch can contain a toxic amount of clonidine even after it has been used for 7 days.

2. Whole bowel irrigation can facilitate passage of transdermal systems.

3. Naloxone may reverse all or none of clonidine's opioid-associated effects.

4. Although rare, naloxone can precipitate hypertension in clonidine-poisoned patients.

REFERENCES:

1. Cada DJ (ed): Clonidine. In Facts and Comparisons. St. Louis, Wolters Kluwer, 2003, p 491.
2. DeRoos F: Miscellaneous antihypertensives. In Goldfrank L, Flomenbaum N, Lewin N, et al (eds): Goldfrank's Toxicological Emergencies, 7th ed. New York, McGraw Hill, 2002, p 776.
3. Segar DL: Clonidine toxicity revisited. J Toxicol Clin Toxicol 40:145-155, 2002.
4. Knapp JF, Fowler MA, Wheeler CA, Wasserman GS: Case 01-1995: A two-year-old female with alteration of consciousness. Pediatr Emerg Care 11:62-65, 1995.
5. Henretig F, Wiley J, Brown L: Clonidine patch toxicity: The proof is in the poop [abstract]. J Tox Clin Tox 33(5):520, 1995.
6. Harris JM: Clonidine patch toxicity. Ann Pharmacother 24:1191-1194, 1990.
7. Wiley JF, Wiley CC, Torrey SB, Henretig FM: Clonidine poisoning in young children. J Pediatr 116:654-658, 1990.

PATIENT 62

A 15-month-old dog with lethargy and red urine

A 15-month-old, spayed, female Maltese dog presents to a veterinary emergency service after exhibiting signs of lethargy, emesis, and dark red discoloration to her urine for 2 days. The owner treated the dog with baby aspirin soon after the onset of clinical signs. The dog is being treated for otitis externa (gentamicin + betamethasone + clotrimazole) by a local veterinarian. There is no other history of significant illness.

Physical Examination: Temperature 36.5° C (normal 37.5–39.0° C), pulse 170/min (80–120/min), respirations 20/min (20–22/min). General: lethargic. HEENT: mucous membranes dry, tacky, and slightly icteric. Chest: clear to auscultation. Cardiovascular: bounding, synchronous pulses; grade III/IV systolic heart murmur. Abdomen: soft. Genitourinary: orange-colored feces, dark red urine.

Laboratory Findings: Hemogram: Hct 7% (normal 38–57%), +2 polychromasia, Heinz bodies, many nucleated RBCs. Serum chemistries: glucose 59 mg/dL (63–109 mg/dL), BUN 122 mg/dL (8.7–30.5 mg/dL), phosphorus 8.2 mg/dL (2.8–6.2 mg/dL), total protein 7.9 g/dL (5.7–7.6g/dL), albumin 3.9 g/dL (2.8–3.8 g/dL), AST 585 U/L (10–32 U/L), alkaline phosphatase 556 U/L (18–94 U/L), GGT 55 U/L (0–6 U/L), total bilirubin 5.5 mg/dL (0–0.23 mg/dL). Urinalysis: dark red color. Parasitology: fecal negative for parasites. Microbiology: fecal negative for *Salmonella* and *Campylobacter*.

Questions: How would you characterize this dog's anemia? What additional study might confirm the toxic etiology?

Diagnosis: Ingestion of U.S. penny coins is the most common cause of Heinz-body hemolytic anemia among dogs. This diagnosis was confirmed with an abdominal radiograph (see figure).

Discussion: Ingestion of zinc-containing pennies is the most common cause of zinc intoxication in dogs. Some pennies minted in 1982 and all pennies minted since 1983 are composed of copper-coated zinc (97.5% zinc). Toxic doses of zinc for dogs have not been definitively determined, but ingestion of one penny is potentially toxic. Most case reports involve dogs weighing less than 30 kg. In dogs, zinc from metallic objects is rapidly solubilized in the acidic environment of the stomach. Zinc-containing metallic objects such as galvanized nuts, cage wiring, nails, staples, zippers, and fence clips are also potentially hazardous. Other products containing zinc include calamine lotion, paints, suppositories, fertilizers, and medications containing zinc salts such as zinc undecylenate (Desenex), zinc oxide, zinc acetate, and zinc sulfate. Zinc is relatively bioavailable irrespective of its form.

Interestingly, ingestion of pennies by young children is *not* considered to present an intoxication hazard. The reason for this difference is unknown but may be related to differences in body weight or dissolution rates of coins in the stomach. However, massive coin ingestions by people can result in zinc intoxication.

The mechanism of toxicity is unknown, although oxidant-induced damage is hypothesized. Red blood cells, liver, kidneys, and the pancreas are target organs. Zinc salts such as zinc chloride are corrosive and their ingestion can cause significant gastrointestinal (GI) damage.

Severe intravascular hemolysis is the most consistent clinical finding in dogs. The onset of clinical signs is variable, ranging from <2 hours to several days. This is dependent on the form and amount of zinc ingested. Initial clinical signs are most often related to GI distress such as anorexia, emesis, and diarrhea. An intravascular hemolysis often follows, characterized by pale or icteric mucous membranes, anemia, hemoglobinemia, hemoglobinuria. Complete blood counts are consistent with hemolysis: icteric serum and a normocytic-macrocytic, hypochromic anemia. A regenerative response ($\uparrow$ nucleated RBCs, basophilic stippling, polychromasia) can be seen later in the intoxication. Serum chemistries often indicate liver, kidney, and pancreatic dysfunction. Kidney impairment may be secondary to a hemoglobinuric nephrosis. Animals are often dehydrated ($\uparrow$ total protein, $\uparrow$ BUN). In some cases, there is radiographic evidence of a metallic object in the GI tract. Objects that exhibit areas of radiolucency are often pennies whose copper coating has begun to dissolve and the underlying zinc is beginning to solubilize. In the Figure, note the round, radiodense object in the upper left. Two radiolucent areas appear within the object.

Zinc intoxication can be confirmed antemortem by measuring serum zinc concentrations; levels are often >10 ppm in confirmed cases. Trace metal free serum tubes should be used to collect and store samples for testing. Liver, kidney, and pancreatic tissues contain elevated zinc concentrations and can be used for analysis postmortem. Differential diagnoses depend on the predominant clinical signs exhibited. If GI signs predominate, acute bacterial, viral, or parasitic infections should

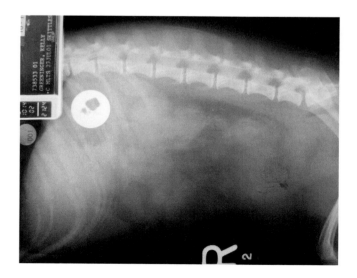

be considered. Other causes of intravascular hemolysis include immune-mediated diseases and onion, garlic, copper, acetaminophen, propylene glycol, and snake venom toxicoses.

Treatment consists of removal of any zinc-containing objects from the GI tract. This is most often done endoscopically. Once the object is removed, serum and tissue zinc concentrations decline rapidly. Whole blood transfusions and intravenous fluids may be necessary to alleviate anemia and dehydration. Antiemetics such as metoclopramide can be used to control emesis. Chelation with calcium disodium EDTA has been suggested to increase zinc excretion, but there are no controlled studies that have investigated its effect on case outcome.

In the present case, the dog vomited a partially digested penny soon after abdominal radiographs were taken. The dog was given a blood transfusion, intravenous fluids, antiemetics (metoclopramide and dolasetron), a gastric mucosal protectant (sulcralfate), and an antioxidant (S-adenosylmethionine). Abdominal ultrasound performed 48 hours after admission was normal. Nausea, emesis, and diarrhea persisted for approximately 5 days. Gradual improvement was noted over the next 2 days as the abnormal hemogram, BUN, and liver enzyme values returned to normal. Serum zinc values declined from 29.6 ppm at initial presentation to 8.3 ppm within 48 hours. The dog was released 1 week after admission and made a full recovery.

Clinical Pearls

1. Abdominal imaging (radiographs, ultrasound) is indicated in any dog presenting with a hemolytic anemia to rule out the presence of a metallic object potentially containing zinc. Radiolucent areas in a round foreign body are consistent with zinc penny ingestion.

2. Zinc concentrations should be determined in appropriately stored serum samples. Rubber stoppers from most blood collection tubes leach zinc, thus artificially elevating serum concentrations. Ideally, trace metal free serum tubes should be used.

3. Once zinc-containing objects are removed from the gastrointestinal tract, serum zinc values fall rapidly. There is no good evidence that chelation treatment alters case outcome.

REFERENCES

1. Gandini G, Bettini G, Peitra M, et al: Clinical and pathologic findings of acute zinc intoxication in a puppy. J Small Anim Pract 43:539-542, 2002.
2. Cahill-Morasco R, DePasquale MA: Zinc toxicosis in small animals. Compend Contin Edu 24:712-720, 2002.
3. Talcott PA: Zinc poisoning. In Peterson ME, Talcott PA (eds): Small Animal Toxicology. Philadelphia, W.B. Saunders, 2001, pp 756-761.
4. Paopairochanakorn C, Warfield S, White S: Zinc toxicity associated with massive coin ingestion. J Toxicol Clin Toxicol 39:553, 2001.
5. White NC: An analysis of 25,394 coin exposures reported to poison centers. J Toxicol Clin Toxicol 38:526, 2000.
6. Llobet JM, Domingo JL, Corbella J: Antidotes for zinc intoxication in mice. Arch Toxicol 61:321-323, 1988.

PATIENT 63

A 13-month-old boy who swallowed a quarter

A mother brings her 13-month-old boy to the emergency department immediately after she witnessed him swallowing a quarter. He coughed and gagged some at the time, but now seems comfortable.

Physical Examination: Temperature 37.1° C, pulse 136/min, respirations 22/min, blood pressure 100/60 mmHg. General: awake, alert, and interactive. HEENT: no foreign body visualized, no drooling. Chest: good aeration of all lung fields without stridor or wheezing. Heart: normal. Abdomen: normal. Extremities: normal. Skin: normal.

Laboratory Findings: Chest radiograph (see below): a circular esophageal foreign body at the level of the thoracic inlet.

Question: When, and by what method, should this esophageal foreign body be removed?

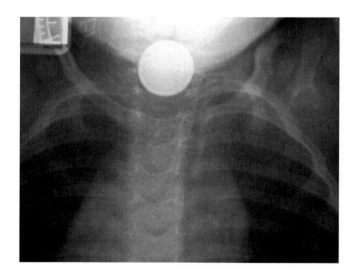

Diagnosis and Treatment: The radiographic shadow around the perimeter of this foreign body suggests it to be a button battery, rather than a quarter. An impacted esophageal button battery calls for emergent endoscopic removal.

Discussion: Coins are the foreign bodies most commonly ingested by children. Most coin ingestions are uneventful, and the proper triage of asymptomatic children with histories of swallowing coins is controversial. Esophageal impaction of an ingested coin is the most frequently encountered complication and, left untreated, may lead to significant morbidity. Most coins lodged within the proximal to mid-esophagus require semielective physical removal, although up to two-thirds of coins trapped at the gastroesophageal junction spontaneously pass within 12 hours. Several techniques for dislodgment of coins have been successful, including balloon-tipped catheter extraction of proximal esophagus coins, bougienage of distal esophagus coins, and endoscopic extraction. Glucagon or diazepam administration has been suggested as a pharmacological maneuver to reduce tone in the lower esophageal sphincter, but clinical effectiveness at passing esophageal coins has not been demonstrated in children.

Disk, or button, batteries may be mistaken for coins. They range in size from 6.8 to 25 mm in diameter and are used to power watches, calculators, cameras, toys, and hearing aids. Over 1500 disk battery ingestion incidents are reported to the American Association of Poison Control Centers Toxic Exposure Surveillance System each year, and many go unreported. It is not known how many of these are initially **misidentified**. The vast majority of ingested button batteries remain asymptomatic, and there is seldom reason for concern once an ingested button battery reaches the stomach.

However, lodgment of a button battery in the esophagus, nose, or ear constitutes a medical emergency. A combination of alkaline or chemical corrosion, generated electrical current, and mechanical pressure may lead to significant injury in these situations. Complications of esophageal impaction of disk batteries can include esophageal burns and perforation, esophagotracheal fistula, esophagoaortic fistula, and death. Injuries observed after button battery impaction within the ear canal or nares include tympanic membrane perforation, otitis externa, ossicle disruption, nasal septum perforation, nasal turbinate destruction, and facial nerve paralysis.

The present patient was initially misidentified as an asymptomatic child with an impacted esophageal quarter. He was admitted to the hospital with a plan to perform endoscopic removal of the coin in the morning if spontaneous passage did not occur. Within 3 hours of hospital arrival, the boy developed stridor and a distressed appearance. On retrospect, the **classic "halo sign"** apparent on the radiograph indicated a disk battery lodged within the esophagus. Emergent rigid endoscopy was performed, during which time a button battery was extracted and circumferential burns to the esophageal mucosa were noted. His recovery was complicated by several exacerbations of stridor and respiratory compromise. Subsequent laryngoscopy revealed granulation of the posterior cricoid and interarytenoid regions. A tracheostomy was employed temporarily to allow for healing, and the boy achieved a full recovery.

Clinical Pearls

1. Many button batteries have a classic double-shadow radiographic appearance, the so-called halo sign, which allows for their proper identification.

2. The radiographs of suspected esophageal coins should be closely inspected to ensure that they are not actually button batteries.

3. Endoscopic removal of impacted esophageal disk batteries is preferred because it allows for visualization of mucosal injury and more controlled extraction.

4. Impacted button batteries should be removed emergently, as tissue injury may occur in only a few hours.

5. The U.S. National Button Battery Ingestion hotline (202-625-3333) or your regional poison control center can help identify a battery and its chemical system.

REFERENCES

1. Cerri RW, Liacouras CA: Evaluation and management of foreign bodies in the upper gastrointestinal tract. Pediatr Case Rev 3:150-156, 2003.
2. Samad L, Ali M, Hasan R: Button battery ingestion: Hazards of esophageal impaction. J Pediatr Surg 34:1527-1531, 1999.
3. Conners GP: A literature-based comparison of three methods of pediatric esophageal coin removal. Pediatr Emerg Care 13:154-157, 1997.
4. Litovitz T, Schmitz BF: Ingestion of cylindrical and button bateries: An analysis of 2382 cases. Pediatrics 89:747-757, 1992.

Amy L. Puchalski, MD
Kevin C. Osterhoudt, MD

PATIENT 64

A 14-year-old girl who ingested acetaminophen

A 14-year-old girl is taken to the emergency department by her mother 3 hours after ingesting approximately 120 tablets of regular-strength Tylenol. She has a history of depression, and the ingestion was intentional.

Physical Examination: Temperature 36.4° C, pulse 83/min, respirations 17/min, blood pressure 129/61 mmHg. General: alert, oriented, and cooperative. HEENT: pupils are symmetrical and reactive. Chest: clear lungs to auscultation bilaterally. Cardiovascular: regular rate and rhythm without murmur, good peripheral perfusion. Abdomen: benign without hepatosplenomegaly. Neuromuscular: intact cranial nerves, normal tone and strength, no asterixis.

Laboratory Findings: Coagulation profile: normal. Serum chemistries: normal (including aminotransferases). Acetaminophen level at 4 hours: 348 µg/mL (possible toxicity range).

Initial Course: The patient receives activated charcoal and an initial dose of oral N-acetylcysteine (NAC), which she vomits within 15 minutes. She receives famotidine, metoclopramide, ondansetron, and trimethobenzamide, none of which relieve her nausea and vomiting to an extent that she can tolerate oral NAC. Attempts at nasogastric administration of NAC fail, and she is now nearly 8 hours postingestion.

Question: Are there any options for her continued treatment?

Diagnosis and Treatment: The patient has ingested enough acetaminophen acutely to potentially injure her liver severely, and she receives treatment with intravenous NAC.

Discussion: Acetaminophen represents one of the most common toxic ingestions reported to poison control centers within North America and accounts for significant poisoning morbidity and mortality. When acetaminophen is ingested and absorbed in therapeutic doses, 90% is metabolized in the liver to inactive compounds through glucuronidation and sulfation. A small amount of that remaining is oxidized by cytochromes to *N*-acetyl-*p*-benzoquinoneimine (NAPQI), which is then reduced by glutathione to a non-toxic metabolite. In the setting of acetaminophen overdose, the rates of NAPQI formation rapidly increase and overwhelm the supply of glutathione. NAPQI then binds to hepatocytes, causing cellular damage and death. NAC is a precursor for reduced glutathione and increases the capacity to detoxify NAPQI. NAC is especially efficacious in the treatment of acetaminophen toxicity *when given within 8 hours of ingestion.*

The **side effects of NAC** include nausea, vomiting, and diarrhea; such therapy may exacerbate any nausea and vomiting related to acetaminophen poisoning. Some patients are also intolerant of the smell and taste of NAC. The incidence of vomiting from acetaminophen toxicity ranges up to 50% among significantly overdosed patients, and, although a frequent problem, there are little data on how often patients vomit after administration of oral NAC. Initially, it is best to keep oral NAC in a closed container to mask the odor, as well as to dilute NAC 1:4 in chilled juice or soda to make it more palatable. For some patients, antiemetic therapy is adequate to make oral NAC tolerable. To date, little evidence exists to compare the efficacy of various antiemetics in this situation. High-dose metoclopromide and ondansetron have both been shown to have some success in reducing NAC-associated emesis. Patients who continue to vomit antidotal NAC despite antiemetic therapy may benefit from slow nasogastric or nasojejunal tube administration. Despite best efforts, vomiting will continue to complicate treatment of a small subset of acetaminophen-poisoned patients.

Intravenous NAC offers an alternative to oral administration, and is the standard of care in Canada and Great Britain. As of 2002, no specific form of intravenous NAC had been approved for use by the United States Food and Drug Administration, but some of the oral formulations are pure enough for parenteral use. Specific situations where the intravenous route may be preferable to the oral route include patients with intractable vomiting, pregnancy, abdominal trauma, fulminant hepatic failure where gastrointestinal bleeding or lactulose therapy may interfere with oral absorption, and coingestion of a substance requiring ongoing gastrointestinal decontamination. One of the more commonly used protocols for intravenous therapy entails administering 140 mg/kg as a 3% solution over 90 minutes followed by 12 doses of 70 mg/kg given every 4 hours over 60 minutes, although even shorter courses have been recommended.

Anaphylactoid reactions, such as rash, angioedema, bronchospasm, hypotension and, rarely, death, may complicate use of intravenous NAC. Most such adverse events occur during infusion of the loading dose and are rate-related. Symptomatic treatment for allergic reactions, along with temporary cessation of the drug infusion, typically allows all patients to complete their course of intravenous NAC. The patient in this case received intravenous NAC therapy. A localized dermatologic reaction to the infusion was treated with diphenhydramine, and she had no further complications. Her peak prothrombin time was 15.4 seconds, and her peak alanine aminotransferase was 21 U/L. Currently, plans are in process to bring an intravenous form of NAC to the U.S. market.

Clinical Pearls

1. *N*-acetylcysteine (NAC) therapy for a single, acute acetaminophen overdose is guided by a serum acetaminophen level in the toxic range on the Matthew-Rumack nomogram and should begin within 8 hours of ingestion for best outcome.

2. In cases of acetaminophen-induced hepatotoxicity, NAC therapy should be continued until objective liver healing begins.

3. Intravenous NAC is an alternative to oral NAC, particularly in cases of:
   Refractory emesis
   Penetrating abdominal trauma
   Fulminant hepatic failure
   Pregnancy
   Coingestants requiring ongoing oral decontamination.

4. The anaphylactoid reactions associated with intravenous NAC are dose, concentration, and rate dependent. They usually can be controlled by knowledgeable medical personnel.

REFERENCES

1. Bizovi KE, Smilkstein MJ: Acetaminophen. In Goldfrank LR, Flomenbaum NE, Lewin NA, et al. (eds): Goldfrank's Toxicologic Emergencies, 7th ed. New York, McGraw-Hill, 2002, pp 480-506.
2. Amizadeh A, McCotter C: The intravenous use of oral acetylcysteine (mucomyst) for the treatment of acetaminophen overdose. Arch Intern Med 162:96-97, 2002.
3. Buckley NA, Whyte IM, O'Connell DL, Dawson AH: Oral or intravenous N-acetylcysteine: Which is the treatment of choice for acetaminophen (paracetamol) poisoning? Clin Toxicology 37(6):759-767, 1999.
4. Yip L, Dart RC, Hurlbutt KM: Intravenous administration of oral N-acetylcysteine. Crit Care Med 26:40-43, 1998.
5. Scharman EJ: Use of ondansetron and other antiemetics in the management of toxic acetaminophen ingestions. Clin Toxicology 36(1-2):19-25, 1998.

PATIENT 65

A 5-year-old female cat with lethargy, weakness, and severe dyspnea

A 5-year-old, mixed breed cat has been vomiting hairballs for 2 days. The cat is anorectic and was given one regular-strength Tylenol tablet (325 mg acetaminophen or *N*-acetyl-*p*-aminophenol [APAP]) by its owner to make the animal feel better. Twenty-four hours after administering APAP, the cat is noted to be tachypneic, severely dyspneic, and cyanotic.

Physical Examination: Temperature 32.5° C (normal 38.3–39.5° C); pulse 120/min (130–140/min); respirations 45/min (20–30/min) and labored. General: lethargic and distressed. HEENT: cyanotic mucous membranes. Chest: auscultation normal, increased respiratory effort. Cardiovascular: grade II/VI systolic murmur. Extremities: edematous face and paws. Endocrine: palpable thyroid nodule.

Laboratory Findings: Hemogram: brown coloration to blood; Heinz bodies present; Hct 23% (25.3–37.5%). Serum chemistries: ALT 2097 U/L (20–107 U/L); AST 2078 (1–37 U/L). Urinalysis: normal. Arterial blood gas: pH 7.28 (7.3–7.4); methemoglobin 45% (0.5–3.0%). T4: 0.5 µg/dL (0.8–4.0 normal). Abdominal radiographs: mild hepatomegaly. Thoracic radiographs: enlarged heart.

Question: What is the likely etiology for methemoglobinemia in this cat?

Diagnosis: APAP intoxication. APAP is *not* typically a cause of methemoglobinemia in humans.

Discussion: APAP is a widely available analgesic and antipyretic contained in many over-the-counter medications intended for human consumption. APAP intoxication in pets, especially cats, is relatively common. In cats, the majority of intoxications are secondary to intentional administration of APAP by their owners. In dogs, exposure is more often due to ingestion following chewing of drug containers. Species sensitivity to APAP is variable; cats are intoxicated by dosages of 50 to 100 mg/kg, while dogs are intoxicated by dosages from 200 to 600 mg/kg. Humans are reportedly intoxicated at dosages of 150 mg/kg or greater. Extensive risk determination guidelines are available to assess human exposures to APAP and the need for antidote administration. Unfortunately, similar guidelines have not been formulated for animals.

Metabolic differences account for the unique sensitivity of cats to acetaminophen (see figures). In most species, APAP is metabolized in the liver via one of three pathways. The parent compound can be conjugated to glucuronide or sulfate via uridine diphosphate (UDP)-glucuronosyltransferase and phenol sulfotransferase, respectively. In addition, it can be metabolized by P450 enzymes to an electrophilic reactive intermediate known as *N*-acetyl-*para*-benzequinoneimine (NAPQI). This reactive intermediate is subsequently detoxified by conjugation with glutathione, cysteine, or mercapturic acid. A small amount of APAP is excreted as parent compound. In humans, the glucuronidation pathway is the most important, accounting for 40–67% of APAP metabolism. Cats are deficient in uridine diphosphate (UDP)-glucuronosyltransferase and are therefore poor at glucuronidation. The primary conjugation pathway for APAP in cats involves sulfation. Both the glucuronidation and sulfation pathways are easily saturated, which can lead to increased production of NAPQI at relatively low dosages of APAP. When endogenous stores of glutathione and other reducing compounds are exhausted, increased quantities of NAPQI interact with multiple cell macromolecules, resulting in cell damage. In addition to limited capacity for glucuronidation, the glutathione conjugation capacity of cats is also limited.

Clinical signs in cats can occur as soon as 1 hour after ingestion, but more commonly occur 6 to 24 hours after exposure. Presenting signs in cats are generally related to hypoxia secondary to methe-

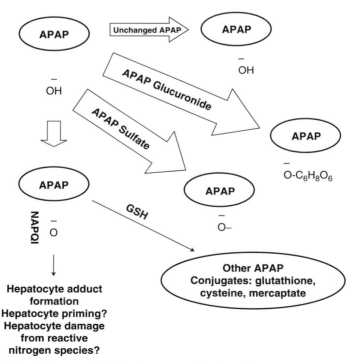

APAP metabolism in humans. (Relative importance of pathway is represented by size of arrow).

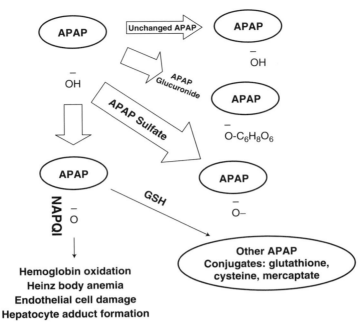

APAP metabolism in cats. (Relative importance of pathway is represented by size of arrow.)

moglobinemia. Mucous membranes are most often a chocolate-brown to blue color, and the cat is dyspneic and tachycardic. While APAP-induced hemoglobin oxidative injury is rarely clinically evident in humans, cat hemoglobin is especially sensitive to oxidative damage, since it has eight reactive sulfhydryl groups compared to only four in dogs. A Heinz body anemia is commonly reported. There is often significant edema of the face, neck, and paws. The pathophysiology of the edema is unknown, but it may be related to damage to endothelial cells. Significant liver dysfunction may or may not be present. Mortality in cats is most often due to hypoxia and not liver damage. In dogs, as in humans, hepatotoxicity is a much more common feature of APAP intoxication. Methemoglobinemia and peripheral edema have also been reported in dogs but are less common than in cats. From a comparative toxicological standpoint, it is interesting to note that damage is not limited to hepatocytes in dogs and cats as it appears to be in humans.

In veterinary medicine, a diagnosis of APAP intoxication relies primarily on a history of APAP ingestion and the occurrence of compatible clinical signs. Analysis of plasma or urine samples for acetaminophen is possible, but results are unlikely to be available quickly enough to influence initial case assessment and need for treatment.

The goals of treatment are to stabilize the patient, decontaminate if appropriate, and administer the antidote N-acetylcysteine (NAC). If dyspneic on presentation, gentle animal handling will reduce stress, and supplemental oxygen should be provided. Nomograms are *not* available for animals, to assist the clinician in determining the need for NAC administration. In veterinary medicine, NAC is given at a loading dose of 140 mg/kg IV, or orally in animals that are not vomiting, and then at 70 mg/kg IV or orally QID for an additional 5 to 7 treatments. Ascorbic acid is a reducing agent that has not been studied extensively. Blood transfusions can be given if anemia is severe, and intravenous fluids are generally recommended.

The present patient was severely dyspneic due to the methemoglobinemia. The patient was placed in an oxygen cage, administered NAC and vitamin C intravenously, and administered fresh whole blood and normal saline. Maintenance doses of NAC were administered for 36 hours. Clinical improvement occurred over the next 2 days, although the cat remained anorectic. Unfortunately, monetary constraints prevented serial serum chemistries being performed to assess liver function. The thyroid nodule was believed to be unrelated to APAP ingestion.

Clinical Pearls

1. There are significant species differences with regard to the toxicity of APAP. Species differences are due to qualitative and quantitative differences in APAP metabolism.

2. APAP-induced hematological (methemoglobinemia, anemia, Heinz body formation) and cardiovascular toxicities (peripheral edema) are common in cats and dogs, but are rare in humans. Mortality in cats is more often due to these effects than to hepatotoxicity.

3. In cats, physiological differences account for the more common occurrence of methemoglobinemia and Heinz body anemia after APAP ingestion. The hemoglobin of cats is much more sensitive to oxidant-induced damage than that of dogs or humans.

4. Treatment of APAP-intoxicated pets parallels that for human intoxications.

REFERENCES

1. Bizovi KE, Smilkstein MJ: Acetaminophen. In Goldfrank LR, Flomenbaum NE, Lewin NA, et al (eds): Goldfrank's Toxicologic Emergencies, 7th ed. New York, McGraw-Hill, 2002, pp 480-506.
2. Sellon RK: Acetaminophen. In Peterson ME, Talcott PA (eds): Small Animal Toxicology. Philadelphia, W.B. Saunders Co., 2000, pp 388-395.
3. Taylor NS, Dhupa N: Acetaminophen toxicity in cats and dogs. Compend Cont Ed Prac Vet 22:160-170, 2000.
4. Aronson LR, Drobatz K: Acetaminophen toxicosis in 17 cats. J Vet Emerg Crit Care 6:65-69, 1996.
5. Savides MC, Oehme FW, Nash SL et al: The toxicity and biotransformation of single doses of acetaminophen in dogs and cats. Toxicol Appl Pharmacol 74:26-34, 1984.

Francis DeRoos, MD

PATIENT 66

A 35-year-old fisherman with an itchy rash

A 35-year-old man presents after 1 day of an itchy rash on his arms. He has no medical problems, is taking no medications, and has no prior history of this rash. Three days ago he went fishing along a nearby creek; he often had to climb over or through plants to access the water.

Physical Examination: Temperature: 37.2° C, pulse 72/min, respirations 16/min, blood pressure 116/74. General: well appearing, in no distress. Skin (see figure) numerous vesicles on erythematous bases clustered on forearms and elbows bilaterally; some vesicles in linear distribution, some evidence of excoriation. Chest: normal. Abdomen: normal.

Laboratory Findings: None

Question: What caused this rash?

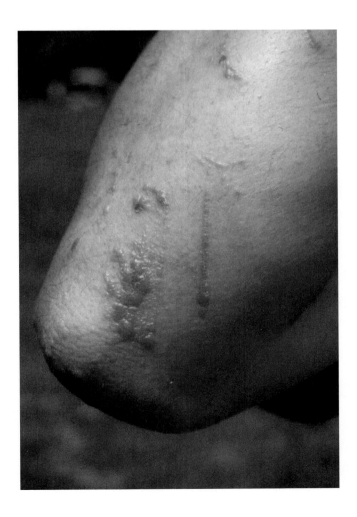

Diagnosis: The linear distribution of the vesicular rash and the fishing history strongly suggest the diagnosis of rhus dermatitis caused by contact with a plant from the genus *Toxicodendron*, such as poison ivy.

Discussion: Each year millions of people develop allergic reactions after coming in contact with plants from the *Toxicodendron* genus, namely poison ivy (*T. radicans;* see figure), poison oak (*T. diversilobum*), and poison sumac (*T. vernix*). *Toxicodendron* is found almost everywhere in the United States except Hawaii and Alaska. The plants may grow either as a shrub or a vine depending on location and species. Poison oak grows predominantly west of the Rocky Mountains and in the Southeast; poison sumac is much less common, growing predominantly in standing water like peat bogs of the far North and the swamps of the South; and poison ivy is the most widely distributed of these plants, found throughout the U.S. except for the Western coastal states. Poison oak and ivy have leaves that grow in clusters of three fostering the old adage, "leaves of three, let them be." Sumac has double rows of smaller leaflets numbering 6 to 13. The leaves tend to be a lively green with almost a sheen on them when they emerge in spring, remain green all summer, and then in fall turn various shades of yellow, red, or brown before shedding. Early in the summer, small bunches of

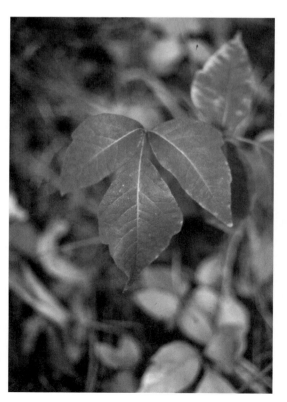

greenish flowers grow off the main stem where the leaves join. Later in the season these will turn into drooping clusters of small, whitish, and waxy berries. Throughout this discussion the use of the term poison ivy refers generically to all three types of plants.

The rash caused by poison ivy is an allergic contact dermatitis to an **oil** called **urushiol** found within all parts of the plant, including the leaves, stems, and roots. This clear to pale-yellow oil escapes whenever the plant is cut or broken. Human exposure is typically from directly brushing against branches or leaves, although indirect exposure from oils that have rubbed off on the fur of pets, outer clothing, or gardening equipment can also occur. Rarely, burning of these plants leads to airborne dermal and pulmonary exposure, which can be life-threatening. Once on the skin, urushiol penetrates and acts as a potent antigen, inducing a cell-mediated (type IV) immunological reaction. With this type of allergy, any re-exposure to urushiol will trigger **"preprogrammed" or sensitized T cells** to release immunological chemicals like histamine and produce the rash, typically within 12 to 48 hours. Over 85% of people, when adequately exposed, will become hypersensitized to urushiol. This allergy tends to decline with age.

In the initial stages of the rash, redness and swelling develop, followed by vesicles and increasing pruritis. After a few days, these vesicular lesions may leak a characteristic clear, honey-yellow fluid that is not contagious; the lesions then become crusted and scaly before healing in about 10–14 days. Any part of the skin can develop this rash if exposed, but areas that are thinner, like the face and genitalia, tend to develop a more pronounced rash sooner, while the soles of the feet and palms of the hands are relatively resistant. Contrary to popular notion, the rash does *not* spread. Rather, the sequential development of the rash (e.g., first the face, then the forearm, and finally the lower leg) after exposure reflects the relative **skin thickness** of these areas and not spreading. If rashes are recurrent, then re-exposure should be strongly considered, particularly from household pets or commonly used clothes like jackets or boots.

After thorough bathing, the main treatment of the poison ivy rash consists of antipruritic therapy such as diphenhydramine, hydroxazine, or chlorpheneramine. The antihistaminic as well as the sedative effects of these drugs will help the patient tolerate the rash until it can heal and will decrease the risk of superinfection by decreasing itching. Other recommended therapies include daily soaks in a bathtub with oatmeal soaps or baking powder to decrease the itching and dry the oozing vesicles. Vesicles should be left open to air as much as possible to promote drying and crusting. Topical lotions like calamine or Burrow's solution may provide some relief, but there is no evidence that topical hydrocortisone 1% cream or ointment provides any benefit. In severe cases, systemic steroids may be valuable. Long-acting agents or taper dosing is often needed to prevent rebound dermatitis.

Prevention of exposure is the best method for minimizing the discomfort associated with this rash. Prevention can be effected through eliminating of any poison ivy from gardens, learning to recognize the characteristics of the plant (leaf color and shape, common habitats), and wearing protective clothing like long-sleeved shirts and pants whenever out in the woods. If an exposed area is washed with soap and water within 30 minutes of contact, the rash will be minimized or even prevented.

Clinical Pearls

1. All parts of the poison ivy plant, whether the leaf, stem, or root, contain urushiol, the oil responsible for producing the allergic rash.

2. Any pruritic, vesicular rash during the summer months, particularly if in a linear pattern, should raise a high suspicion for a contact dermatitis from poison ivy.

3. Standard treatment includes soaking baths with drying solutions like oatmeal soaps or baking soda, diphenhydramine to decrease itching, and systemic steroids in patients with severe or extensive reactions.

4. The main complication of this allergic dermatitis is superinfection secondary to excoriating and opening these pruritic vesicles.

REFERENCES
1. Lee NP, Arriola ER: Poison ivy, oak, and sumac dermatitis. West J Med 171:354-355, 1999.
2. Fisher AA: Poison ivy/oak dermatitis. Part I: Prevention—soap and water, topical barriers, hyposensitization. Cutis 57: 384-386, 1996.

Robert G. Hendrickson, MD

PATIENT 67

A 56-year-old man with AIDS and metabolic acidosis

A 56-year-old man with a history of AIDS, hepatitis C, and hypertension presents with a 1-week history of increasing dyspnea on exertion, nausea, and fatigue. He is hospitalized for presumed *Pneumocystis carinii* pneumonia, treated with intravenous trimethoprim-sulfamethoxazole, and continued on his maintenance medications which include nelfinavir, lamivudine, nevirapine, and clonidine. After 3 days of gradual improvement in his symptoms, significant dyspnea and tachypnea develop.

Physical Examination: Temperature 37.3° C, (rectal), pulse 130/min, respirations 30/min, blood pressure 100/50 mmHg. General: sitting up in bed with significant respiratory distress. HEENT: normal. Neck: normal. Chest: scattered rhonchi. Cardiaovascular: tachycardia with regular rhythm and no murmur. Abdomen: normal. Skin: normal.

Laboratory Findings: Hemogram: WBC 14,200/μL with 84% neutrophils and no bands, hemoglobin 9 mg/dL, MCV 105. Serum chemistries: sodium 132 mEq/L, potassium 4.8 mEq/L, choride 85 mEq/L, bicarbonate 13 mEq/L (anion gap 34 mEq/L), blood urea nitrogen 64 mg/dL, creatinine 3.9 mg/dL, glucose 129 mg/dL, AST 2040 IU/L, ALT 550 IU/L, total bilirubin 1.2 mg/dL, alkaline phosphatase 100 IU/L, lipase 50 IU/L. Arterial blood gas (50% Fio_2): pH 7.06, $Paco_2$ 16 mmHg, Pao_2 166 mmHg, arterial lactate 19 mmol/L. CPK 398 IU/L, MB mass 21.7, troponin 10.9 ng/mL. Serum salicylate: none detected. Serum ketones: normal. EKG: Sinus tachycardia 134/min, no ischemic changes. Chest radiograph: no infiltrate.

Question: What is the cause of this patient's lactic acidosis?

Diagnosis and Treatment: An acute wide anion gap metabolic acidosis and hyperlactatemia may be caused by end-organ hypoperfusion or by poisoning with several medications, including iron, metformin/phenformin, isoniazid, salicylates, cyanide, theophylline, toluene, or nucleoside analogue reverse transcriptase inhibitors. In the present case, all of these causes—except nucleoside analogue—induced lactic acidosis—may be eliminated based on lack of availability of medications, symptomatology, or serum levels.

Discussion: Nucleoside analogue–induced lactic acidosis is a disorder that may occur among patients chronically treated with nucleoside analogues. Patients may develop an asymptomatic hyperlactatemia or develop constitutional symptoms for several months. These mild symptoms may be followed by an abrupt onset of acidosis, hyperlactatemia, and multiple organ failure.

Lactic acidosis develops when normal aerobic metabolism is disrupted, as may be caused by poor tissue oxygen supply from shock, arterial occlusion, or hypoxemia. This is predominantly effected by increased conversion of pyruvate to lactate. Lactic acidosis may also develop if there is disruption of normal functioning of the mitochondria (a mitochondriopathy), the site of aerobic metabolism. This is the mechanism by which nucleoside analogue reverse transcriptase inhibitors are thought to produce a lactic acidosis.

Nucleoside analogue reverse transcriptase inhibitors are a group of medications, including didanosine (Videx), lamivudine (3TC, Epivir), stavudine (d4T, Zerit), zalcitabine (ddCC, Hivid), zidovudine (AZT, ZDV, Retrovir), used to treat patients infected with HIV. They function by interfering with viral reverse transcriptase and thereby inhibiting viral replication. As a side effect, these medications also inhibit **mitochondrial DNA polymerase gamma**, but not eukaryotic DNA polymerase alpha and beta. This inhibition of DNA polymerase gamma may lead to an inefficient production of mitochondrial enzymes, including the cytochromes a and a3, which are essential components of the electron transport chain. Decreased numbers of these cytochromes leads to less aerobic metabolic capacity and a decrease in the $NAD/NADH_2$ ratio.

Accumulation of $NADH_2$ in the mitochondria shunts pyruvate into lactate rather than allowing it to enter the tricarboxylic acid cycle (seen when the $NAD/NADH_2$ ratio is high). The accumulation of $NADH_2$ by nucleoside analogues in some individuals can lead to **hyperlactatemia** with or without acidosis. Under normal cellular metabolism, hydrogen ions that are generated by hydrolysis of ATP are "buffered" by the electron transport chain and hydrogen ion–specific ATPase channels or pores. In a cell with nucleoside-induced abnormal mitochondrial function, these mechanisms are impaired or blocked.

Asymptomatic hyperlactatemia may occur in a small percentage of patients who are chronically taking nucleoside analogues, with less than 1% developing serum lactate levels more than twice normal. *Symptomatic* hyperlactatemia is noted in as many as 0.8% of HIV-infected patients who are treated with nucleoside analogues. Symptoms generally include fatigue, weakness, lipoatrophy, weight loss, nausea, or dyspnea on exertion and persist for many weeks to months. However, as in the present patient, the acute onset of profound dyspnea secondary to a rapidly developing lactic acidosis has also been reported. Symptomatic hyperlactatemia only develops after long-term therapy (typically longer than 1 year) and is not seen after acute overdoses. Patients with symptomatic hyperlactatemia may develop hepatic macrovesicular steatosis due to inhibition of mitochondrial fatty acid beta-oxidation, as well as pancreatitis and multiple organ failure.

The treatment of hyperlactatemia in asymptomatic patients without acidosis requires only removal of the drug. Symptomatic patients, however, may benefit from close monitoring and supportive care. Severe acidosis should be aggressively treated with a bicarbonate infusion, or hemodialysis with a bicarbonate buffer in the case of renal failure or fluid overload. Riboflavin, L-carnitine, and thiamine have been suggested as therapeutic agents, and while none have proven efficacy, they may be reasonable adjuncts in treating this serious condition.

Unfortunately, in the present patient, multiple organ failure, worsening severe acidosis, and hepatitis developed in the face of appropriate treatment including discontinuation of all his nucleoside analogue, early mechanical ventilation, bicarbonate infusion, thiamine, and l-carnitine. After 4 days of this aggressive therapy, his acidosis resolved, and he recovered fully.

Clinical Pearls

1. Constitutional symptoms in a patient treated with chronic nucleoside analogue therapy should prompt testing for hyperlactatemia and acidosis.

2. Nucleoside analogue–induced lactic acidosis is caused by inhibition of multiple mitochondrial enzymes.

3. Nucleoside analogues may induce a syndrome of severe acidosis, hyperlactatemia, and multiple organ failure.

4. Treatment of severe nucleoside analogue–induced lactic acidosis involves supportive care, bicarbonate, and possibly L-carnitine, riboflavin, and thiamine.

REFERENCES

1. Coghlan ME, Sommadossi JP, Jhala NC, et al: Symptomatic lactic acidosis in hospitalized antiretroviral-treated patients with human immunodeficiency virus infection: A report of 12 cases. Clin Infect Dis 33:1914-1921, 2001.
2. Boubaker K, Flepp M, Sudre P, et al: Hyperlactatemia and antiretroviral therapy: The Swiss HIV Cohort Study. Clin Infect Dis 33:1931-1937, 2001.
3. Carr A, Miller J, Law M, et al: A syndrome of lipoatrophy, lactic acidaemia and liver dysfunction associated with HIV nucleoside analogue therapy: Contribution to protease inhibitor–related lipodystrophy syndrome. AIDS 14:F25-F32, 2000.
4. Gerard Y, Maulin L, Yazdanpanah Y, et al: Symptomatic hyperlactatemia: An emerging complication of antiretroviral therapy. AIDS 14:2723-2730, 2000.
5. Claessens YE, Cariou A, Chiche JD, et al: L-carnitine as a treatment of life-threatening lactic acidosis induced by nucleoside analogues. AIDS 14:472, 2000.
6. Roy PM, Gouello JP, Pennison-Besnier I, et al: Severe lactic acidosis induced by nucleoside analogues in an HIV-infected man. Ann Emerg Med 34:282-284, 1999.
7. Sundar K, Suarez M, Banogon P, et al: Zidovudine-induced fatal lactic acidosis and hepatic failure in patients with acquired immunodeficiency syndrome: Report of two patients and review of the literature. Crit Care Med 25:1425-1430, 1997.

PATIENT 68

An 11-year-old boy with vomiting, weakness, and neck mass

An 11-year-old boy with blindness and mental retardation is evaluated for vomiting, weight loss, and a neck mass. Three weeks ago he began vomiting several times each day. The vomitus is neither bloody nor bilious. Despite antiemetics and dietary manipulation prescribed by a family physician, occasional vomiting persists. Two weeks ago a midline neck mass appeared, and the child has become easily fatigued and anorexic. Over the past 3 days severe vomiting has recurred, and the neck mass appears larger. By the time of presentation, his mother estimates that a 5- to 10-lb. weight loss has occurred over the preceding 3 weeks.

The child was the product of a twin gestation, complicated by breech delivery, perinatal hypoxia, and low Apgar scores. His early developmental milestones were very delayed, and he is severely visually handicapped and developmentally retarded with autistic features. He lives at home with his family and attends a special school for the blind. There are no other medical conditions and he takes no medications.

Physical Examination: Temperature 37° C; pulse 120/min, respirations 24/min, blood pressure 110/70 mmHg. General: thin, quiet, obviously functionally blind; moderately dehydrated with dry mucous membranes and slightly sunken eyes. Neck: 5×6 cm, firm, nontender mass, butterfly-shaped and positioned at the anterior midline. Chest: normal. Cardiovascular: normal. Abdomen: mild hepatomegaly. Neuromuscular: roving eye movements. Cardiac, pulmonary, and remainder of exam: unremarkable.

Laboratory Findings: Hemogram: WBC 6600/μL (normal differential), hemoglobin 19.2 g/dL, Hct 54.6%, platelets 288,000/μL. Serum chemistries: Na^+ 134 mEq/L; K^+ 4.1 mEq/L; Cl^- 104 mEq/L; bicarbonate 13 mEq/L; BUN 8 mg/dL; creatinine 0.3 mg/dL. Urinalysis: specific gravity 1.025; pH 5.0; negative blood, protein, glucose. Venous blood gas (in room air): pH 7.36, P_{CO_2} 27 mmHg, P_{O_2} 44 mmHg. Thyroid function tests pending.

Initial Hospital Course: The child is admitted with diagnoses of thyroid disorder and dehydration with pseudo-polycythemia and begun on intravenous fluid therapy. The next morning his vomiting worsens, and a gallop rhythm develops. The serum bicarbonate falls to 11 mEq/L, while the hemoglobin remains 19 g/dL. Chest radiograph reveals cardiomegaly, and abdominal ultrasound notes slight hepatomegaly. EKG is notable for sinus tachycardia and an axis of $-77°$, with normal intervals. Echocardiogram demonstrates normal anatomy, mildly dilated left ventricle, and decreased shortening fraction of 25%. With thyroid function tests still pending, the complex of thyromegaly, cardiomegaly, and persistent tachycardia is interpreted as mild congestive heart failure secondary to hyperthyroidism. Thus, the patient is begun cautiously on propranolol. However, he fails to improve. Vomiting and metabolic acidosis persist, and his heart failure seems to worsen. Thyroid function tests return with *hypothyroid* values: thyroxine 2.4 μg/dL and TSH 26 μIU/mL. Propranolol is discontinued, and several consultations are sought.

Questions: What additional diagnostic tests are indicated? Is there a unitary diagnosis for the complex of vomiting, metabolic acidosis, polycythemia, congestive heart failure, and hypothyroidism?

Diagnosis: Cobalt toxicity. The persistent vomiting prompted an abdominal radiograph (see figure). The large radiopaque mass proved to be the explanation for this rare poisoning in a child, when at surgical removal it was discovered to be a matted clump of 51 cobalt-containing magnets, apparently ingested by this developmentally and visually handicapped child. The serum cobalt level was 4.1 μg/dL (normal 0.35–1.7), and the urine cobalt excretion was 1700 μg/24 hrs (normal 1–7).

Discussion: Cobalt has a fascinating therapeutic and toxicological history. It is an essential mineral, contained in cyanocobalamin (vitamin B_{12}). It has been used in the past as a hematinic and was often quite efficacious in the treatment of anemias such as those due to chronic renal failure and sickle cell disease. Unfortunately, its usefulness in this context was compromised by its tendency to produce clinically significant hypothyroidism as an adverse effect.

Cobalt salt toxicity has been described mostly as a chronic intoxication causing "beer-drinker's cardiomyopathy." In the mid-20th century, many beer manufacturers added cobalt salts to beer to enhance and stabilize the beer's foam ("head"). This produced a typical tetrad of metabolic acidosis, polycythemia, goiter, and cardiomyopathy—all features precisely reproduced in our patient! Cobalt is also a component of hard metals, and occupational exposures to hard metal dust may result in asthma or severe alveolitis that can progress to pulmonary fibrosis.

The mechanisms of cobalt's toxicity are not fully understood. It inhibits conversion of pyruvate to acetyl CoA and blocks certain Krebs cycle enzymes resulting in metabolic acidosis. Its hematinic effect and the subsequent polycythemia is due to stimulation of erythropoietin production. Cobalt blocks thyroid iodine uptake and may inhibit tyrosine iodinase, leading to functional hypothyroidism and goiter. Lastly, cobalt appears to deposit in the myocardium and impairs myocardial contractility.

There is little experience with specific therapy of cobalt toxicity beyond cessation of exposure, as was typically employed in the treatment of affected beer drinkers. Unfortunately, despite the removal of the magnets, the patient's signs, symptoms, and laboratory abnormalities improved little over the next few days. Some animal data on enhanced cobalt excretion with the use of chelating agents had been published, but to our knowledge there were no human case reports available to guide chelation therapy decisions at the time (1987) of this child's presentation. Based on some evidence of enhanced excretion in animals, and our familiarity with its use in the common clinical problem of lead poisoning, calcium disodium edetate (EDTA) was chosen for a trial of therapy. Thus, on hospital day 12, the patient began treatment with EDTA at 50 mg/kg/day in four divided doses for 5 days. Urinary cobalt excretion increased four-fold during chelation, and serum cobalt dropped to 1.2 μg/dL, with concomitant increased alertness, loss of bicarbonate requirement, normalization of cardiac function, and ability to tolerate full diet. He was discharged on hospital day 20, on outpatient thyroxine replacement therapy with close endocrine and cardiac follow-up. One animal study published subsequently to this patient's presentation suggested that *N*-acetylcysteine might be a more effective chelator than Ca Na_2 EDTA or dimercaptosuccinic acid.

Of note, the patient's school was the source of his access to magnets. Apparently, blind children are sometimes taught spelling by learning to identify by touch plastic Braille letters backed by magnets. These are then affixed in sequence to a metallic surface.

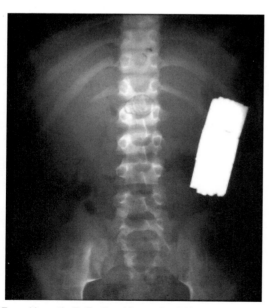

From Henretig F: Further history. Int J Med Toxicol 1(2):15, 1998; with permission.

Clinical Pearls

1. Complex clinical syndromes require careful history taking, an effort to account for each major finding, and an open mind.

2. Sometimes those "hoofbeats" are from "zebras," especially if the senior clinicians involved in the patient's care are stumped!

REFERENCES

1. Barceloux DG: Cobalt. J Toxicol Clin Toxicol 37:201-216, 1999.
2. Henretig F, Shannon M: An 11-year-old boy develops vomiting, weakness, weight loss and a neck mass. Int J Med Toxicol 1(2):13-15, 1988.
3. Henretig F, Joffe M, Baffa G et al: Elemental cobalt toxicity and effects of chelation therapy [abstr]. Vet Hum Toxicol 30: 372, 1988.
4. Duckham JM, Lee HA: The treatment of refractory anaemia of chronic renal failure with cobalt chloride. Q J Med 45: 277-294, 1976.
5. Rona G, Chappel CI: Pathogenesis and pathology of cobalt cardiomyopathy. Recent Adv Stud Cardiac Struct Metab 2: 407-422, 1973.
6. Alexander CS: Cobalt-beer cardiomyopathy. A clinical and pathologic study of 28 cases. Am J Med 53:395-417, 1972.
7. Schirrmacher UO: Case of cobalt poisoning. Br Med J 1:544-545, 1967.

Diane P. Calello, MD
Fred M. Henretig, MD

PATIENT 69

A 4-year-old boy with somnolence

A 4-year-old boy cannot be awakened from his nap. He had been well earlier in the day. He has no prior medical history. Medications in the household include acetaminophen, ibuprofen, and carbamazepine. His mother states that it is very unlikely he could have taken any medications, as all pills in the home are out of reach. Naloxone (2 mg intravenously) is administered without clinical response.

Physical Examination: Temperature 37.0° C, pulse 110/min, respirations 15/min, blood pressure 100/60 mmHg. General: obtunded, withdraws to painful stimuli. HEENT: pupils equal and sluggishly reactive, 3–4 mm; mucous membranes moist. Chest: normal. Cardiovascular: normal. Abdomen: normal active bowel sounds. Skin: warm and dry. Neuromuscular: obtundation, normal cranial nerve function.

Laboratory Findings: EKG: normal sinus rhythm.

Question: What additional laboratory study will most likely reveal the toxic cause of this child's illness?

Diagnosis: The serum carbamazepine level is 23 µg/mL. Additional toxicological testing was unremarkable: urine drug immunoassay is negative for amphetamine, barbiturates, benzodiazepines, cannabis, cocaine, and opioids.

Discussion: Carbamazepine is a first-line agent in the management of seizures as well as for a number of other neuropsychiatric conditions, and its widespread use parallels its frequency of overdoses each year. Recent poison center data notes that carbamazepine accounts for approximately 6000 overdoses each year and comprises 18% of all anticonvulsant overdoses, even as newer anticonvulsant agents are coming into use. Although many consequential carbamazepine overdoses are in adults (and therefore usually suicidal), exploratory pediatric cases like this one also occur frequently.

The structure of carbamazepine, an iminostilbene derivative, closely resembles that of the tricyclic antidepressants (TCAs). Its anticonvulsant mechanism of action seems largely due to inactivation of voltage-gated sodium channels in the brain, preventing repetitive firing and propagation of epileptiform discharges. In addition, it appears to modify glutamatergic and cholinergic neurotransmission, and to have some impact on adenosine receptors as well. These diverse targets of action help to explain the varied clinical consequences of carbamazepine overdose.

Available only in oral form, carbamazepine undergoes slow and erratic absorption from the gastrointestinal (GI) tract. This is due to its lipophilicity as well as its tendency to induce an ileus and form pharmacobezoars in the stomach. It is largely protein bound (approximately 70%) in therapeutic dosing, but in overdose it is present in significant quantity as free drug. In addition, its metabolism via the hepatic cytochrome oxidase system generates an active metabolite, carbamazepine-10,11-epoxide (CBZE) which has the same toxicity, and is measurable, but is unaccounted for in standard carbamazepine level measurements. It is therefore very difficult to predict a correlation between the dose ingested, serum drug levels, time to peak effect, and extent of toxicity. As a rule, while peak drug levels are reached within 4–8 hours in therapeutic dosing, and in even shorter time in patients on chronic therapy with induction of hepatic metabolism, *peak levels may be delayed as long as 70 hours after overdose.*

The primary toxicity of acute carbamazepine overdose is central nervous system (CNS) depression. As in this patient, somnolence is common, with the potential for respiratory depression and coma in severe cases. Due to the erratic absorption characteristics of the drug, **"cyclic coma"** (fluctuations in consciousness) is often described.

Nystagmus, ataxia, dysarthria, dystonic reactions, and movement disorders may occur. The pupillary exam is variable. There is a paradoxical propensity for seizures in these overdose patients, even those without preexisting seizure disorders; fortunately, status epilepticus is uncommon. Rare fatalities from carbamazepine overdose usually occur as a result of apnea, coma, and seizures.

The structural similarity of carbamazepine to the TCAs imparts similar pharmacological action and helps to predict some other aspects of its toxicity. Anticholinergic symptoms are often noted, with at least some of the classic toxidromal features; this anticholinergic activity may contribute to carbamazepine's proconvulsant activity in overdose. In addition, at high levels the drug loses selectivity for CNS sodium channels and can affect cardiac sodium channels, altering action potential propagation and generating dysrhythmias. Although sinus tachycardia is by far the most common finding (likely owing to anticholinergic effect), bradycardia, AV block, widened QRS and QT intervals, and ventricular dysrhythmias do occur, especially in the elderly. Fortunately, these cases are unusual, and most cardiac effects of carbamazepine are of little consequence. Other clinical effects (see table) of carbamazepine in overdose include disorders of taste and smell, syndrome of inappropriate antidiuretic hormone secretion (SIADH), acute tubular necrosis, and elevation of transaminases.

There is a separate constellation of clinically important effects of carbamazepine toxicity when taken chronically. These include agranulocystosis, milder hematological derangements, hepatotoxicity which is also usually mild, acute interstitial nephritis, and potentially life-threatening anticonvulsant hypersensitivity syndromes. Fortunately, these are not of concern in the patient with acute overdose.

Although patients may experience toxicity at "therapeutic" levels (4–12 ug/mL), a serum level of >40 ug/mL has correlated with seizures, coma, and ventricular dysrhythmias. However, children appear to have greater toxicity at lower levels, possibly due to enhanced hepatic cytochromes and more rapid generation of the active epoxide metabolite. Therefore, a lower threshold for concern (27–35 µg/mL) has been suggested for the pediatric population. Serial drug levels should be monitored until it is clear they are trending down, as absorption may continue hours after ingestion. Note that serum levels provide some guidelines for these patients, but they are *an adjunct to the*

Clinical Effects of Carbamazepine Overdose

Neurological
  Somnolence, lethargy, coma, apnea
  "Cyclic coma"
  Nystagmus
  Ataxia
  Dysarthria
  Dystonic reactions
  Hypo/hyperreflexia
  Seizures
  Diplopia
  Ophthalmoplegia
  Abnormal papillary exam (mydriasis, sluggish
    or absent light reflex)
  Chorea, dyskinesia, myoclonus, other
    movement disorders
Cardiovascular
  AV block, bradycardia, prolonged QRS/QTc,
    premature ventricular contractions, ventric-
    ular tachycardia
  Cardiac arrest (rare)
  Hypotension
  Ventricular dysfunction/congestive heart
    failure
Other
  Anticholinergic symptoms (hyperthermia,
    tachycardia, ileus, urinary retention)
  Elevated transaminases
  Disordered taste, smell
  Hyponatremia/SIADH
  Emesis

patient's clinical exam and should *not* solely dictate management decisions.

Attention to airway patency, adequacy of breathing, and circulatory status are paramount. **Activated charcoal** binds well to carbamazepine and should be considered as a decontamination strategy. Because of carbamazepine's anticholinergic properties, which will slow gastric emptying, charcoal administration may be beneficial beyond the 2 hours postingestion typically invoked regarding care of poisoned patients. In addition, multiple-dose activated charcoal has been shown to speed drug elimination, and may decrease time to recovery. However, this therapy must be undertaken cautiously, as the combination of multiple-dose charcoal in a patient with an ileus can lead to intestinal obstruction. For this reason, whole bowel irrigation with polyethylene glycol solution may be more beneficial with less risk.

Seizures may be managed with benzodiazepines; phenytoin shares some pharmacological action with carbamazepine and, therefore, is *not* the drug of choice. Cardiac conduction abnormalities may respond to intravenous sodium bicarbonate, but there is little data to confirm benefit.

The effectiveness of hemodialysis in carbamazepine overdose is impeded by the drug's lipophilicity and propensity for protein binding. However, charcoal hemoperfusion and/or high-efficiency dialysis have been demonstrated to dramatically decrease carbamazepine elimination half-life. In general, these invasive methods are indicated in severely ill patients with refractory seizures, hypotension, or dysrhythmias; they may also be considered in patients expected to have prolonged coma or for whom the carbamazepine level, or the sum of the carbamazepine plus CBZE level, is greater than 60 µg/mL.

In the present patient, one dose of charcoal was given in the emergency department, and three subsequent doses were given upon admission to the intensive care unit. By the next morning his mental status had significantly improved. On repeat examination, he had some residual ataxia and nystagmus. He did not experience seizures or dysrhythmias. He continued to improve and was discharged home 2 days after admission.

Clinical Pearls

1. Carbamazepine's primary toxicity in overdose is CNS depression and seizures.

2. Toxicity and drug levels may fluctuate for many hours after overdose, so careful monitoring and serial drug levels are necessary—even in the patient showing clinical improvement.

3. Serum carbamazepine levels provide some guidelines but do not directly predict the extent of toxicity.

4. Activated charcoal binds carbamazepine well and should be instituted early in overdose patients. Multiple-dose charcoal reduces the drug half-life and may accelerate recovery.

REFERENCES

1. Litovitz TL, Klein-Schwartz W, Rodgers GC, et al: Annual Report of the American Association of Poison Control Centers Toxic Exposure Surveillance System, 2001. Am J Emerg Med 20:391-452, 2002.
2. Lifshitz M, Gavrilov V, Sofer S: Signs and symptoms of carbamazepine overdose in young children. Pediatr Emerg Care 16:26-27, 2000.
3. Schuerer DJE, Brophy PD, Maxvold NJ et al: High-efficiency dialysis for carbamazepine overdose. J Toxicol Clin Toxicol 38:321-323, 2000.
4. Apfelbaum JD, Caravati EM, Kerns WP et al: Cardiovascular effects of carbamazepine toxicity. Ann Emerg Med 25:631-635, 1995.
5. Stremski ES, Brady WB, Prasad K, Hennes HA: Pediatric carbamazepine intoxication. Ann Emerg Med 25:624-630, 1995.
6. Bridge TA, Norton RL, Robertson WO: Pediatric carbamazepine overdoses. Pediatr Emerg Care 10:260-263, 1994.
7. Wason S, Baker RC, Carolan P, et al: Carbamazepine overdose-the effects of multiple-dose activated charcoal. J Toxicol Clin Toxicol 30:39-48, 1992.

Rebecca Guest, MD
James R. Roberts, MD

PATIENT 70

A 36-year-old stone mason with cramping muscle pain, nausea, and diaphoresis

A 36-year-old man was repairing a dilapidated stone wall. He felt a slight pinprick sensation on the top of his right hand, but continued working because it was only minimally painful and then went away. Within 30-45 minutes severe muscle cramping developed in that arm, with rapid progression to the abdomen and back. Shortly thereafter nausea and diaphoresis developed.

Physical Examination: Temperature 37.4° C, pulse 120/min, respirations 22/min, blood pressure 185/100 mmHg. Pulse oximetry: 99% in room air. General: very restless, complaining of severe pain in abdomen and back HEENT: diffusely diaphoretic, bilateral conjunctivitis, and rhinorrhea. Chest: clear breath sounds bilaterally with good air movement. Cardiovascular: sinus tachycardia. Abdomen: firm, nondistended, with normal bowel sounds and no specific area of tenderness. Back: normal. Extremities: central macule with a 2-cm surrounding erythematous ring on dorsum of right hand; two small red spots in the center of lesion.

Laboratory Findings: Hemogram: WBC 12,000/μL, hemoglobin normal, platelets normal. Serum chemistries: normal. Cardiac enzymes: normal. Urinalysis: normal. EKG: normal. Abdominal radiographs: normal.

Question: What envenomation caused this clinical scenario?

Diagnosis and Treatment: This envenomation is from the bite of a black widow spider, producing the clinical syndrome known as latrodectism.

Discussion: Black widow spiders (see figure) belong to the phylum Arthropoda, the class Arachnida, and the genus *Latrodectus*. There are five species in this genus, the *Latrodectus mactans* being the widow spider whose female has the characteristic red hourglass mark on her ventral surface. These spiders live in temperate and tropical latitudes and they are most toxic in the summertime. They typically reside in dark, dry areas such as stone walls, woodpiles, outhouses, basements, and garages. Envenomation from a female spider's bite is more dangerous than that of the male because her neurotoxin is more potent, and because her larger fangs facilitate her poison's penetrating a victim's skin. The female spider is shiny black and about 10 mm long.

The neurotoxic venom of the black widow spider is thought to bind to presynaptic receptors causing a cascade of events, including persistent opening of sodium influx channels, the release of acetylcholine and norepinephrine into the synapses, and the inhibition of their reuptake. The excess of these neurotransmitters at the neuromuscular junction is thought to be responsible for the autonomic features of the latrodectism syndrome. While quite distressing and painful, this envenomation is not usually fatal, except rarely in children and the elderly.

When the spider bites her victim, there is an initial pinprick sensation or sharp pain. The local reaction can progress over the next 30 to 120 minutes to an erythematous wheal and increased pain at the site with progression of pain up the envenomated limb may be experienced. Often the site of envenomation appears relatively benign. Even when the bite site is classic in appearance, the **dramatic systemic symptoms** usually draw attention away from the local site (see table).

Signs and Symptoms of Latrodectism

Local
Pain at bite site (resolves quickly)
Erythema
Fang marks (two red spots)
Target lesion
Edema
Urticaria
Piloerection
Progressive limb pain
Local adenopathy (sometimes painful)

Systemic (general)
Facies latrodectismica (contorted, grimaced face muscles)
Generalized weakness (may persist for weeks)
Diaphoresis
Nausea
Vomiting
Anxiety, restlessness, confusion
Flushed skin
Conjunctivitis/chemosis
Rhinitis
Pavor mortis (fear of death)
Priapism (rare)
Salivation
Urinary retention (rare)
Peripheral edema

Neuromuscular
Severe muscle cramps: thighs, abdomen, chest, back
Muscle rigidity
Fasciculations
Contractions (rigid abdomen)
Tremor

Cardiopulmonary
Bronchorrhea
Hypertension (sometimes severe)
Tachycardia

Laboratory
Leukocytosis, hyperglycemia, elevated creatinine phosphokinase
No test is diagnostic

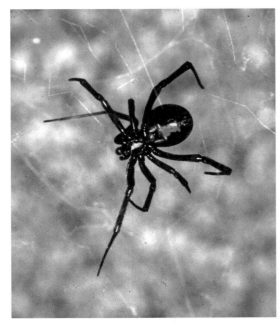

Courtesy of Rick Vetter, Department of Entomology, University of California, Riverside, CA.

219

Erythema, edema, a characteristic "target" lesion, and local tender lymphadenopathy may be seen. Two small, red fang marks may be identified in the center of the lesion.

Skeletal muscle cramping may extend from the location of the bite to other skeletal muscle groups, characteristically including those of the abdomen, thighs, back, chest, and/or face. The abdominal musculature may be rigid. Fasciculations and muscle rigidity may develop in all skeletal muscles. Hypertension and tachycardia are common. The degree of hypertension may occasionally be severe. Other autonomic nervous system symptoms include nausea, vomiting, and diaphoresis. A red flush may be seen over the entire body. Conjunctivitis, chemosis, tearing, and rhinitis may be seen. The patient may exhibit a contorted, grimaced face. The pulmonary system is usually unaffected, but bronchorrhea has occurred. Rarely, tremor, hyperreflexia, or seizures occur. The patient often appears restless and agitated and may be confused. Rare clinical manifestations of latrodectism are priapism, urinary retention, and sweating on the upper lip or tip of the nose. Peripheral edema may be seen. Without treatment, the acute symptoms typically last 2 to 4 days. There are no long-term sequelae of black widow spider envenomation; however, malaise, generalized weakness, and muscle spasms may persist for several weeks. The differential diagnosis of latrodectism is wide (see table), and without a history of a bite or a characteristic lesion, the diagnosis may be quite difficult.

Initial management is consistent with standard emergency care principles, with focus on airway, breathing, and circulation. Clean the local wound site, and give tetanus boosters when indicated. Supportive care may include intravenous (IV) fluid hydration.

Analgesia with adjunctive anxiolysis is the cornerstone of treating the victim of a black widow spider bite. When pain is severe, as it often is, give parenteral **opioids** at full therapeutic doses. Hypertension and tachycardia frequently resolve with adequate pain control. Use **benzodiazepines** generously when clinically indicated. Calcium gluconate was used for years as a first-line treatment of severe envenomations because it was believed to provide symptomatic relief, but its efficacy is now questionable. It has been shown that the combination of IV opioids and benzodiazepines is more effective than calcium gluconate.

Lactrodectus antivenom may dramatically control pain and other systemic symptoms. Since it is rapidly curative (20–30 minutes after infusion), it should be considered in patients with severe or persistent systemic symptoms, cardiovascular toxicity, or pain unrelieved by parenteral opioids. Antivenom may be effective as long as 48–72 hours after envenomation. Because it is a horse serum–derived product, the antivenom can cause hypersensitivity reactions, including anaphylaxis. Serum sickness can be noted after a single vial (the usual dose). Contraindications include known horse serum allergy and, possibly, the concomitant use of beta-blockers. Horse serum skin testing, prior to antivenom administration, is controversial. A single vial of antivenom is infused over 10 minutes in a controlled monitored setting. Some clinicians pre-treat with antihistamines and corticosteroids.

The decision to admit or discharge envenomated patients is determined by the severity of the patients' symptoms and the patients' underlying medical conditions. The severity of latrodectism varies depending upon the season; the sex and size of the spider; and the victim's age, size, and co-morbidities. Those at greatest risk are individuals with underlying heart disease or other chronic illnesses, the elderly, pregnant women, and small infants. All patients with severe pain or other symptoms requiring parenteral medication should be hospitalized. Patients receiving skin-testing and antivenom should be closely observed and then admitted to a monitored environment.

Differential Diagnosis for Signs and Symptoms of Black Widow Spider Envenomation

Perforated abdominal viscus / peritonitis
Heat cramps
Pancreatitis
Ischemic bowel
Aortic dissection
Toxic ingestion (sympathomimetic)
Hypertensive crisis

Clinical Pearls

1. A black widow spider bite may mimic a surgical abdomen, heat cramps, hypertensive crisis, vascular catastrophe, or sympathomimetic drug overdose.

2. The bite site may be quite benign in light of the systemic symptoms; therefore, look carefully for the characteristic local findings.

3. Autonomic instability is common following black widow envenomation, and hypertension may be severe.

4. Antivenom is rapidly curative but carries the risk of anaphylaxis and serum sickness.

5. Pain control is difficult without narcotic analgesics, and benzodiazepines are often beneficial in controlling severe anxiety and agitation.

6. Antivenom is rapidly curative and should be given for severe envenomations. It may be effective for 72–90 hours after bite.

REFERENCES

1. Grishin EV: Black widow spider toxins: The present and the future. Toxicon 36:1693-1701, 1998.
2. Suntorntham S, Roberts JR, Nilsen GJ: Dramatic clinical response to the delayed administration of black widow spider antivenom. Ann Emerg Med 24:1198-1199, 1994.
3. Clark RF, Werthern-Kestner S, Vance MV, Gerkin R: Clinical presentation and treatment of black widow spider envenomation: A review of 163 cases. Ann Emerg Med 21:782-787, 1992.
4. Moss HS, Binder LS: A retrospective review of black widow spider envenomation. Ann Emerg Med 16:188-191, 1987.

PATIENT 71

A 26-year-old man who ingested 26 venlafaxine tablets

A 26-year-old man states that he ingested 26 tablets of venlafaxine (Effexor) just prior to calling 911. Upon arrival to the emergency department the patient is agitated and diaphoretic.

Physical Examination: Temperature 37.8° C, pulse 124/min, respirations 18/min, blood pressure 139/94 mmHg. HEENT: pupils 7 mm bilaterally and reactive. Chest: normal. Cardiovascular: normal. Neuromuscular: slight rigidity of upper extremities, marked rigidity of lower extremities, 3-beat ankle clonus bilaterally, patella and achilles reflexes 3+ bilaterally. Skin: diffuse diaphoresis.

Laboratory Findings: Serum chemistries: normal. Serum acetaminophen, salicylate, alcohol: negative. Urine immunoassay for drugs of abuse: negative.

Questions: How might this patient's clinical status be characterized? What is the treatment?

Diagnosis and Treatment: This patient is suffering from the serotonin syndrome. Treatment is mainly supportive with consideration for the use of sedative-hypnotic agents (e.g., benzodiazepines) and serotonin antagonists (e.g., cyproheptadine).

Discussion: The serotonin syndrome occurs in the setting of drug therapy that results in excessive stimulation of specific postsynaptic serotonin receptors in the brain and spinal cord (see table). Usually two or more serotonergic drugs given concurrently induce this syndrome. It may occur following the intake of high therapeutic doses or overdoses of a single serotonergic agent. Finally, the serotonin syndrome may occur following the discontinuation of one serotonergic agent and the initiation of another prior to complete elimination of the first.

Excessive postsynaptic serotonin receptor stimulation may produce neuromuscular symptoms, cognitive-behavior symptoms, and dysfunction of the autonomic nervous system. The *neuromuscular symptoms* associated with serotonin syndrome include restlessness, resting tremor, clonus, and isolated rigidity of the lower extremities. The *cognitive-behavioral symptoms* include anxiety, confusion, agitation, coma, and seizures. *Autonomic nervous system dysfunction* seen with serotonin syndrome includes diaphoresis, hyperthermia, hypertension, tachycardia, and mydriasis. Severe complications of serotonin syndrome include rhabdomyolysis, renal dysfunction, metabolic acidosis, and death.

The treatment of serotonin syndrome is mainly supportive care. Agitated patients may need physical restraints and chemical sedation (e.g., benzodiazepines). Hyperthermic patients should undergo rapid external cooling. The causative serotonergic agents or agents should be identified and withheld. Most cases of serotonin syndrome resolve in less than 24 hours. There are case reports of successful adjunctive treatment of the serotonin syndrome with cyproheptadine, an antihistamine agent with serotonin antagonist action.

The present patient was admitted to the hospital and given cyproheptadine 4 mg by mouth every 8 hours. Over the next 24 hours the patient's agitation, rigidity, clonus, and diaphoresis all resolved. He was able to ambulate without difficulty. The patient was discharged approximately 36 hours after the ingestion and was referred for subsequent outpatient psychiatric counseling.

Serotonergic Drugs

Amitriptyline	Lithium
Amphetamines	L-Tryptophan
Buspirone	Meperidine
Clomipramine	Methadone
Cocaine	Nefazodone
Codeine derivatives	Nortriptyline
Desipramine	Paroxetine
Dextromethoraphan	Phenelzine
Doxepin	Selegiline
Fluoxetine	Sertraline
Fluvoxamine	Sumatriptan
Imipramine	Tranylcypromine
Indoles (e.g., LSD)	Trazodone
Isocarboxazid	Venlafaxine

Clinical Pearls

1. Serotonin syndrome typically occurs following the concurrent use of two or more serotonergic agents or following excessive use/overdose of one serotonergic agent.

2. Serotonin syndrome may occur following the discontinuation of one serotonergic agent and the initiation of another prior to complete elimination of the first.

3. Serotonin syndrome typically produces neuromuscular findings including tremor, hyperreflexia, and rigidity. Often the lower extremities are more involved than the upper extremities.

4. Treatment of serotonin syndrome is mainly supportive and focuses on resuscitation, external cooling, and chemical sedation.

REFERENCES
1. Kolecki P: Isolated Venlafaxine-induced serotonin syndrome. *J Emerg Med* 15:4:491-493, 1997.
2. Mills KC: Serotonin syndrome. *Am Fam Physician* 25:1475-1482, 1995.

PATIENT 72

A 17-month-old boy who ingested a Christmas plant

A 17-month-old boy was found on the living room floor with a handful of poinsettia leaves. The parent inspected his mouth and found that he had chewed an unknown number of leaves. His mouth was cleaned out and 911 was called. He arrives to the emergency department (ED) playful and in no distress. The ED triage nurse contacts the Poison Control Center to see what the course of treatment should be for this toddler.

Physical Examination: Temperature 36.9° C, pulse 99/min, respirations 12/min, blood pressure 96/50 mmHg. Neurological: normal. Neck: supple, no adenopathy Eyes: pupils 2–3 mm, briskly reactive to light. Skin: warm, well perfused. Respiratory: breath sounds clear bilaterally, pulse oximetry 100% on room air. Gastrointestinal: abdomen soft, non-distended, bowel sounds present.

Question: What are the first steps in the treatment of this toddler?

Answer: Confirm the identity of the ingested plant and ascertain whether any other plants may have been ingested as well.

Discussion: Poinsettia (*Euphorbia pulcherrima*) is a nontoxic plant. At most, it may cause gastrointestinal (GI) upset. Other nontoxic holiday plants include pine cones and Christmas cactus (*Schlumbergera bridgesii*). However, there are several toxic holiday plants.

Yew (*Taxus canadensis*) is a tree or shrub and contains an arrhythmogenic alkaloid, taxine. All parts are toxic except for the red, fleshy globe which surrounds a hard seed. Symptoms are unlikely if this seed is swallowed whole because the seed coat is resistant to digestive enzymes. If small quantities are ingested, GI symptoms are possible. However, if eaten in large quantities or the seeds are chewed, there is risk for cardiac arrhythmias and seizures.

Small ingestions of holly berries (*Ilex* species) can cause mild to moderate gastritis and possibly mild drowsiness. If large amounts of berries are eaten, more serious and prolonged GI distress can occur. The exact toxin is unknown, but it is suspected that saponins are responsible for the GI effects. The leaves are nontoxic; however, the sharp spines are a choking hazard and can cause damage to skin and mucous membranes.

Jerusalem cherry (*Solanum pseudocapsicum*) is a plant that contains solanocapsine in the leaves and solanine in the berries. Depending on the quantity consumed, symptoms ranging from GI upset to cardiovascular effects such as tachycardia can occur.

Boxwood (*Buxus sempervirens*) is an evergreen shrub used for ornamental purposes. Typically an ingestion of boxwood leaves or twigs cases GI irritation. It is only in large quantities that symptoms such as convulsions and coma may result. The toxins involved are buxene, an alkaloid, and galactobuxin, a flavonoid glycoside.

Ingestion of three or fewer mistletoe (*Phoradendron flavescens*) leaves or berries produces at most, a mild gastroenteritis. Packaged mistletoe may be artificial. Christmas trees include pine, spruce, juniper, fir, and cedar varieties. Large ingestions can cause severe gastroenteritis. However, the primary concern is the risk of the sharp needles becoming lodged in the esophagus.

Poison control centers provide written information on poison prevention and give advice on how to manage poisonings when they occur. With a national toll-free number, poison control centers are available 24 hours a day, 7 days a week, to callers from both the public and healthcare settings. Their services help to keep relatively benign or non-toxic exposures out of emergency departments by providing appropriate at-home treatment advice.

In the present case, confirmation was obtained that only poinsettia had been ingested. Thus, the ingestion was nontoxic, and there was no role for gastric decontamination or laboratory studies. GI symptoms did not develop, and the patient was discharged to home. His parents were given some basic poison prevention advice along with the poison control center phone number. If an individual is asymptomatic after ingesting a plant, a poison control center should be called to determine if the plant is toxic and whether symptoms can be watched for at home or a visit to the emergency department is necessary.

Clinical Pearls

1. It is a common myth that ingestion of the Poinsettia plant is dangerous. In large amounts, minor GI upset may result. There have been scant reports of the plant causing oral irritation.

2. The seeds of the yew are not toxic if swallowed whole as the seed coat resists digestive enzymes.

3. Mistletoe is relatively nontoxic when ingested in small quantities. At one time, the plant's leaves and berries were thought to cause serious toxicity, even in small doses. However, it is the ingestion of *large* quantities that is worrisome and warrants emergency department evaluation.

REFERENCES

1. Der Marderosian A, Liberti L. Holly. In Der Marderosian A(ed): The Review of Natural Products. Facts and Comparisons, St. Louis, 1996.
2. Cummins RO, Haulman J, Quan L, et al: Near-fatal yew berry intoxication treated with external cardiac pacing and digoxin-specific FAB antibody fragments. Ann Emerg Med 19:38-43, 1990.
3. Hall AH, Spoerke DG, Rumack BH: Assessing mistletoe toxicity. Ann Emerg Med 15:1320-1323, 1986.
4. Rodrigues TD, Johnson PN, Jeffrey LP: Holly berry ingestion: Case report. Vet Hum Toxicol 26:157-158, 1984.
5. Edwards N: Local toxicity from a poinsettia plant: A case report. J Pediatrics 102:404-405, 1983.

Philip R. Spandorfer, MD

PATIENT 73

A 3-week-old girl with hypernatremia

A 3-week-old girl is having seizures. In the emergency department, these seizures are unresponsive to benzodiazepine therapy. She was the product of a full-term uncomplicated pregnancy. The mother reports that the child has only been drinking 1.5 ounces of milk-based formula every 3 hours for the past day instead of her usual 3 ounces per feed. Aside from gassiness, which the mother is treating with a home remedy, there are no other complaints. Of note, there has been no fever, vomiting, diarrhea, or symptoms of an upper respiratory infection.

Physical Examination: Temperature 38.8° C, pulse 180/min, respirations 68/min, blood pressure 50/24 mmHg. Pulse oximetry: 98% in room air. General: ill-appearing and irritable (see figure). HEENT: Dry mucous membranes, sunken fontanelle, sunken eyes, absent tears, otherwise normal. Chest: tachypneic, mild intercostal retractions, clear to auscultation. Cardiovascular: no murmur. Abdomen: liver 1 cm below costal margin. Genitourinary: normal female genitalia. Extremities: capillary refill at 3 seconds. Skin: no rash. Neuromuscular: hypotonic.

Laboratory Findings: Hemogram: WBC 15,000/µL, hemoglobin 12.0g/dL, platelets 484,000/µL. Serum chemistries: Na^+ 193 mEq/L, K^+ 4.3 mEq/L, Cl^- 114 mEq/L, CO_2 40 mmol/L, glucose 243 mg/dL, Ca^+ 6.3 mg/dL. Capillary blood gas (100% FiO_2): pH 7.53, $PaCO_2$ 51 mmHg, PaO_2 25 mmHg, base excess +18 mmol/L.

Question: What is the probable cause of her seizures?

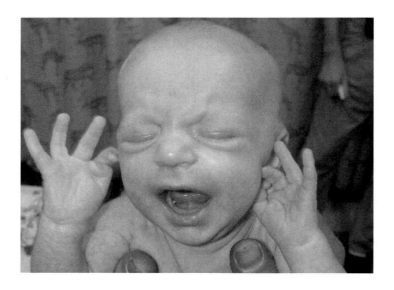

Diagnosis: Hypernatremia from sodium bicarbonate poisoning

Discussion: Ill-appearing, febrile infants pose an interesting differential diagnosis. The most important diagnoses to consider include bacterial infections such as meningitis, bacteremia, pneumonia, and urinary tract infections. Viral syndromes, congenital heart defects, congenital adrenal hyperplasia, and metabolic disorders are also important diagnoses to consider during the evaluation of such infants. Poisoning is unusual in this age range, but can occur with improper formula preparation or through malicious intent of a caretaker.

An important clue to this child's diagnosis is that she is markedly hypernatremic with an impressive metabolic alkalosis. Serum sodium levels that are 150 mEq/L or greater are considered hypernatremic. Levels greater than 160 mEq/L should be considered critically elevated. Antidiuretic hormone increases water reabsorption in the kidneys to help maintain serum sodium levels in the normal physiological 135 mEq/L to 145 mEq/L range. To counterbalance the effect of long-term elevations of extracellular osmolarity, brain cells can produce idiogenic osmoles. These idiogenic osmoles serve to raise intracellular osmolarity in order to draw free water back into the cell and maintain cellular integrity.

Hypernatremia can arise from three main mechanisms: **hypotonic fluid loss, free water deficit**, or **excessive sodium intake** (see Table). Typically, hypernatremia is due to a water imbalance rather than sodium overload. Water imbalance can be thought of as either increased loss of water or decreased intake of free water. Both forms of hypernatremic water imbalance will yield decreased total body water and total body sodium concentrations, but the water loss is greater than the sodium loss. Excessive free water losses occur with diarrheal illnesses and renal concentrating defects. Free water deficits can occur when the patient has restricted access to water, such as the case for an infant or a bed-ridden patient. Free water deficit is also an issue for patients with central or nephrogenic diabetes insipidus. Although rare, hypernatremia due to sodium excess does occur, particularly in young infants who are being fed sodium. The sodium can come from table salt (sodium chloride) or baking soda (sodium bicarbonate). It is critical to ask the parents of infants to describe how they prepare the formula. Often, there are subtle errors in the manner in which it is prepared. However, on rare occasions, a grievous error is discovered and may be the primary cause of the child's symptoms. Administration of sodium bicarbonate during medical cardiovascular resuscitation is another potential source of excessive sodium that can lead to hypernatremia. Toxins can result in hypernatremia either through a direct sodium load or as a cause of diabetes insipidus (see Table).

Clinically, the presentation of a patient with hypernatremia is that of early neurological irritability with a relative preservation of the circulatory status. In hypernatremic states, water will passively diffuse across cell membranes to follow sodium ions. The heart rate and blood pressure do not accurately reflect the total body fluid deficit since there is a relative preservation of the extracellular volume where the "extra" sodium resides; hence, the dehydration is disproportionately intracellular. Patients will be irritable and lethargic, and are often hyperthermic. Furthermore, due to the intracellular dehydration, the brain shrinks

Etiologies of Hypernatremia

Hypotonic fluid loss
   Diarrhea
   Congenital renal disease
Water deficit
   Central diabetes insipidus
   Nephrogenic diabetes insipidus
   Excessive sweating
   Diabetes mellitus
   Increased insensible losses
   Lack of thirst (adipsia)
Excess sodium intake
   Salt poisoning
   Improper formula preparation
   Seawater ingestion
   Sodium bicarbonate administration
     (e.g., resuscitations)

Toxins Causing Hypernatremia

Drugs that cause diabetes insipidus:

Amphotericin	Lobenzarit disodium
Colchicine	Methoxyflurane
Demeclocycline	Mesalazine
Ethanol	Propoxyphene
Foscarnet	Rifampin
Glufosinate	Streptozotocin
Lithium	

Antacids
Cathartic abuse (sorbitol)
Lactulose therapy
Mannitol
Sodium salts (bicarbonate, chloride, citrate, hypochlorite)
Valproic acid (divalproex sodium)

away from the skull and places tension on the bridging veins, which may lead to intracranial hemorrhage. Coma and seizures may also develop. Although the mechanism is unclear, hyperglycemia and hypocalcemia are frequently seen.

Treatment focuses on slowly lowering the serum sodium while maintaining the hemodynamic status. The therapeutic goal is to lower the serum sodium by 0.5 mEq/L per hour. This slow correction will help prevent the development of cerebral edema. The free water deficit should be replaced over 48 hours. The free water deficit can be calculated as 4 mL/kg for every mEq/L the serum sodium is greater than 145 mEq/L. Maintenance fluids and ongoing losses should also be provided. Avoidance of insulin is important since rapid decrease in serum glucose levels may be associated with cerebral edema.

Prognosis from hypernatremia is variable. There is at least a 10% mortality rate. The degree of neurological recovery does not correlate well with the severity of the hypernatremia. However, the development of new neurological deficits is greater when the serum sodium is greater then 160 mEq/L.

The present patient was found to have been receiving exogenous sodium bicarbonate. The mother had been adding significant amounts of baking soda to the girl's formula to help with the gassiness for the previous week. As many as 11% of inner city mothers report having heard of giving infants baking soda for gassy colic, and almost 1 in 20 claim that they have added it to their infant's formula. Standard formula has 70.8 mEq of sodium per liter; the formula this girl was receiving had 240.9 mEq/L. For comparison, ocean water has approximately 480 mEq of sodium per liter. The patient was admitted to the intensive care unit for 3 days until her serum sodium corrected to 145 mEq/L. An MRI of her head revealed bilateral parietal infarcts and a right temporal infarct (see figure). She failed her visual evoked responses and was felt to be cortically blind. Cultures of her cerebrospinal fluid, blood, and urine were negative.

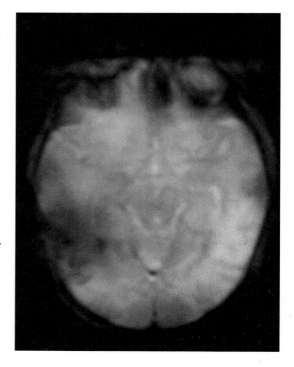

Clinical Pearls

1. When caring for ill infants, a careful dietary history is important.

2. Consider metabolic or electrolyte abnormalities among patients with seizures recalcitrant to benzodiazepine therapy.

3. The hallmark of hypernatremic dehydration is early neurological irritability with relative preservation of the extracellular volume.

4. Slow correction of hypernatremia will reduce the risk of cerebral edema.

REFERENCES
1. Spandorfer PR, Alessandrini EA: Sugar and spice and everything nice. Pediatric Annals 30(1): 603-606, 2001.
2. Selbst SM: The septic appearing infant. In Fleisher GR, Ludwig S (eds): Textbook of Pediatric Emergency Medicine, 4th ed. Philadelphia, Lippincott Williams & Wilkins, 2000, pp 565-572.

Diane P. Calello, MD

PATIENT 74

A 15-year-old boy with altered mental status and ventricular bigeminy

A 15-year-old boy presents to the emergency department with ataxia and lethargy after a suicidal ingestion. A number of empty pill bottles were found in his home, including containers for clonazepam, hydroxyzine, a multivitamin, and Midrin, an antimigraine medication containing acetaminophen, isometheptene (a sympathomimetic), and dichloralphenazone, a chloral hydrate derivative. An empty bottle of tequila was also found.

Physical Examination: Temperature 35.6° C rectally, pulse 85 beats/min, respirations 15/min, blood pressure 130/92 mmHg. General: obtunded, responsive to painful stimuli. HEENT: pupils small, minimally reactive; mucous membranes moist. Remainder of exam is noncontributory.

Laboratory Findings: Serum chemistries and complete blood count: normal. EKG: ventricular bigeminy (see figure).

Question: What sedative ingestion could explain this patient's clinical presentation?

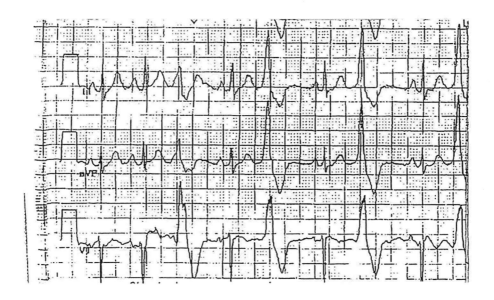

Diagnosis: Chloral hydrate overdose

Discussion: Chloral hydrate is the oldest sedative-hypnotic available, first synthesized in 1832. Its sedative-hypnotic action arises from activation of the GABA$_A$ receptor, much like benzodiazepines, and from inhibition of the NMDA receptor. In addition, it is a halogenated hydrocarbon (see figure below), which imparts some myocardial toxicity. Therapeutic doses for sedation and anxiolysis range from 25 mg/kg to 100 mg/kg in children and adults, and are usually given orally. Toxicity has been reported with therapeutic doses, but usually occurs in adults around 2–3 g; fatal overdoses usually involve 10 g or more.

$$Cl-\overset{\displaystyle Cl}{\underset{\displaystyle Cl}{C}}-\overset{\displaystyle H}{\underset{\displaystyle Cl}{C}}-OH$$

The metabolism of chloral hydrate is notable for its influence on, and susceptibility to influence by, the metabolism of other substances. The parent compound is rapidly absorbed and converted quickly into trichloroethanol (TCE) via alcohol dehydrogenase (ADH). TCE, an active metabolite, has a much longer half-life than chloral hydrate, and is largely responsible for therapeutic and toxic effects. Under normal circumstances, the TCE is then converted via dehydrogenases to trichloroacetaldehyde, an inactive metabolite, which is then further conjugated and excreted by the kidneys. Metabolism of medications such as furosemide and coumarin are altered via changes in protein binding. The popular combination of chloral hydrate and ethanol, the infamous "Mickey Finn" or knockout drops, arises from the intertwined metabolism of these two substances, which increases the effect of both. This takes place via four mechanisms: (1) Ethanol drives the conversion to TCE via the formation of NADH, a substrate for alcohol dehydrogenase. (2) Chloral hydrate competes with ethanol for ADH, thereby prolonging the half-life of ethanol. (3) TCE further inhibits the conversion via ADH of ethanol to acetaldehyde. (4) Ethanol inhibits the oxidation of TCE to trichloroacetaldehyde (see figure, *bottom*).

Chloral hydrate has a unique toxicity profile which helps to distinguish its clinical presentation in the context of an unknown ingestion. After overdose, patients exhibit rapid onset of **CNS depression** and coma, and may have the distinct "pear-like odor" often cited. The pupillary exam is much like that in barbiturate coma, beginning with miosis which progresses to mydriasis as coma deepens; other autonomic abnormalities include hypotension and hypothermia. Chloral hydrate is a mucosal irritant, so symptoms ranging from minor gastritis to esophageal strictures and gastric perforation have been observed. Hepatic and renal injury may also occur. The most significant cause of morbidity however, and the cause of mortality in most fatal cases of overdose, is **ventricular dysrhythmia** and cardiac arrest.

The combination of CNS depression and dysrhythmias in a patient with an unknown ingestion should raise the suspicion of an overdose with chloral hydrate. Given this patient's list of potential medications, it is clear that this was the cause of his clinical presentation.

The arrhythmogenic properties of chloral hydrate are similar to those of other halogenated hydrocarbons, such as halothane. In addition to decreasing myocardial contractility, it alters

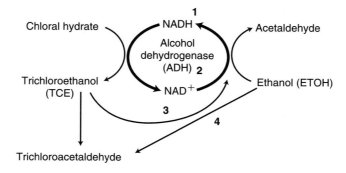

Interaction of chloral hydrate and ethanol metabolism: (1) ETOH generates NADH excess, favoring production of active TCE; (2) CH competes for ADH, slowing ethanol conversion to acetaldehyde; (3) TCE further inhibits ETOH conversion to acetaldehyde; (4) ETOH inhibits conversion of TCE to inactive trichloroacetaldehyde.

Beyond ACLS: Unique Resuscitation Modalities in the Management of Poisoned Patients

Overdose	Treatment
Tricyclic antidepressants, other drugs causing cardiac sodium channel blockade	Sodium bicarbonate
Beta-antagonists (propranolol, esmolol)	Glucagon, calcium, insulin/glucose
Calcium-channel antagonists	Calcium, insulin/glucose (+/− glucagon)
Clonidine	Naloxone
Chloral hydrate	Propranolol, other beta-antagonists

myocardial repolarization, shortening the refractory period and creating a milieu conducive to reentrant circuits. As a result, the myocardium develops a heightened sensitivity to endogenous catecholamines, which may induce a premature ventricular contraction and trigger dysrhythmias that include, but are not limited to, torsades de pointes, ventricular tachycardia, and ventricular fibrillation.

Because of the contribution of catecholamines to this cascade, administration of commonly used exogenous catecholamines, such as dopamine and epinephrine, is not helpful and has been reported to worsen ectopy in these patients. Lidocaine has been used with variable success. However, beta-receptor antagonists, specifically propranolol and esmolol, have successfully abolished or suppressed arrhythmias in the majority of reported cases. The use of beta-blockade in this scenario is one of

many interesting examples in which the management of poisoned patients differs from the standard of care under Advanced Cardiac Life Support (ACLS) resuscitation guidelines (see table).

The recommended adult dosage for propranolol is a 1 to 2-mg IV bolus (which can be given in 0.5-mg aliquots titrated for heart rate), followed by an infusion of 1–2 mg/hr. In children a 0.01 to 0.1-mg/kg bolus should be followed by an infusion of the same dose over an hourly rate. Esmolol has also been effective, at 500-µg/kg/dose bolus (for adults and children), and a subsequent infusion of 25- to 100-µg/kg/min.

The present patient was given a 1-mg bolus of IV propranolol, after which his bigeminy resolved. No further ectopy developed, and so an infusion was not started. Hours later his mental status improved, and he was discharged to psychiatric care 2 days after admission.

Clinical Pearls

1. Chloral hydrate overdose can be life-threatening not only from CNS depression, but also as a result of ventricular dysrhythmias.

2. The effect of chloral hydrate is significantly enhanced by ethanol, due to the metabolism of each.

3. Because the dysrhythmias caused by chloral hydrate are a result of catecholamine sensitivity, typical antiarrhythmic therapy is often not successful; however, propranolol and other beta-antagonists have been effective in most cases.

REFERENCES
1. Pershad J, Palmisano P, Nichols M: Chloral hydrate: The good and the bad. Pediatr Emerg Care 15:432-435, 1999.
2. Zahedi A, Grant MH, Wong DT: Successful treatment of chloral hydrate cardiac toxicity with propranolol. Am J Emerg Med 17:490-491, 1999.
3. Lee DC, Vassalluzzo C: Acute gastric perforation in a chloral hydrate overdose. Am J Emerg Med 16:545-546, 1998.
4. Ludwigs U, Divino Filho JC, Magnusson A, Berg A: Suicidal chloral hydrate poisoning. Clin Tox 34:97-99, 1996.
5. Graham SR, Day RO, Lee R, et al: Overdose with chloral hydrate: A pharmacological and therapeutic review. Med J Aust 149:686-688, 1988.
6. Young JB, Vandermolen LA, Pratt CM: Torsade de pointes: An unusual manifestation of chloral hydrate poisoning. Am Heart J 119:181-183, 1986.

PATIENT 75

A 16-year-old girl who has been "dipping"

A 16-year-old girl is found unconscious on her street. Upon arrival to the emergency department, she is awake but intermittently agitated. She denies any specific complaints but is slow in answering questions, and it is difficult to obtain any information. She admits to "dipping" tonight at a party, but denies any other drug use.

Physical Examination: Temperature 36.8° C, pulse 96/min, respirations 20/min, blood pressure 144/92 mmHg. General: awake and alert but intermittently agitated. HEENT: pupils mid-position, vertical and horizontal nystagmus. Neck: supple. Chest: normal. Cardiovascular: normal. Abdomen: normal. Neuromuscular: cranial nerve function intact, poorly cooperative, agitated to external stimuli.

Laboratory Findings: Hemogram: normal. Serum chemistries: normal. Urine immunoassay for drugs of abuse: positive for phencyclidine (PCP) and cannabinoids.

Question: What is "dipping"?

Diagnosis: Dipping is one of a number of terms for smoking tobacco or marijuana cigarettes after dipping them in "embalming fluid," the street term for a solution of phencyclidine in formalin (or other solvent).

Discussion: The diagnosis and treatment of patients who use illicit drugs often requires the physician to have an understanding of the slang terms and drug usage techniques currently being used in the community. One of the more recent and varied slang terminologies has developed around the use of phencyclidine, also known as PCP. Confusion among physicians, the lay press, and even the drug users and dealers has developed concerning the **liquid form of PCP** known as embalming fluid (see figure).

The history of the association between embalming fluid and PCP is not completely clear. The drug has been sold in liquid, powder, and tablet form with various names, the most familiar being angel dust. During the 1970s, embalming fluid was simply one of many slang terms for PCP itself, but today it appears the term has evolved to describe any solvent in which PCP is dissolved. While commercial embalming fluid may contain a number of substances, including formaldehyde, methanol, ethanol, and glutaraldehyde, in most instances of dipping, other potentially less toxic solvents are used. **Tobacco or marijuana cigarettes** are dipped into the PCP-containing solvent and then smoked. The marijuana or tobacco may

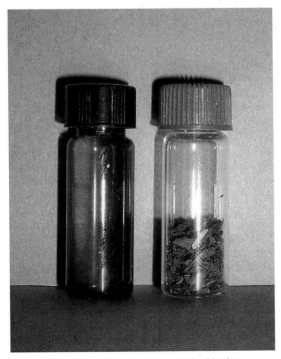

Left, PCP solution. Right, tobacco soaked in the solution.

also be soaked in the solution prior to purchasing or smoking it. Common terms for these activities and substances include dipping, wet, fry, amp, illy, and dank. This slang terminology often differs significantly from one city or region to another.

Several publications from the 1980s and 1990s reflect confusion concerning the active ingredient of these preparations. Some authors, as well as interviewed users and dealers, suggested that the embalming fluid itself was the cause of the strong effects—there was no mention of PCP. However, the small amounts of solvents in embalming fluid are not likely to result in any significant toxicity, particularly if these substances evaporate or burn. In our clinical experience, when screened, patients who present intoxicated after using wet or dipping have positive phencyclidine assays.

PCP is referred to as a **dissociative anesthetic agent**. Its effects are similar to the pharmaceutical sedative/dissociative anesthetic ketamine, which is commonly used for procedural sedation but is also recreationally abused. While these have complex and incompletely understood mechanisms of action, the most significant effect seems to be noncompetitive antagonism of the excitatory neurotransmitter glutamate at the *N*-methyl-D-aspartate (NMDA) receptor. The major metabolite of dextromethorphan possesses similar activity at this site, and consequently this common cough suppressant has become a popular recreational drug as well.

The clinical effects of PCP intoxication are variable. Most significantly, a state of dissociation from the environment and disordered thinking occur. Subanesthetic doses generally result in decreased perception of pain, distorted body image, feelings of numbness, and depersonalization. Hostility or other inappropriate behavior may result from misinterpretation of external stimuli. The classically described violent, uncontrollable PCP-intoxicated patient with seemingly superhuman strength does occur, but is clearly a minority of patients. Intoxication may cause agitation or catatonia. Higher doses may produce a comatose appearance, as was likely the case during this patient's initial unresponsive state. Some patients, particularly those with underlying psychiatric disorder or after a large dose of the drug, may develop a psychosis that is indistinguishable from schizophrenia, and this state may (though rarely) be persistent.

On physical examination, mild hypertension, tachycardia, tachypnea, and hyperthermia (rare) may be present. One of the most common physical findings, as was witnessed in the presented patient, is **nystagmus**. This nystagmus may be vertical, horizontal, and/or rotatory. Much less common are hypersalivation, diaphoresis, urinary retention, increased muscle tone, and motor disturbances such as acute dystonic reactions. Laboratory studies may reveal elevated creatine kinase indicative of rhabdomyolysis, elevated liver transaminases, hypoglycemia, leukocytosis, and a positive urine immunoassay drug screen for PCP. A negative result on the urine test does not necessarily rule out PCP intoxication, and a positive result could be related to ketamine, dextromethorphan, or a PCP analogue.

The treatment of the PCP-intoxicated patient depends on the degree of agitation and associated trauma or illness. Violent patients are clearly a danger to themselves and others, and benefit from both physical and chemical restraint. However, many patients may be managed by simply placing them in a quiet area for observation, as the duration of intoxication may be only a few hours. The choice of chemical restraint is open to some debate. The intravenous benzodiazepines are generally considered the safest choice in managing the agitated patient, although intramuscular administration may be needed in the severely agitated patient in whom intravenous access cannot be obtained. Some clinicians advocate the use of antipsychotic agents, such as droperidol or haloperidol, alone or in combination with a benzodiazepine for more rapid and more prolonged sedation.

The present patient was intermittently agitated, but not exhibiting any violent behavior. She was placed in a quiet room for observation and given a small dose of lorazepam (1 mg) intravenously. Within 30 minutes she was much more calm, and within 6 hours she was cooperative and no longer exhibiting any signs of intoxication. Repeat physical examination revealed no signs of trauma, and the patient was discharged home under her family's care.

Clinical Pearls

1. A current trend in drug use involves the use of PCP dissolved in embalming fluid or other solvents.

2. Drug users may be unaware that the active ingredient in the "embalming fluid" or "wet" is PCP and not the solvents themselves.

3. Numerous slang terms exist, differing by geographic region, for the current formulations of PCP, including wet, fry, amp, dank, sherm, illy, hydro, dip, hog, and many others.

4. Benzodiazepines are the safest drugs for use in sedation of the agitated PCP-intoxicated patient.

REFERENCES

1. Morocco AP: Getting wet from recreational use of embalming fluid. Pediatr Case Rev 3:111-113, 2003.
2. Olmedo R: Phencyclidine and ketamine. In Goldfrank LR, Flomenbaum NE, Lewin NA, et al (eds): Goldfrank's Toxicologic Emergencies, 7th ed. New York, McGraw-Hill, 2002, pp 1034-1041.
3. Elwood WN: "Fry": A study of adolescents' use of embalming fluid with marijuana and tobacco. Austin, TX, Texas Commission on Alcohol and Drug Abuse, 1998.
4. Holland JA, Nelson L, Ravikumar PR, Elwood WN: Embalming fluid-soaked marijuana: New high or new guise for PCP? J Psychoactive Drugs 30:215-219, 1998.
5. Javitt DC, Zukin SR: Recent advances in the phencyclidine model of schizophrenia. Am J Psychiatry 148:1301-1308, 1991.
6. Spector I: AMP: a new form of marijuana. J Clin Psychiatr 46:498-499, 1985.
7. McCarron MM, Schulze BW, Thompson GA, et al: Acute phencyclidine intoxication: Incidence of clinical findings in 1,000 cases. Ann Emerg Med 10:237-242, 1981.
8. Petersen RC, Stillman RC: Phencyclidine (PCP) abuse: An appraisal. Rockville, MD, National Institute of Drug Abuse, 1978.

PATIENT 76

An infant with hyponatremia

A 7-week-old girl presents with several days of intermittent low-grade fevers, cough, emesis, and progressively increased work of breathing. Her respiratory distress is treated with albuterol administered by nebulization, and blood, urine, and cerebrospinal fluid are obtained in an evaluation for occult bacterial infection. Unexpected laboratory results are encountered.

Physical Examination: Temperature 36.3° C, pulse 160/min, respirations 66/min, blood pressure 82/46 mmHg. Oxygen saturation of hemoglobin: 92% in room air. General: lethargic. HEENT: sunken anterior fontanelle, dry mucus membranes. Chest: subcostal and intercostal retractions, coarse breath sounds bilaterally with scattered rales. Cardiovascular: regular rate and rhythm, no murmur or gallop, good distal pulses. Abdomen: soft, nondistended. Extremities: warm. Skin: clear. Neuromuscular: symmetric reflexes, decreased tone globally.

Laboratory Findings: Hemogram: WBC 12,800/μL with 27% neutrophils. Serum chemistries: sodium 118 mEq/L, potassium 7.8 mEq/L, chloride 94 mEq/L, bicarbonate 11 mEq/L, BUN 17 mg/dL, creatinine 0.4 mg/dL, glucose 44 mg/dL. Nasal aspirate: positive fluorescent antibody test for respiratory syncytial virus.

Question: What was the poison responsible for this infant's hyponatremia? (Hint: this case exemplifies the famous toxicology quote offered below.)

What is there that is not poison? All things are poison and nothing [is] without poison. Solely the dose determines that a thing is not a poison.

—Paracelsus

Diagnosis: Water. Gastrointestinal sodium loss and water intoxication are the most common causes of hyponatremia in the young infant. With a more directed history, it was discovered that the patient's mother had administered an excess of dietary water.

Discussion: Hyponatremia exists when the serum sodium concentration falls below 130 mEq/L. Regulation of serum sodium levels depends upon a delicate balance between total body water, natriuretic elements, hormonal signals, obligate fluid losses, and oral intake. Given the intricate interplay of factors that determine the serum sodium concentration, there is a wide range of disease states that may contribute to abnormal sodium levels. The most common etiologies of hyponatremia include medication side effects, congestive heart failure, renal failure or nephrosis, liver disease, excessive gastrointestinal losses, and hyperglycemia (see table). Drugs that may be toxic to sodium balance include any medication that stimulates antidiuretic hormone (ADH) secretion, causing syndrome of inappropriate secretion of ADH; products such as lithium that produce a salt-wasting syndrome; or silver nitrate, which draws sodium out of the extracellular space and into its hypotonic medium. Uncommonly, water intoxication resulting from the consumption of excessive amounts of free water creates a similar electrolyte imbalance (see table). This is seen most commonly in patients with psychogenic polydipsia or, as in this case example, in young infants whose families dilute infant formulas inappropriately.

Infants 3 to 6 months of age are most commonly discovered to be symptomatic from excess water intake for a number of physiological and social reasons. Young children have low glomerular filtration rates, limiting their ability to waste excess free water. In addition, infants do not readily discriminate between foods offered to them and will drink what is provided when they are hungry. Finally, efforts to make a supply of expensive infant formula last longer may lead families to dilute the milk with water.

The clinical manifestations of hyponatremia relate both to the rate of decline of serum sodium levels from baseline and to the absolute serum sodium level. Rapid changes in sodium levels create more pronounced symptomatology, including anorexia, nausea, lethargy, agitation, muscle cramps, and acute respiratory failure. On examination, patients typically demonstrate an altered sensorium, decreased tendon reflexes, hypothermia, seizures, Cheyne-Stokes respirations, and/or

Differential Diagnosis of Hyponatremia

- Normal total body water and sodium (hyperosmolar hyponatremia)
  Hyperglycemia
  Mannitol administration
- Increased total body water and sodium (edema-forming states)
  Heart failure
  Liver failure
  Renal failure
- Decreased total body water and sodium (hypovolemic states)
  Renal losses
  Diuretics
  Renal tubular acidosis
  Mineralocorticoid deficiencies
  Extrarenal losses
  Third-space losses (ascites, burns, pancreatitis, peritonitis)
  Gastrointestinal losses (vomiting, diarrhea, fistulas)
- Increased total body water but normal total body sodium
  Syndrome of inappropriate antidiuretic hormone secretion (SIADH)
  Water intoxication
  Emotional or physical stress
  Miscellaneous (reset osmostat, hypothyroidism, glucocorticoid deficiency)
- Pseudohyponatremia
  Extreme hyperlipidemia or hyperproteinemia

Toxins Causing Hyponatremia

Agents that cause SIADH:
  Diuretics
  Tricyclic antidepressants (TCAs)
  Monoamine oxidase inhibitors (MAOIs)
  Antineoplastic agents (e.g., vincristine, vinblastine, cisplatin, cyclophosphamide)
  Phenothiazines
  Antidiabetic agents (e.g., sulfonylureas, diazoxide, biguanides)
  Selective serotonin reuptake inhibitors (SSRIs)
  Methylenedioxymethamphetamine (MDMA)
  Nicotine
Angiotensin-converting enzyme (ACE) inhibitors
Lithium
Nonsteroidal anti-inflammatory drugs (NSAIDs)
Silver nitrate
Water

pseudobulbar palsy. These findings most commonly occur with sodium levels below 120 mEq/L.

In medically stable patients, the treatment of hyponatremia due to water intoxication is water restriction to 25–50% of maintenance requirements. Individuals experiencing CNS depression, seizure activity, or respiratory insufficiency may require a more rapid correction of serum sodium concentrations through administration of 3% sodium chloride. In these patients, a bolus of hypertonic saline, calculated to correct the sodium level to 125 mEq/L, restores sodium homeostasis. The volume (mL) of 3% sodium chloride (0.5 mEq/mL) required is derived from the following equation:

[desired sodium (mEq/L) – actual sodium (mEq/L)] × 0.6 (constant representing total body water) × weight (kg)

Care must be taken to avoid too expeditious of a correction, as an increase in the serum sodium level by more than 2 mEq/L per hour has been associated with an osmotic demyelination syndrome (central pontine myelinolysis).

This infant's mother reported that she had been diluting the baby's formula with twice as much water as was appropriate in an effort to stretch the formula supply given to her through government aid. It was calculated that she had been giving her an excess of 6 ounces of free water each day. This baby was treated with dextrose in response to her hypoglycemia, and was given a bolus of intravenous normal saline (10 mL/kg). She was subsequently restricted to 80 mL/kg of fluids per day in the form of D5NS. Twenty-four hours after her admission to the neonatal intensive care unit, her sodium was 139 mEq/L.

Clinical Pearls

1. Even water, which is a requirement for life, can be poisonous in a high dose.
2. Too rapid of a correction of hyponatremia (>2 mEq/L per hour) may cause irreversible neurological dysfunction (central pontine myelinosis).
3. Water restriction is the treatment for hyponatremia due to water intoxication.

REFERENCES

1. Hoffman R: Fluid, electrolyte, and acid-base principles. In Goldfrank L, Flomenbaum N, Lewin N, et al (eds): Toxicologic Emergencies, 7th ed. New York, McGraw Hill, 2002, pp 364-380.
2. Cronan K, Norman, M: Renal and electrolyte emergencies. In Fleisher G, Ludwig S (eds): Textbook of Pediatric Emergency Medicine, 4th ed. Philadelphia, Lippincott Williams Wilkins, 2000, pp 811-858.
3. Bruce R, Kliegman R. Hyponatremic seizures secondary to oral water intoxication in infancy: Association with commercial bottled drinking water. Pediatrics 100:E4, 1997.
4. Berry P, Belsha C. Hyponatremia. Pediatr Clin North Am 37:351-363, 1990.

INDEX

Page numbers followed by *f* denote figures and *t* denote tables

Anticholinesterase toxicity, nicotinic activity and, 89
Anticoagulant rodenticide, 164
Anticoagulant toxicity, 164
Antidotal therapy, 2
    verapamil ingestion and, 79
Antidysrhythmias
    sodium channel antagonists and, 105
    suicidal ingestion of, 104
Antiemetic drugs, mushroom poisoning and, 149
Antihistamines
    ACEI-induced angioedema and, 58
    serum sickness and, 22, 23
Anti-muscarinic toxidrome, 102
Antiphylaxis, black widow spider bite and, 221
Antipruritic therapy, poison ivy and, 206
Antivenin Polyvalent (ACP). *See also* Crotalidae
        Polyvalent Immune Fab
    rattlesnake envenomation and, 22
Antivenom. *See also* Envenomation
    black widow spider bite and, 221
    rattlesnake and, 22
Anxiety, LSD and, 161
APAP (Tylenol) intoxication, 204
    household pets and, 202
    human metabolism of, 202f
APAP-induced hemoglobin oxidative injury
    dogs and, 203
Arsenic poisoning. *See* Acute arsenic intoxication
Arterial blood gas. *See* ABG
Arterial catheter, hydrofluoric acid and, 143
Asbestos bodies, asbestosis and, 189
Asbestos taxonomy, 189t
Asbestosis, 188, 188f, 189
Ascending paralysis, ticks and, 108
Aspiration pneumonitis, 72, 72f, 73
Aspirin, cocaine and, 64
Atrial fibrillation, ma huang and, 70
Atropine, muscarinic toxicity and,
        90, 131
    mushroom poisoning and, 148
    sodium channel antiarrhythmic poisoning
        and, 106

B
Bacillus anthracis, 117
Baclofen, bradycardia and, 18
Bad trip, LSD and, 160
BAL. *See* Dimercaprol
Barbiturates
    alcoholism and, 44
    overdose of, 18
Benzene exposure, 166, 167
Benzodiazepine toxidrome, bradycardia and, 18
Benzodiazepines
    black widow spider bite and, 221
    body packers and, 41
    carbamazepine overdose and, 216
    cocaine and, 64
    cocaine-associated chest pain and, 65
    LSD and, 161
    mushroom poisoning and, 148
    neuroprotective agents and, 90
    NMS and, 177
    PCP intoxication and, 234

Benztropine, acute dystonia and, 183
Beta blockade, cocaine and, 64, 65
Beta-adrenergic blocking agents
        inhalant abuse and, 86
Beta-antagonists, chloral hydrate overdose and, 231
BIG. *See* Botulism immune globulin
Bleeding
    ginkgo biloba and, 70
    warfarin and, 163
Blood flow, fingertip pain and, 83
Blood glucose, poisoned patient and, 2
Blood-brain barrier, p-glycoprotein and, 123
Bodifacoum, 163
Body packing (drugs), 40, 40f, 41
Body stuffers (drugs), body packers v., 41
Bone marrow, benzene exposure and, 166, 167
Bone marrow transplant, benzene exposure and, 167
Botulism, food-borne, infant botulism v., 180
Botulism immune globulin (BIG)
    infants and, 181
Bowel, body packers and, 41
Boxwood *(Buxus sempervirens),* 225
Bradycardia
    case study and, 17
    clonidine overdose and, 191
    toxidrome and, 5
Bradydysrhythmias, sodium channel antiarrhythmic
        poisoning and, 106
Bradykinins, ACEI-induced angioedema and, 57
Brain, lead neurotoxicity and, 53
Breathing
    carbamazepine overdose and, 216
    poisoned patient and, 2
Bruising, poisonous bite and, 20
Bundle branch blockade, sodium channel blockade
        and, 105
Burns, sulfur mustard and, 115
Button battery, medical emergency for, 197

C
CA. *See* Cyclic antidepressants
CaEDTA. *See* Calcium disodium edathamil
Calcium channel blocker (CCB), children and, 79
Calcium disodium edathamil (CaEDTA), lead
        poisoning and, 54
Calcium disodium edetate (EDTA)
    cobalt toxicity and, 212
    zinc poisoning and, 195
Calcium gluconate gel, hydrofluoric acid and, 143
Calcium oxalate crystals, plant toxicity and, 111, 112
Calcium salts, digoxin toxicity and, 120
Calomel teething powder, mercury and, 9
Captopril therapy, ACEI-induced angioedema and, 57
Carbamates
    anticholinesterase activity and, 89
    toxicity of, 89
Carbamazepine, 215, 216t
    indications for, 215
Carbon monoxide toxicity, 25-26
Carboxyhemoglobin (COHb), toxicity and, 25
Cardiac arrhythmias, SSD and, 86
Cardiac glycoside poisoning, digoxin-specific Fab
        fragments and, 120, 120t
Cardiac glycosides, 119, 119f

Ethylene glycol poisoning, 60
  hemodialysis in, 61, 61f
  laboratory studies in, 61
  sever wide anion gap metabolic acidosis
      and, 60
External pacing, digoxin toxicity and, 120
Extracorporeal life support, verapamil ingestion
      and, 81
Extracorporeal membrane oxygenation (ECMO),
      lamp oil and, 73
Eye, raphides and, 111

F

Famotidine, ACEI-induced angioedema and, 57
Feces, botulism identification in, 180
Ferrous sulfate, pediatric overdose mortality and,
      156-157
Fetus
  COHb and, 25, 26
  hepatic necrosis in, 75
Fever, NMS and, 178
Finger pain, 82, 82f, 142, 142f
Flashbacks, LSD and, 161
Fluids, sulfur mustard and, 115
Fomepizole, ethylene glycol poisoning and, 61

G

GABA. *See* Gamma-aminobutyric acid
Gamma-aminobutyric acid (GABA)
  alcohol and, 44
  CNS and, 18
  moxidectin and, 123
  seizures and, 35
Gamma-hydroxybutyrate. *See* GHB
Gas chromatography, ibuprofen and, 146
Gastric erosion, inorganic mercury ingestion
      and, 9
Gastroenteritis, 93
  arsenic intoxication and, 93, 93t
Gastroenteritis, early-onset, mushroom poisoning
      and, 148
Gastrointestinal decontamination therapy, exploratory
      drug ingestion and, 11
Gastrointestinal (GI) system
  carbamazepine and, 215
  ibuprofen and, 146
  lead in, 53
  lithium toxicity and, 136
  mercury and, 10
  mushroom poisoning and, 148
  organic mercury compounds and, 9
  poinsettia plant and, 225
  VPA and, 174
  zinc intoxication and, 195
GC/MS analysis, cyproheptadine and, 126, 127f
G-CSF. *See* Granulocyte colony-stimulating factor
GHB (gamma-hydroxybutyrate), 18, 19
GHB (gamma-hydroxybutyrate) abstinence
      syndrome, 19
Ginkgo biloba, 70
Ginkgolides, 70
Glucose, neurological disability and, 2
Glucose-6-phosphate dehydrogenase, methemoglobin
      and, 68

Glyburide
  children and, 152
  metformin combined with, 38
Glycopyrrolate, muscarinic activity and, 90
Gouty arthritis, colchicine and, 140
Granulocyte colony-stimulating factor
      (G-CSF), colchicine and, 141
Guillain-Barré syndrome, arsenic intoxication
      and, 93

H

Hair spray inhalation, 85, 85f
Hallucinations, auditory, 49, 49f
Hallucinogens, 160
Halo sign
  body packers and, 41
  esophagus and, 197
Haloperidol
  dystonia with, 183
  LSD and, 161
Hazardous materials
  chemical attacks and, 169t
HBO. *See* Hyperbaric oxygen therapy
HD. *See* Hemodialysis
Headache, poisoning syndrome and, 4
Health care workers, sulfur mustard decontamination
      and, 114
Heart worm medication, dogs, toxicity of, 123
Heinz-body hemolytic anemia, dogs, penny coin
      ingestion and, 193, 194, 194f
Hematological system, lithium toxicity and, 136
Hemodialysis (HD)
  chronic toluene abuse and, 186
  ethylene glycol poisoning and, 62
  lithium toxicity and, 137, 138
  metformin overdose and, 39
  salicylate intoxication and, 50
Hemodynamic collapse, colchicine and, 141
Hemoglobin, toxicity and, 25
Hemolytic anemia, zinc poisoning and, 195
Hemorrhages, intracranial, ginkgo biloba and, 70
Hepatic failure, L-carnitine supplementation and,
      174-175
Hepatic injury, acetaminophen overdose and, 75
Hepatotoxicity, VPA and, 175
Herbal supplements, cardiac dysrhythmias and, 69
Heroin
  blood-brain barrier and, 154
  body packing and, 41
HIV-protease inhibitors, St. John's wort and, 72
Holly berries, toxicity of, 225
Holocyclotoxins, ticks and, 108
Hydrocarbon pneumonitis, vomiting and, 73
Hydrocarbons, 134
  children and, 73
Hydrofluoric acid (HF), 143
  management of, 143
Hydrogen sulfide poisoning, cyanide poisoning
      v., 95
Hydroxyzine, poison ivy and, 206
Hyperammonemia, L-carnitine supplementation and,
      174-175
Hyperbaric oxygen therapy (HBO)
  toxicity and, 26, 26f

Other Titles in the Pearls Series®

Duke	**Anesthesia Pearls**	1-56053-495-8
Carabello & Gazes	**Cardiology Pearls, 2nd Edition**	1-56053-403-6
Sahn & Heffner	**Critical Care Pearls, 2nd Edition**	1-56053-224-6
Sahn	**Dermatology Pearls**	1-56053-315-3
Baren & Alpern	**Emergency Medicine Pearls**	1-56053-575-X
Greenberg & Amato	**EMG Pearls**	1-56053-613-6
Jay	**Foot and Ankle Pearls**	1-56053-445-1
Concannon & Hurov	**Hand Pearls**	1-56053-463-X
Danso	**Hematology and Oncology Pearls**	1-56053-577-6
Jones *et al.*	**Hypertension Pearls**	1-56053-583-0
Cunha	**Infectious Disease Pearls**	1-56053-203-3
Heffner & Sahn	**Internal Medicine Pearls, 2nd Edition**	1-56053-404-4
Mercado & Smetana	**Medical Consultation Pearls**	1-56053-504-0
Waclawik & Sutula	**Neurology Pearls**	1-56053-261-0
Gault	**Ophthalmology Pearls**	1-56053-498-2
Heffner & Byock	**Palliative and End-of-Life Pearls**	1-56053-500-8
Inselman	**Pediatric Pulmonary Pearls**	1-56053-350-1
Lennard	**Physical Medicine & Rehabilitation Pearls**	1-56053-455-9
Kolevzon & Stewart	**Psychiatry Pearls**	1-56053-590-3
Silver & Smith	**Rheumatology Pearls**	1-56053-201-7
Berry	**Sleep Medicine Pearls, 2nd Edition**	1-56053-490-7
Eck *et al.*	**Spine Pearls**	1-56053-571-7
Schluger & Harkin	**Tuberculosis Pearls**	1-56053-156-8
Resnick & Schaeffer	**Urology Pearls**	1-56053-351-X